Sports Ophthalmology

Bruce M. Zagelbaum, M.D.
Corneal and External Disease

North Shore University Hospital
New York University School of Medicine
Manhasset, New York

Nassau County Medical Center
East Meadow, New York

Clinical Instructor in Ophthalmology
Cornell University Medical College
New York, New York

Team Ophthalmologist,
St. John's University Department of Athletics

Principal Investigator: National Basketball Association Eye Injury Study
Principal Investigator: Major League Baseball Eye Injury Study

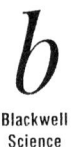

Blackwell
Science

Blackwell Science

EDITORIAL OFFICES:
238 Main Street, Cambridge, Massachusetts 02142, USA
Osney Mead, Oxford OX2 0EL, England
25 John Street, London WC1N 2BL, England
23 Ainslie Place, Edinburgh EH3 6AJ, Scotland
54 University Street, Carlton, Victoria 3053, Australia
Arnette Blackwell SA, 1 rue de Lille, 75007 Paris, France
Blackwell Wissenschafts-Verlag GmbH
   Kurfurstendamm 57, 10707 Berlin, Germany
   Feldgasse 13, A-1238 Vienna, Austria

DISTRIBUTORS:
USA
Blackwell Science, Inc.
238 Main Street
Cambridge, Massachusetts 02142
(Telephone order: 800-215-1000 or 617-876-7000)

Canada
Copp Clark, Ltd.
2775 Matheson Blvd. East
Mississauga, Ontario, Canada L4W 4P7
(Telephone orders: 800-263-4374 or 905-238-6074)

Australia
Blackwell Science Pty Ltd
54 University Street
Carlton, Victoria 3053
(Telephone orders: 03-347-0300 fax: 03-349-3016)

Outside North America and Australia
Blackwell Science, Ltd.
c/o Marston Book Services, Ltd.
P.O. Box 87
Oxford OX2 0DT
England
(Telephone orders: 44-1865-791155)

Acquisitions: James Krosschell
Development: Debra Lance
Production: Ellen Samia
Manufacturing: Lisa Flanagan
Printed and bound by Braun-Brumfield, Inc.

©1996 by Blackwell Science, Inc.
Printed in the United States of America
96 97 98 99 5 4 3 2 1

All right reserved. No part of this book may be reproduced in any form or by any electronic or mechanical means, including information storage and retrieval systems, without permission in writing from the publisher, except by a reviewer who may quote brief passages in a review.

Notice: The indications and dosages of all drugs in this book have been recommended in the medical literature and conform to the practices of the general medical community. The medications described do not necessarily have specific approval by the Food and Drug Administration for use in the diseases and dosages for which they are recommended. The package insert for each drug should be consulted for use and dosage as approved by the FDA. Because standards of usage change, it is advisable to keep abreast of revised recommendations, particularly those concerning new drugs.

Library of Congress Cataloging-in-Publication Data

Sports ophthalmology / [edited by] Bruce M. Zagelbaum.
   p.   cm.
   Includes bibliographical references and index.
   ISBN 0-86542-365-2
   1. Sports ophthalmology.   I. Zagelbaum, Bruce M.
   [DNLM: 1. Eye Injuries—prevention & control.   2. Athletic Injuries.   WW 525 S794 1996]
RE827.S662   1996
617.7'008'8796—dc20
DNLM/DLC
   for Library of Congress   95-42108
                                                            CIP

Contents

Preface v
Contributors vii
Dedication x

1. Introduction 1
   Paul F. Vinger

2. Baseball 23
   Bruce M. Zagelbaum

3. Basketball 43
   Chad Starkey and Bruce M. Zagelbaum

4. Hockey 56
   Robert C. Pashby and Thomas J. Pashby

5. Racket and Court Sports 72
   Michael Easterbrook

6. Boxing 90
   Vincent J. Giovinazzo

7. Football 108
   John B. Jeffers

8. Golf and Soccer 119
   Wayne I. Larrison

9. Shooting and Water Sports 132
   M. Lisa McHam and Bradford J. Shingleton

10 Anatomy 154
    Brian S. Biesman and Albert Hornblass

11 Anterior Segment Injuries 184
    *Roopinder K. Grewal, Deepinder K. Dhaliwal,
    Peter S. Hersh, and Bruce M. Zagelbaum*

12 Posterior Segment Injuries 210
    Stephanie A. Skolik, D. Virgil Alfaro, and Peter E. Liggett

13 Medicolegal Aspects 224
    John G. Classé

14 Visual Training 240
    David B. Granet and Richard W. Hertle

Index 261

Preface

My goal in putting together "Sports Ophthalmology" has been to produce a comprehensive yet easily understood textbook that would fill a specific void in the medical literature. Sporting events today are a major attraction with millions of spectators and close media attention. The eyecare/medical provider may thus be faced with situations in which an athlete sustains an eye injury and team management is anxious to have their athlete back into action as quickly as possible. Whether in the playground or at a professional sporting arena, our role is to rapidly formulate a diagnosis, treatment, and management plan that would result in the best ultimate outcome for the athlete involved.

While this book places an emphasis on sports-related eye trauma and treatment, preventive measures are constantly stressed. I have included areas that will give the reader the necessary information for appropriately managing and treating all forms of eye injuries where indicated, including when to refer to the specialist. Specific recommendations have been made that I believe are most likely to help the injured athlete.

I have been most fortunate in being able to assemble the known experts within the field, some of whom have donated a great percentage of their time in the prevention and treatment of sports-related eye injuries. Each contributor was selected primarily for his or her expertise in the area covered. Although I am grateful to all of the contributors, a special thanks goes to Paul Vinger, Michael Easterbrook and Thomas Pashby. These dedicated ophthalmologists are recognized worldwide for their accomplishments and have been a major influence in my becoming involved in this field.

With an array of experienced contributors, I hope to provide an extensive text that is a complete reference relating to sports and the eye. Since professional athletes today are looked at by youngsters as role models, it is essential that they be made aware of injury prevention in order to convey the message to the general public. Kareem

Abdul-Jabbar, one of the greatest players ever to play the game of basketball, will always be remembered wearing those famous goggles.

I hope that this book will be useful to ophthalmologists, optometrists, opticians, emergency room physicians and ancillary staff, sports educational institutions, athletic trainers, and students. The text has been divided into various sections with each sport treated individually to allow the reader to select his or her area of interest, or to be used as a reference for the practitioner, whether in the office or on the field of play. The ever important topic of medicolegal issues has been addressed as well as the basics of visual training.

I am indebted to Ellen Samia, Debra Lance and Mike Snider for their assistance with editing this project. I would also like to thank Tod Turiff, Michael Arnolt, Alan Ashare and Jess Heald for their valuable input. I am also grateful to Ron Linfonte and Steve Pritchard of St. John's University, Stephen Lombardo of the National Basketball Association, and William Bryan, David Dines and Fred Hina of Major League Baseball, for their confidence in me. Lastly, a special thank you to Peter Hersh, who has always been instrumental in guiding me in the proper direction.

Bruce M. Zagelbaum

Contributors

D. Virgil Alfaro, MD
Assistant Professor of Ophthalmology
Uniformed Services University of the Health Sciences
F. Edward Hebert School of Medicine
Bethesda, Maryland

Brian S. Biesman, MD
Assistant Professor of Ophthalmology
Tufts University School of Medicine
Director, Eye Plastics and Orbit Service
New England Eye Center
Boston, Massachusetts

John G. Classé, OD, JD
Associate Professor, School of Optometry
University of Alabama at Birmingham
Member of the State of Alabama Bar
Birmingham, Alabama

Michael Easterbrook, MD
Associate Professor of Ophthalmology
University of Toronto
Team Ophthalmologist, Toronto Maple Leafs
Team Ophthalmologist, Toronto Raptors
Toronto, Ontario
Canada

Vincent J. Giovinazzo, MD
Assistant Professor of Ophthalmology
State University of New York, Health Science Center
Brooklyn, New York
Medical Advisory Board, New York State Athletic Commission
New York, New York

David B. Granet, MD
Assistant Adjunct Professor of Ophthalmology
University of California at San Diego
Director, Abraham Ratner Children's Eye Center
La Jolla, California

Richard W. Hertle, MD
Assistant Professor of Ophthalmology
University of Pennsylvania School of Medicine
Children's Hospital of Philadelphia
Philadelphia, Pennsylvania

Peter S. Hersh, MD
Chief, Cornea and Refractive Surgery
UMDNJ-New Jersey Medical School
Hackensack University Medical Center
Newark, New Jersey

Albert Hornblass, MD
Director of Ophthalmic Plastic Surgery
Manhattan Eye Ear and Throat Hospital
New York, New York
Clinical Professor of Ophthalmology
State University of New York, Health Science Center
Brooklyn, New York

John B. Jeffers, MD
Clinical Assistant Professor of Ophthalmology
Jefferson Medical College
Director of Residency Education and Emergency Services
Wills Eye Hospital
Team Ophthalmologist, Philadelphia Eagles
Team Ophthalmologist, Philadelphia 76ers
Philadelphia, Pennsylvania

Wayne Larrison, MD, MS
Connecticut Retinal Consultants, P.C.
New Haven, Connecticut
Yale University School of Medicine
New Haven, Connecticut

Peter E. Liggett, MD
Private Practice
Hamden, Connecticut

M. Lisa McHam, MD
Clinical Instructor of Ophthalmology
Tufts University School of Medicine
Boston, Massachusetts

Robert C. Pashby, MD
Assistant Professor of Ophthalmology
University of Toronto
Don Mills, Ontario
Canada

Thomas J. Pashby, MD
Associate Professor Emeritus
Department of Ophthalmology
University of Toronto
Don Mills, Ontario
Canada

Bradford J. Shingleton, MD
Associate Clinical Professor of Ophthalmology
Tufts University School of Medicine
Assistant Clinical Professor of Ophthalmology
Harvard Medical School
Boston, Massachusetts

Stephanie A. Skolik, MD
Assistant Professor of Ophthalmology
Marshall University School of Medicine
Huntington, West Virginia

Paul F. Vinger, MD
Associate Clinical Professor, Ophthalmology
Tufts University School of Medicine
Boston, Massachusetts

I would like to dedicate this book to Alice, Matthew, Jennifer and Andrew for their love and support.

CHAPTER 1

Introduction

Paul F. Vinger

The publication of this book is another step toward the realization that ophthalmologists, optometrists, and opticians have a vital role in sports visual performance, prevention of sports injuries, and treatment of athletes with rapid return to normal sports activity a prime concern.

When I first became interested in sports ophthalmology in 1971, my attention was caught by the devastating eye injuries caused by ice hockey. The only ophthalmologist whom I could find that was truly involved in sports performance and safety was Thomas Pashby, who had been a motivating force in Canada and then internationally for over three decades. The list of involved ophthalmologists began to grow as Michael Easterbrook, Jack Jeffers, and Louis Pizarello took leadership roles. As this group ages, it is with great relief that a new generation of interested ophthalmologists, including Bruce Zagelbaum, Richard Orlando, Peter Hersh, and Vincent Giovinazzo, are becoming involved. The aging cadre salutes and wishes great success to the energetic and resourceful second wave.

I apologize to those I have not named, but the point is that one can really list those who are involved in this tiny field. The older crew realizes that involvement means donating about 20% of one's time, with no hope of grant money or compensation, to an effort for which the only motivation is self-fulfillment, doing a necessary job in which interesting people are met and real goals are accomplished.

The role of ophthalmology is essential. We know the mechanisms and best means of treating and preventing injury. We must look critically at those who use the elite athlete as a means to increase their own professional status rather than the best interests of the athlete. We must seek honest answers to questions such as, Is visual training helpful to athletic performance? Should an athlete subject himself or herself to globe weakening radial keratotomy? Does excimer laser for myopia degrade or improve performance? Ophthalmologists must work together with optometrists and opticians to assist in developing protocols to answer valid questions on vision as it relates to visual performance and the best means to prevent eye injuries without degrading performance or removing the fun or appeal from the sport.

Sports-Related Eye Injuries

Ophthalmology, as a discipline, recognizes that eye injuries pose a substantial and preventable risk. Yet preventing traumatic eye injuries is not taken seriously enough by organized ophthalmology and funding agencies. Epidemics as widespread and costly in terms of ocular disability and social costs from other causes, such as acquired immunodeficiency syndrome or diabetes, generate effective study and action by our profession. Despite the fact that the average ophthalmologist sees many patients with sports-related eye injuries for each new melanoma or gyrate atrophy, the literature and research funds overwhelmingly emphasize the rarer diseases. Research directed toward the prevention of traumatic eye injuries is considered "applied," thus unworthy of funding, whereas that directed toward disease etiology or treatment is considered "basic" and therefore worthy. Why? Perhaps because ophthalmologists are trained to treat disease and feel more comfortable with diseased eyes than with healthy eyes that have only the potential of pathology. As primary eyecare providers, our responsibility in discussing injury prevention cannot be denied. Eyecare specialists, by educating their patients about the risks of eye injuries in various sports and the benefits and availability of protective equipment, have the potential to prevent injury to well over 100,000 eyes each year.

The ideal scenario for a sports (or any other) eye injury is prevention. Prevention, effective in terms of both injury reduction and cost savings to society, should be part of the core curriculum of any professional who prescribes, manufactures, or dispenses eyewear, as well as those in the capacity of formulating and implementing rules in the athletic or work environment.

Data Collection

Without knowledge of the incidence and severity of sports-related eye injuries, it would be impossible to attempt injury reduction because there would be no way to determine whether preventive methods were indicated or whether they had an adverse or beneficial effect. A major potential pitfall is that the epidemiologic data obtained may reflect only the risk of the sport and not the benefits that justify the risk. The objective is to reduce preventable eye injuries to the minimum consistent with retaining the benefits of fun and appeal that draw participants into the sport. It is possible to achieve this goal most of the time after the accurate incidence and mechanism of eye injuries are ascertained and athletes, coaches, referees, officials, and the medical profession meet to solve the problems and to strive for minimal interference with the sport.

Unfortunately, the true incidence of eye injuries in sports is unknown at this time because there is no data collection system that is reliable, fast, and complete for sports or any other form of eye trauma. Lacking knowledge of the exact incidence of eye injuries in each sport, we must rely on other incomplete, and often specially designed, methods of collecting data to ascertain where problems exist and to follow the effects of intervention in a meaningful manner. The currently available data-gathering systems are not as efficient or complete as desired.

The National Safety Council system and state data-collecting systems have been of little value in the study of sports-related eye injuries because their data are difficult for others to obtain and are often inconsistent. Gathering of statewide data from hospital records is often impeded by the characteristics of hospital record keeping, which often fails to identify the cause of injury or the circumstances surrounding the injury.

The National Athletic Injury/Illness Reporting System (NAIRS) has in the past obtained useful data by following injury rates in participating schools. However, because of lack of funding, the data pool is shrinking and the future of NAIRS is uncertain.

The National Electronic Injury Surveillance System (NEISS) was established under a 1973 congressional mandate that formed the Consumer Product Safety Commission (CPSC) to protect the public from unreasonable risks of injury and death associated with consumer products. NEISS is limited in that only emergency room visits related to injuries caused by products are recorded as the basis for projections of a national probability sample of 91 hospital emergency rooms. Because specialty eye hospitals and private ophthalmologists' offices, where most of the sports-related eye injuries are seen, are greatly underrepresented in the sample, NEISS data must be viewed with caution. For example, the extreme eye injury hazard of boxing is not apparent from NEISS data. Yet national trends are often apparent from these data.

The National Eye Trauma System (NETS) is a consortium of approximately 50 regional eye trauma centers that prospectively gather information on the etiology, treatment, and final results of penetrating eye injuries. NETS can optimally report on the subset of penetrating injuries and help to establish management protocols. However, most sports-related injuries are caused by blunt objects and do not perforate the globe and thus are not recorded. Despite these unrecorded sports-related injuries, it is astounding that 14.1% of all injuries in the NETS database are from sports. As expected, injuries caused by projectiles (38.1% of reported recreational injuries were due to BB and air guns) lead the NETS list of perforating injuries due to sports.

The United States Eye Injury Registry (USEIR), which began with the 1982 Eye Injury Registry of Alabama, is now a federation of 39 state registries, representing 226 million people, each endorsed by its state ophthalmologic society. The USEIR collects and disseminates comprehensive data on the statewide occurrence of serious (involving permanent or significant structural or functional changes to the eye) ocular injuries. They can optimally document population-based data on the broad spectrum of eye injuries to include blunt trauma and chemical injuries, which are frequently seen only in ophthalmologists' offices. The USEIR has been influential in controlling fireworks-related eye injuries. It is hoped that the database will be expanded to be useful in future study of sports-related eye injuries and that there will be areas of congruence with NETS for a more effective database.

National data collected by the cooperating ophthalmologists of the Canadian Ophthalmological Society (COS) under the leadership of Tom Pashby and Mike Easterbrook are the most useful national data currently available for following trends in sports-related injury and the results of intervention with rule changes or protective devices. COS, which freely shares its data, has maintained the longest prospective database of sports-related eye injuries and has played a vital role in the prevention of these injuries.

Records from private offices, hospitals, and clinics usually give rise to the clinical impression that a potential problem, which requires further investigation, exists. For specific studies, data collected from sports organizations, which involve cooperation among athletes, coaches, officials, and doctors, are usually the most specific. Data collection is frequently the most frustrating and difficult aspect of preventing eye injuries in sports, yet despite the lack of an ideal data-collecting system, it is possible to ascertain the eye injury potential of specific sports and follow the results of intervention with rule changes or protective equipment by means of limited specifically designed studies.

It is hoped that the National Society to Prevent Blindness (NSPB) subcommittee recommendations on sports-related eye injury data gathering will fulfill the following criteria: 1) permit population-based comparisons involving a known denominator, 2) record demographic data and details of the injury at the time of presentation to the medical facility, 3) record the diagnosis of the physician at the time of examination, and 4) record the final outcome of the injury. It is the accurate combination of clinical and epidemiologic data that will result in effective proposals for injury prevention.

Economics

The social cost of eye trauma, the most common ophthalmic indication for hospitalization, is enormous. National projections estimate annual U.S. hospital charges of $175 to $200 million for 227,000 eye trauma hospital days. Because essentially all sports-related eye injuries are preventable, the potential economic savings resulting from the prevention of sports eye injuries are great. There is no question that prevention of traumatic sports eye injuries is cost effective. In 1980 dollars, the hockey face protector saves society $10 million a year by preventing approximately 70,000 eye and face injuries in 1.2 million protected players.

Sports-related injuries are not accidents but, like most other injuries, are predictable events that can be studied according to the basic epidemiologic factors of time, agent, host, and environment and are shown to have definite patterns with nonrandom characteristics that can be modified with rule changes or protective devices.

In the past, there has been minimal expenditure for the prevention of eye trauma, and the likelihood for improvement in the near future is slim. Of the proposed $360 million 1993 National Institute of Health fiscal budget, there is no specific mention of eye trauma prevention as a funding sector. It is time that funding agencies realize that simple preventive measures can save huge amounts of money.

Safety Standards and Protector Design

In two decades of active involvement writing safety standards as a member of the American Society for Testing and Materials (ASTM), I am enormously impressed by the technical expertise and capabilities of engineers and designers. I am equally impressed with their need for help for the visual needs of the athlete and the importance of the eyecare professional as part of the standards writing team. Protectors will be worn only if they are comfortable and do not degrade performance. Our input on optics, field of view, transmission of forces, and comfort is essential to the development of a standard, which is the basic tool for protective devices designed for the ultimate goal of reducing eye injuries.

A protective device should prevent damaging forces from reaching the eyes by dissipating potentially harmful forces over time and area. This theory is simple enough, but the practical application can be difficult. As soon as design is begun on a protective device for a sport with an ocular hazard, many problems arise. What forces are involved in this sport? Are they high velocity, low mass (hockey puck); low velocity, high mass (player sliding into a goal post); or a combination of high velocity and high mass (bicycle racer collision)? Does a protector have to be designed differently for each type of force? How? Where on the head will the forces be transmitted, and how will it be done? Will the player be killed or suffer brain damage if the force is transmitted to his or her brain through the protective device rather than being dissipated into broken facial or orbital bones, as was the case before the protector? Will the protector change the form or appeal of the game? What about the design, player acceptance, expense, weight, interference with vision, product liability, and full disclosure to the consumer?

These questions cannot be answered by any one individual, because expertise at many levels and different areas of interest is required. The best way to design and build a protective device is by the development of a performance standard to which the protector will be made. Such standards require input from players, coaches, engineers, manufacturers, physicians, and possibly lawyers and economists. A protective device is effective only when worn by the player.

Even the best designed protective device, if it does not appeal to the taste of the player, will remain on the dealer's shelf.

It is clear to those who write standards that one cannot tell how a protector will perform until it is tested under dynamic conditions that approximate game conditions. If those who write standards and test protectors cannot tell how a protector will perform until the protector is tested, it is obvious that the untrained consumer will be unable to determine by inspection in the retail shop which products will provide adequate protection with minimal impact on performance. The problem of severe eye injuries in sports can be solved by writing performance standards that specify the protector's energy attenuation and visual requirements followed by certification of the protective equipment produced by manufacturers. Sports regulatory bodies must mandate the use of equipment that passes the standard requirements, and governing bodies must legislate against uncertified products gaining access to the marketplace.

Most ophthalmologists and optometrists are familiar with standards that bear the seal of the American National Standards Institute (ANSI), which publishes standards for use in the ophthalmologic/optometric field. The Z80 series gives standard specifications for prescription ophthalmic lenses and frames, contact lenses and lens solutions, sunglasses and fashion eyewear, intraocular lenses, and low vision aids; the Z87 series is for industrial eyewear, and the Z136 series is for lasers. ANSI has standard Z86 for scuba diving masks and Z90 for protective headgear, including bicycle helmets.

Most sports eyewear standards writing comes under the jurisdiction of the ASTM. The largest of the approximately 400 standards-writing bodies in the United States, the ASTM is neither a government nor a manufacturer organization, but a nonprofit corporation organized in 1898 for development of voluntary standards arrived at by consensus among all interested parties.

ASTM committee F-8 on sports safety standards and sports safety was formed in 1968 to address the sharp increase in head and neck injuries in football. ASTM F-8 now has subcommittees that write standards for many sports, including gymnastics, golf, archery, wrestling, fencing, racket sports, hockey, and baseball, as well as for activities including the use of trampolines and fitness products. These subcommittees also write standards for groups concerned with the more general problems of medical aspects and biomechanics, playing surfaces, headwear, footwear, padding, statistics, warning labels and signs, the female athlete, and eye safety.

The ASTM standards-writing committees are groups of volunteer experts (producers, users, ultimate consumers, those representing the general public interest) who are representative of those in the community that have an interest in the development and/or use of protective devices for a particular sport. With such diversity, marked differences of opinion frequently require resolution in a fair and democratic manner. In writing standards, strict ASTM guidelines for due process are followed.

The best sports standards are performance standards that specify how a protector must perform (e.g., visual fields, impact resistance, distribution of forces) rather than design standards that contain certain design elements that may or may not relate to performance. By and large, design standards are unnecessarily restrictive, tend to stifle the introduction of better, more innovative protector designs, and are less desirable from an antitrust perspective.

The standard methodology used by the ASTM eye safety subcommittee in testing protective devices has been to test with real objects (e.g., squash ball, racket, hockey puck) under conditions that simulate actual game conditions and have an impact as close as possible to the actual game conditions. Before any laboratory testing of protective devices is started, the potential injury-producing forces are analyzed, and then test procedures are established to ascertain that products will protect the eyes and face under actual game conditions.

Performance standards serve as the minimum safety floor for sports eye protective devices. Well-written standards have eliminated over half of the "eye protective devices" sold for various sports that were poorly designed and not adequate to prevent most eye injuries in the intended sport. Testing a sports eye/face protector to the requirements of a performance standard is the only means to assure the consumer that the protective device is adequate.

Standards are designed to be revised as experience is gained. No matter how well the protector performs on paper or in the testing laboratory, it is only the use by thousands of players and continued injury monitoring that prove the protective value or demonstrate the failures of a particular design. For this reason, the ASTM mandates review of all published standards every 5 years. Other standards organizations (e.g., Canadian Standards Association [CSA], ANSI, Deutsches Institut für Normung, International Organization for Standardization) operate under various bylaws.

The international community is now working on standards for eye protection in the racket sports. It would be more efficient to recognize one standard that would allow manufacturers to make protectors with the worldwide market in mind. Toward this effort, the United States and Canada are working toward similarity in standards. When a united standard is achieved, this will be presented to other countries for their consideration.

Equipment Certification Councils

The Sports Equipment Certification Council (SECC) is composed of coaches, participants, scientists, physicians, manufacturers, and administrators. Its purpose is to seek out and select codes and standards, including test methods and procedures, for equipment used in athletic, sporting, recreational, and leisure time activity. In addition, the council identifies and publishes all factors associated with safety, whether the factor is protective equipment, playing surfaces, rules, attitudes, officiating, training, conditioning, or administration. The SECC usually has a seal that manufacturers affix to a protective device that is assurance to the consumer that a product meets a performance standard and that the manufacturer meets quality control criteria.

The Hockey Equipment Certification Council (HECC) is an independent nonprofit organization established in 1978 through the joint efforts of the Amateur Hockey Association of the United States and a number of interested volunteers. HECC selects codes and standards to certify playing equipment and facilities, monitors the effectiveness of its certification program, and promotes research pertaining to the prevention and/or reduction of ice hockey injuries. HECC is extremely effective in fulfilling its mandate of reducing injuries in hockey.

Certification councils can be extremely difficult to establish. After 4 years of attempting to structure a third-party certification program for racket sport protectors in the United States, the NSPB abandoned the effort because of lack of support from the manufacturers and distributors of sports products. The reasons for this lack of participation included the cost and testing of certification, the use of only one testing laboratory, and duplicity testing and certifying in both the United States and Canada. There is also the possibility that some manufacturers may have had the hidden agenda of not wanting a certification council so that the quality of their products would not be subjected to the close scrutiny of the test methods of a true certification council. It seems that the solution to the racket sport certification problem will be the development of a North American, followed by an international, standard, then the mandating of labeling as to whether the product was tested to the standard by an independent testing laboratory or by an organization such as the CPSC, and then education of officials and consumers to purchase only those products tested to the standard by an independent testing laboratory.

Protective equipment is obsolete when it no longer provides adequate protection; cannot be purchased under normal circumstances; is no longer in the newest style; is unreconditioned "hand-me-down" equipment; or is worn out, broken, or ill-fitting. As injury data result in standard modification, certification councils must publish a list of equipment that has become obsolete by newer advances, and this obsolete equipment must be discarded.

Guidelines for Athletic Participation

The classification of sports into three main categories (contact and collision, limited contact and impact, and noncontact) by the American Academy of Pediatrics is more appropriate to the musculoskeletal and neurologic systems than to the eye. Whereas musculoskeletal injuries and cerebral concussions are inevitable in contact and collision sports (such as rodeo) and rare in noncontact sports (such as golf), eye injuries may be more common and severe in the "safer sport." It is apparent that more realistic guidelines for participation in sports by people with various ocular handicaps and ocular diseases must be devised.

The One-Eyed Athlete

For the purpose of recommending extra safety precautions, a person is functionally one-eyed when loss of the better eye would result in a significant change in lifestyle because of the poor vision in the remaining eye. An athlete certainly should be considered one-eyed if his or her best corrected vision in the involved eye is 20/200 or less, with the other eye found normal by an ophthalmologist. On the other hand, most of us would function fairly well with 20/40 or better vision in the remaining eye. More difficult is advising patients with between 20/40 and 20/200 best corrected vision in the affected eye. The inability to drive a vehicle legally in most states would be a handicap to most people and would significantly interfere with the jobs available to a youngster when he or she is older. Also, studies would be more difficult throughout the school years. Therefore, we could safely conclude that a child is effectively one-eyed when the best correctable vision in the poorer eye is less than 20/40 and consider an adult effectively one-eyed if he or she believes the level of vision in the poorer eye would interfere with his or her life or livelihood if the better eye were lost. Functionally one-eyed athletes (and their parents in the case of minors) must be well informed of the potential long-term consequences if the good eye is lost. They should also be informed of the risks of injury (without and with various eye protectors) and the possibility of repair of injuries typically seen with the sport in question.

As protective devices improve and effective sports eye protectors are developed, more and more sports become quite safe even for the one-eyed athlete. The outright ban by some schools for one-eyed participation in collision and contact sports while the one-eyed students are permitted to play more dangerous (to the remaining eye) sports, such as badminton, is not prudent and should be re-evaluated. With proper protection, the one-eyed athlete may participate in most sports.

The medical and school committees should specify that the one-eyed athlete wear sports eye protectors that meet the ASTM or CSA racket sport standard for all sports with risk of eye injury for all games and practices. These eye protectors must be worn under the face mask of those sports that usually require a face mask (e.g., hockey, football, lacrosse). Baseball face protectors should be used for batting and base running. Face protectors should be required for women's lacrosse (already required for men's lacrosse) and field hockey.

For daily wear, off the athletic field, one-eyed people should wear polycarbonate lenses mounted in a sturdy streetwear frame (a good compromise between safety and cosmetic acceptance most of the time to protect the good eye). This is especially true of young active people who are subject to injury on or off the athletic field. The eyecare professional should emphasize the important role of proper eyewear as a protective device, with lateral protection if there is potential exposure to fragments.

If the athlete is informed of the need for protection and also given specific advice by the ophthalmologist, optometrist, optician, and ocularist, there is a far greater likelihood of protection compliance.

Blind Patients and Sports

The U.S. Association for Blind Athletes (USABA), established in 1976, enables blind and partially sighted athletes to participate in competition on a national level. Events include track and field; gymnastics; wrestling; the 10-km run; and goal ball, a fast-paced game developed especially for blind athletes in which a 4.5-pound ball containing bells is rolled on a 30 × 60-foot mat, past opposing players, across an end. To eliminate the advantage the partially sighted may have over the totally blind, all players, including the totally blind, wear blindfolds in the game. Athletes of all ages are divided by vision into three groups: class A, totally blind or light perception with no acuity, with less than 3 degrees of visual field; class B, 20/400 or less with 3 to 10 degrees of visual field; and class C, less than 20/200 and/or between 10 and 20 degrees of visual field.

Because of encouragement from organizations such as the USABA, the blind are participating in more active sports, such as beep baseball, tandem cycling, golf, downhill and cross-country skiing, skating, wrestling, judo, track, and swimming, in addition to the usual activities of the blind such as bowling, nature hikes, boating and fishing, picnics, and dances. Beep ball was invented by the Telephone Pioneers of America and uses a sound-emitting softball with sound-emitting bases. All players wear head, face, and chest protection. The sport is so popular that the National Beep Baseball Association drew a crowd of 1200 spectators at a national tournament. The U.S. Blind Golfers Association is the oldest organization that promotes an organized sport for totally blind athletes. Ski for Light, the Blind Outdoor Leisure Development, and the American Blind Skiing Foundation promote skiing for the blind.

The sports achievements of the blind are impressive. Harry Cordellos, blind from diabetes, completed the Boston Marathon in under 3 hours with the help of a sighted companion. An example of the ultimate trust in a sighted helper is that given by Tom Sullivan, who pulls the rip cord at the signal (by helmet radio communication) from his sighted sky-diving companion. Tom O'Connor completed a triathlon in the remarkable time of 3:49:06 without being tethered to a guide. For the 0.9-mile swim, he swam in a lane formed by 20-foot tubes pulled by a kayak, he ran 6.2 miles with a guide, and cycled 25.1 miles guided only by verbal commands shouted from a guide car—a true ordeal.

It is important that eyecare professionals encourage patients who become partially sighted or blind to pursue sports activities through one of the many organizations with expertise in promoting active sports that are challenging, safe, and especially, fun.

Contact Lenses in Sports

Contact lenses offer advantages for many sports, especially for high ametropes: better visual field, no fogging, and staying in place with rapid motion. New lens technologies that combine the excellent visual acuity of rigid gas permeable contact lenses with the comfort and retention characteristics of soft lenses are preferred by many athletes, especially those with astigmatism. Large-diameter (15.5-mm) soft lenses are available for athletes who cannot wear standard soft or rigid gas permeable lenses because of decentration with sports activity.

Many sports offer environments that make contact lens wear more difficult because of increased exposure to water, wind, sun, dust, and dirt. The use of wraparound polycarbonate sunglasses over the contact lenses frequently allows the highly ametropic mountain bicycle racer to have the benefits of contact lens vision in the face of wind and debris. For sports in which low humidity may be encountered, such as ice hockey, low water, low soiling, low dehydrating, larger diameter, thin, soft contact lenses, replaced approximately every 3 months, seem to give satisfactory results for most players. Wind, dry air, ultraviolet (UV) light, and decreased oxygen at high altitude often cause punctate keratitis in skiers. Skiers who wear contacts should be encouraged to wear goggles that absorb UV rays and break the wind. If contact lens wear becomes impossible, spectacles could save an otherwise ruined performance.

Contact lenses are becoming more popular for the water sports, but probably should be used only where vision is critical and spectacles are impractical, such as in surfing or windsailing. Pool swimmers retain lenses better if several drops of distilled water are placed onto the contact lens several minutes before entering the pool. It probably is safer for swimmers to remove contact lenses before swimming for several reasons. Despite use of distilled water, which may not be sterile and thus may be a source of potential corneal ulceration, the lens still may be lost. Chlorine or other pool contaminants may remain in the contact lens and cause punctate keratitis. Contact lenses could be dislodged, especially in a scuba diving emergency, and could be the source of more problems in an already difficult situation. Contact lenses probably should not be worn for deep prolonged dives, because of the possibility of keratitis and corneal edema from lack of oxygenation. Despite the fact that soft contact lenses become less adherent to the cornea in hypertonic solutions, such as ocean water, the loss rate is quite low among surfers, provided precautions are taken to close the eyes on submersion and not to rub the eyes. Ametropic surfers are probably better off with large soft lenses that tend not to get lost and help to view incoming swells and select waves. Also, surfers who see better can avoid obstacles and other surfers and can maintain orientation in the water with respect to landmarks on the shore.

Because contact lenses offer no protection from impact, it must be stressed to patients that protective devices, where indicated, should be worn in addition to the contacts. Patients who want contact lenses for sports use deserve a few minutes of discussion of injury prevention.

Sports Sunglasses

Many athletes, such as mountaineers, skiers, sailors, and lifeguards, are exposed to large doses of UV light, often in situations where there is the potential for injury from impact, in adverse conditions of high wind or dust. The inability to see well because of UV keratitis, windburn, corneal foreign bodies, or traumatic injury from shattered spectacles may be life threatening as well as eye threatening. Other athletes are concerned about the long-term effects of chronic UV exposure and wish to prevent future eye problems with proper sunglasses. Dark sunglasses permit one to be comfortable in bright light without squinting. However, one must be certain that the reduction in the protective effect of squinting by dark sunglasses that have poor absorption in the toxic UV and blue light ranges does not cause ocular injury. Skiers should be advised that the reflection from the front surface of mirrored sunglasses may result in severe sunburn to the nose unless extra protection is used. Reflected UV light also must be considered. Fresh snow reflects about 80% and older snow over 50%. Clean white sand reflects about 30%, water reflects 5%, and earth and grass reflect less than 5%. Thus, the greatest UV exposure occurs at high altitude on a field of fresh snow.

The visible spectrum includes wavelengths between 400 and 700 nm. UV radiation is divided into bands depending on the wavelength. The differentiation into bands varies according to authors. ANSI definitions state UVB includes wavelengths from 290 to 315 nm and UVA from 315 to 380 nm; others specify UV as UVC, 200 to 286 nm; UVB, 286 to 320 nm; A_1, 320 to 340 nm; and A_2, 340 to 400 nm. The stratospheric ozone layer absorbs wavelengths below about 285 nm, corneal tissue absorbs most radiation below 295 nm, and the wavelengths below 380 nm are almost completely absorbed by anterior segment structures. In adults, less than 1% of radiation below 340 nm and 2% of radiation between 340 and 360 nm reach the retina. At 400 nm, 10% of the incident light is transmitted to the retina in the phakic patient. In phakic individuals, light from 400 to 1400 nm reaches the retina. In a normal phakic adult, for 365-nm near-UV radiation, 25% is absorbed by the cornea, 11% by the aqueous humor, and 64% by the lens; less than 1% reaches the retina.

As early cataract surgery becomes more common, the UV effect on the retina is not trivial. Removal of the lens exposes the retina to wavelengths above approximately 300 nm. At 325 to 350 nm, the retina is approximately six times more sensitive to damage than to short wavelength visible radiation of 441 nm. Untreated polymethylmethacrylate intraocular lenses (IOLs) absorb UV radiation only below approximately 300 to 320 nm. Because many IOLs classified as "ultraviolet protective" offer less than optimal protection and because it is not known how long the UV filter on UV-absorbing IOLs lasts, it is prudent for all aphakic and pseudophakic athletes to wear sunglasses that absorb 99% of light between 470 and 500 nm.

Both acute and chronic UV exposure are cause for concern. Pterygium, climatic droplet keratopathy, and nuclear cataract are associated with exposure to the broad band of UVA and UVB, whereas photokeratitis, sunburn, and cortical and posterior subcapsular cataract are mostly caused by the shorter, more biologically active wavelengths of the "erythema" UVB band. Despite the fact that the absorption of glass spectacle lenses drops to 30% at 330 nm, the incidence of nuclear sclerotic cataracts is lower in eyeglass wearers than in emmetropes.

Cumulative exposure to UVB causes basal and squamous-cell carcinomas in white persons, whereas intense exposure causing blistering sunburns in childhood is more commonly associated with cutaneous malignant melanoma. The effect of sunlight on ocular melanoma is controversial. Some believe that the short wavelength range of 400 to 470 nm may be phototoxic to the retina. There is no increased association of age-related macular degeneration with exposure to UV light, but high levels of exposure to blue or visible light may be related to the development of age-related macular degeneration. Even relatively brief exposure to viewing the sun when high in the sky (zenith above 60%) may result in solar retinitis due to photochemical injury from intense short wavelength (blue light) and UV radiation. Many clinicians have the impression that herpes simplex keratitis may be precipitated by exposure to UVB.

Athletes who wish maximum UV protection should wear a hat with a brim, which reduces ocular exposure by half, and close-fitting sunglasses that absorb both UVA and UVB when in conditions in which they could get sunburned. The amount of UVB is highest between 10 a.m. and 2 p.m. during the summer. One problem is choosing sunglasses from the retailer's shelf. Although several inexpensive clip-on sunglasses offer excellent UV protection, some sunglasses are poor in their ability to absorb UV. Sunglasses with labels such as "meets ANSI cosmetic UV requirements" may have their 1% cutoff (longest wavelength at which the sunglass transmits no more than 1% of the incident light) as low as 303 nm, whereas others labeled "UV protection up to 400 nm" may have their 1% cutoff at 348 nm. This is especially dangerous in children's sunglasses because children frequently spend more time in the sun; damage to the lens (and possibly retina) from UV light is cumulative, and the crystalline lens of children transmits more short-wavelength visible radiation and UV light to the retina than does that of the adult.

Even with darkly tinted glasses, there is no way to predict by gross visual inspection which lenses effectively filter reasonable quantities of near-infrared light (700 to 800 nm) and near-UV light (300 to 400 nm), which are not visible to the human eye. Cost, color, and lens composition are unreliable indicators of adequate filtration. Fifty-three percent of glass and 11% of plastic lenses have an unfavorably high near-UV transmission peak greater than 25%. Eighty percent of the amount of infrared light present in daylight is transmitted to the retina. Although the infrared light present in daylight is not toxic in itself, some believe that it may help facilitate damage from UV light and lower wavelength light and may contribute to ocular discomfort. Because infrared light contains no useful visual information, it is probably wise to filter it out. UV light absorption is quite different for various lens materials.

Most sunglasses sold for sports use are deficient in impact resistance. Sports sunglasses should prevent rather than contribute to injury. The combination of lens and frame must prevent ocular contact by either the missile or the sunglass lens. Manufacturers should state the sport(s) for which the sunglasses are intended. Racket sports sunglasses should meet the impact requirements of ASTM F803; a softball should not shatter sunglasses designed for all-purpose recreational use nor should the lens pass through the frame under expected sports impact. Impact performance standards for sports sunglasses that test the lens-frame combination under realistic conditions on anatomic headforms are needed.

It is essential that manufacturers are required to provide the following information, in a statement easily understood by the consumer, on all sunglasses sold for use in sports:

- the percent of visible light transmitted through the lens
- the percent of UV light and infrared light (wavelengths specifically stated) transmitted through the lens
- additional treatments or coatings (e.g., polarization) to reduce glare
- the specific sports standards to which they conform and the sports for which the sunglasses have adequate impact resistance as well as the sports for which the sunglasses are definitely not recommended

The ideal sports sunglasses should have the following:

1. UVB (280 to 315 nm) less than 5% transmittance and less than 1% transmittance for wavelengths less than 310 nm.
2. UVA (315 to 400 nm) less than 10% transmittance and absolutely less than maximal visible light transmittance; for aphakes, less than 1% transmittance.
3. Blue light (400 to 500 nm) less than 10% transmittance and absolutely less than the maximal visible light transmittance. A blue light transmittance of 25% to 50% of the peak visible transmittance would be desirable.
4. Long wavelength visible light (500 to 760 nm) less than 15% transmittance for bright conditions, such as sand or snow.
5. Infrared (above 760 nm) filtration desirable but not essential.
6. Color discrimination sufficient to recognize traffic signals.
7. Side shields and either a rim across the top or used in conjunction with a brimmed hat to protect against oblique incident radiation in very bright conditions.
8. The option of polarization to prevent glare from water for fisherman and boaters.
9. Aerodynamic efficiency to combat the drying effects of wind in speed and wind sports (cycling, yachting, mountaineering, skiing).
10. Lightweightness. Heavy sunglasses will tend to fly off the face with rapid changes in head position.

11. Cosmetic acceptability.
12. Impact resistance.

These conditions lead to dark amber polycarbonate lenses (although lighter shade lenses could be used if one wore a brimmed hat).

Athletes With Prior Eye Surgery or Eye Disease

Several situations make the eye more prone to significant injury or rupture on impact. Conditions such as high myopia, previous injury or infection, or prior surgery that have altered the intraocular structures may increase the risk of serious ocular injury by a lesser force than would be necessary to injure the normal eye. Any corneal incision results in a scar that does not have the same tensile strength as the original cornea.

There is no question that penetrating keratoplasty, intracapsular and extracapsular cataract surgery, glaucoma filtering procedures, and radial keratotomy significantly weaken the eye and make rupture of the globe more likely. It is also possible, although not yet proven, that procedures that thin the cornea, such as keratomileusis and laser surgery for myopia, may weaken the globe to some degree. It seems reasonable that phacoemulsification through clear cornea may cause more weakness than that performed through a scleral tunnel. The effects of scleral buckling, strabismus surgery, or scleral thinning from high myopia or prior bouts with scleritis are unknown, but it should be assumed that the eye is weakened at least to some degree by these conditions or procedures.

Weakening of the globe is of concern because the prognosis for return of vision is diminished by rupture of the globe after blunt trauma. Athletes with conditions that weaken the structure of the globe should not be discouraged from sports but should be given advice as to the best means of injury prevention in the desired sport and a specific prescription for protective eyewear. The practice of promoting refractive surgery (radial keratotomy) as a means to play sports without glasses and the depiction of athletes, such as tennis players, playing without protective eyewear should cease. All athletes who are contemplating refractive surgery should be given a clear warning that the eye is weakened, probably for life, by the procedure and that, rather than removing glasses, the athlete is more in need of protective eyewear after the procedure than before.

Sports Visual Training

Considering the fact that a good deal of athletic performance is related to how well the brain coordinates patterns of muscular response to anticipation of the future position of objects, such as balls, by the brain, ophthalmologists and optometrists should be aware of the need to study other parameters of vision in addition to the usual visual acuity and contrast sensitivity measurements (see Chapter 14).

The controversy surrounding visual training and athletic performance does not center around whether or not other visual parameters are important for athletic performance; they clearly are. The matter of contention is the claim, by some, that visual training can improve athletic performance. It is intuitive that training of the entire reflex–vision–muscular pathway must take place primarily under actual performance conditions. Although visual training may improve some elements of perception, the key question remains: Will equivalent time spent with a good coach or instructor under actual game or performance conditions result in better final performance than equivalent time spent with visual training? The proponents of visual training must be certain they are causing no harm by depriving athletes of more exposure to actual game conditions by the time spent doing visual training.

The use of visual training to improve athletic performance is increasing in popularity as more practitioners (mostly optometrists) enter the field. Most ophthalmologists are unaware of the terms and techniques used by visual training practitioners and are doubtful of claimed results. Can the sports vision specialist really improve a player's overall athletic success by improving certain aspects of visual performance or are the claims exaggerated and unproven?

In any field that is young, there is a rash of cases that claim extraordinary results, use unstandardized test methods, and report results in a way that does not permit statistical validation. The excesses of some practitioners should not cloud the work that is in progress by many optometrists and psychologists to help answer many questions concerning the role of visual function that is not routinely tested by most ophthalmologists and optometrists.

Standardized test methods, normal values, and controlled studies, all lacking at this time, are needed. We should keep an open mind on this active area. Practitioners and researchers in the area of visual training should continue to develop standardized tests and gather data on the normal range of values. Controlled studies, such as those proposed by the Vision Performance and Safety Committee of the

United States Olympic Committee, should be funded and performed. Not only may visual training prove a valuable technique for improving athletic performance, but the techniques learned may also help in other areas, such as macula disease and field loss.

Legal Implications of Sports-Related Eye Injuries

Prescribing and/or dispensing eyewear for athletes is fertile ground for litigation because there is significant potential for injury and the sale of a product is frequently involved. Thus, legal claims can be directed on the grounds of negligence as well as those of product liability. Negligence awards for the plaintiff have arisen from failure to prescribe the lens material of choice and failure to warn of the differences in impact resistance between various lens materials. Manufacturers of sunglasses and protective eyewear have had product liability judgments against them for defects in design that resulted in an otherwise preventable injury. It would be legally imprudent for anyone writing a prescription or dispensing eyewear to athletes not to prescribe polycarbonate lenses or to be certain that prescribed sports eyewear meets applicable safety standards. The dispenser should beware of the stylish sunglasses with the CR39 or glass lens that could shatter if struck with a tennis ball or softball. It is apparent that malpractice negligence and product liability suits will remain a significant factor in sports-related eye injuries.

Although suits against ophthalmologists for improperly prescribing optical devices are rare at this time, they certainly will increase in frequency as lawyers become aware of advances in eyewear protection that the professional should advise for athletic patients exposed to specific risks. Another area of significant liability risk appears to be failure to warn radial keratotomy patients of the extra need for eye protection against traumatic rupture of the globe likely to occur from the energy in many sports. The optician, dispensing optometrist, and ophthalmologist must take a sports, industrial, and hobby history and advise appropriate protective eyewear. Manufacturers must participate in the voluntary standard-setting process and test their products before release to the general public. Devices that are advertised as protective but that fail to give adequate protection will result in litigation.

Athletic administrators, coaches, doctors, and equipment manufacturers realize that injuries cannot be entirely eliminated from sports. They are working to at least minimize the risk of serious injury. The best defense in a legal suit seems to be the ability to demonstrate that all concerned were acting responsibly, using state-of-the-art protective devices, playing surfaces, and conditioning and training techniques to protect the athlete to an acceptable level of risk considering the nature of the sport.

Roles of Professionals in Sports Safety and Performance

National ophthalmology, optometry, and optician organizations should give more emphasis to prevention as an important part of eyecare practice. Ophthalmologists and optometrists can get patients to protect their eyes by having an office prevention plan, giving simple handouts, and writing a specific prescription. Opticians should be part of the protection team. The optician is usually the last person who interacts with the player. Part of every optical shop should be a display of sports and industrial eyewear that meets applicable standards, as well as handouts that give specific advice on eye protection for various activities. School committees should be sensitive to their responsibility to properly educate their interscholastic coaches and provide athletic trainers. Certified athletic trainers are invaluable in monitoring the athletes for fitness and ensuring that protective equipment fits properly and is maintained. The athletic trainer is the bridge between the medical staff and the athlete.

Because it is only the coach who is with the athlete before, during, and after both practices and games, the coach assumes the role of everyman. In addition to producing winning teams and teaching proper playing techniques, the coach is expected to keep the athletes healthy and injury free. Because certified athletic trainers and physicians are not present at every game, the coach should have a basic knowledge of injury prevention, recognition, and first aid. Forty states have specific standards for coaches that include a coaching philosophy that places the well-being of the athlete above all other considerations, planning and instructional skills, emergency first aid, psychology of coaching, principles of training and conditioning, legal aspects of coaching, awareness training in drug and alcohol education, human growth and development, and an understanding of the principles and policies of the state associations and the interscholastic sports programs. It is important that the ophthalmologist realizes that most athletic directors, trainers, and coaches are skilled professionals and part of the health care team. It is only by working in harmony with these professionals that we can develop and maintain meaningful athletic vision performance and safety programs.

Many of our patients are active in sports, even into the "golden years." We can help them by improving vision when possible, encouraging the visually impaired, and promoting safety.

Reference

Vinger PF. The eye and sports medicine. In: Tasman W, Jaeger EA, eds. Duane's clinical ophthalmology. vol. 5. Philadelphia: Lippincott, 1994:1–103.

CHAPTER 2

Baseball

Bruce M. Zagelbaum

Baseball, America's favorite pastime, is one of the most popular sports played throughout the world. Its popularity as an Olympic sport has done much to promote the game internationally. At last count, baseball was being played on an organized level in 65 countries throughout the world. Although there is much speculation regarding the origin of baseball, it is believed that the modern day game was invented by Abner Doubleday in 1839 at Cooperstown, New York.

In the United States there are approximately 5 million youngsters who participate in baseball each year, of which 2.7 million belong to Little League teams. The incidence of injury in baseball is estimated at 2% to 8% of participants per year (1). Of the 900,000 baseball-related injuries each year, 170,000 are facial (2). Most of these injuries are soft-tissue trauma; however, deaths have also occurred from direct impact to the head or chest.

Each year, baseball is the number one cause of sports-related eye injuries among the 5- to 14-year-old age group (3). Overall, in all age groups combined, baseball is usually first or second in order of causing the most sports-related eye injuries in the United States. The Consumer Product Safety Commission estimates that in 1993, hospital emergency departments treated over 41,000 eye injuries that were sports or recreation related; baseball accounted for 6136 (14.9%) (3). Most reported injuries occur in less skilled beginners and amateurs, especially where play is not well controlled. For individual age groups, baseball was the most common cause of eye injuries in the 5- to 14-year-olds (3150 injuries), second to basketball among 15- to 24-year-olds (1407 injuries), and third among 25- to 64-year-olds (1185 injuries), after basketball and racket and court sports.

Studies have been conducted concerning eye injuries in baseball. Larrison et al (4) conducted a 1-year study of 202 sports-related eye injuries and found that baseball accounted for 19.8% of all injuries. In their population, 52% described their level of expertise as intermediate, 30% as beginner, and 17% as expert. According to Morehouse, the younger the batter, the greater the risk of being hit by a pitched ball, because of lower skill levels, slower reaction times, wide variations in skill levels, and differences in physical maturity (5). Mills (6) believes that ocular injuries were more likely to happen to weekend athletes, who are not in top physical condition, and to school-age competitors, who may have more enthusiasm than skill.

Zagelbaum et al (7) reported on a prospective study among major league professional baseball players. The incidence of ocular injury was 1.9 eye injuries per 100,000 player innings. Most injuries were minor in nature, and 55% were caused by a batted ball. Common diagnoses included lid/periorbital contusions and lacerations, corneal abrasions, and traumatic iritis. One injury was to a pitcher who was hit by a line drive and sustained a hyphema, eyelid abrasion, subconjunctival hemorrhage, and traumatic iritis.

Players hit by a batted ball are almost always infielders or those on the sidelines. Players in the on-deck circle and dugout are especially susceptible because numerous high velocity foul balls are hit toward these areas. The players in these two areas are usually attentive and need to exhibit extraordinary reflexes, for any delay in reaction time may result in injury. In addition, errant throws to first or third base may go into the dugout. Bahill et al (8) concluded that professional baseball players have faster smooth-pursuit eye movements, have better head-eye coordination, and are very adept at suppressing the vestibulo-ocular reflex, all of which may contribute to their ability to avoid injury.

The Batter

A pitcher generally stands 60 feet away from home plate; in youth leagues, it is 40 feet. The batter sees the initial trajectory of the pitched ball and within fractions of a second must predict its final course and decide whether to swing. The start of the swing, therefore, must be before the ball arrives (Fig. 2.1). It is believed that a baseball player attempting to hit a pitched ball is one of the most difficult visual and physical coordination efforts that the human sensorimotor system can perform (8,9). The eyes send signals to the brain, which in turn sends signals to the muscles to react. As a pitch is being delivered, the batter "steps into" the approaching pitched ball, attempting to hit it. While all this is happening, a batter must also be ready to "bail out" or "hit the dirt" if it is believed that the ball will hit him or her. A natural instinct is to get out of the way of an approaching high velocity object. Naturally, there is always fear. Although the instinct to get out of the way is seen in youngsters and weekend players, professionals have learned to adjust better to the fear of getting hit.

The interval from the time the ball leaves the pitcher's hand to the

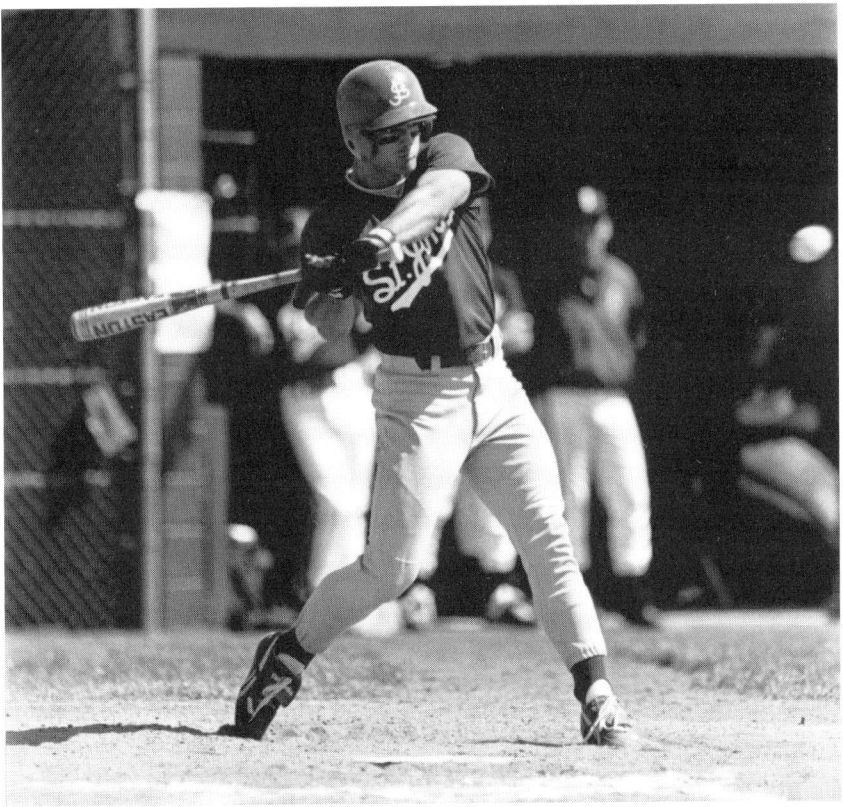

Figure 2.1 *The batter's swing must start before the ball arrives. Note that the batter's eyes are on the ball as he is "stepping into" the pitched ball.*

moment it crosses home plate is 400 ms (four-tenths of a second) (9). Because the batter needs 200 ms to initiate the swing, bringing the bat across the plate, a decision must be made in the first 200 ms based on the speed and path of the pitched ball. At this point, the baseball is still 30 feet away from home plate. Ted Williams, one of the greatest hitters of all time, was supposedly able to see the baseball actually strike his bat. Nonetheless, he still had to start his swing sooner.

Weather conditions also play a role in the batter's ability to clearly see the oncoming pitched ball. A batter may actually stand in a shadow cast from the surrounding stadium while the pitcher is still standing in direct sunlight. In stadiums that have centerfield bleachers, a batter may encounter difficulty in initially picking up the pitcher's delivery because the white baseball may blend in with spectators wearing white shirts.

The Pitch

Whether it is a rising fastball, a dipping curve, a swerving screwball, a sinking split-fingered fastball, or an out of control knuckleball, there is always the potential of a batter being struck in the eye or face by a pitch. One can imagine being at bat and having a 95-mph fastball sail right by one's head. Many professional pitchers today are capable of throwing a baseball at speeds in excess of 90 mph, and a few can throw over 100 mph. Although 12-year-old pitchers generally pitch at velocities of 40 to 50 mph (Seefeldt, VD, unpublished data, 1993), some have the capabilities of throwing over 70 mph (10).

In strategic maneuvers, a pitcher may throw a ball close to the batter (high and tight), in an attempt to back him or her off the plate, or throw down and away. In trying to keep the batter guessing, the pitcher throws an assortment of pitches, including the curve ball, which may seem to be headed for a batter's head until the last instant in which it curves away. The curve ball, while rotating, creates different air pressure on each side of the ball, allowing it to travel in a curved path. If a pitcher is having a bad inning, it appears that "throwing at" the batter may be a retaliation.

After the pitch is made, the follow-through may put the pitcher off balance for a split second. Keeping in mind that a pitch can come in at 100 mph and a batted ball can travel even faster, pitchers must keep an eye on the ball at all times, for if a line drive is hit back toward them, reflexes alone may not save them from getting hit.

The Catcher

The catcher is the field sergeant, ordering pitches and aligning the fielders. It is the most difficult and dangerous of positions. Before 1875, the catcher stood alone without mit or mask. Then, in the late 1870s, the first masks were used (Figs. 2.2 and 2.3).

Catchers need to see everything around them. Masks that earlier resembled wire cages were altered in the 1920s and 1930s to provide protective crossbars that afford greater visibility.

Catchers today are as safe as modern equipment can provide (Fig. 2.4), yet the ball still comes toward them at a full speed of 1.5 miles/min and base runners still hit them head on at plays at the plate. Helmet and mask combinations are a must to prevent foul tips from striking the face. Major league players swing their bat through the strike zone at an average of 70 mph. The swing is in close proximity to the catcher's face.

The Fielder

Third basemen usually stand closest to home plate and on occasion make plays by blocking the ball with their body. Line drives may be hit sharply down to the third or first basemen, who must keep their eyes on the ball and have quick reflexes. The shortstop and second basemen stand further from home plate and have more time to react to a batted ball.

Outfielders have the least chance of getting hit by a batted ball because of the large distance between the batter and themselves. At times, the bright sunlight or stadium lights may cause them trouble in seeing an oncoming ball. Collisions may also be seen between the fielder and another fielder, a base runner, or a wall (i.e., outfielders sprinting after a batted ball who collide with the outfield wall). All of these have the potential to create injury.

The Base Runner

The player going around the bases is running at full speed to get to the next base. Frequently throughout a game, players are attempting to "steal" a base. Within the past few years, the "headfirst" slide has

28 Sports Ophthalmology

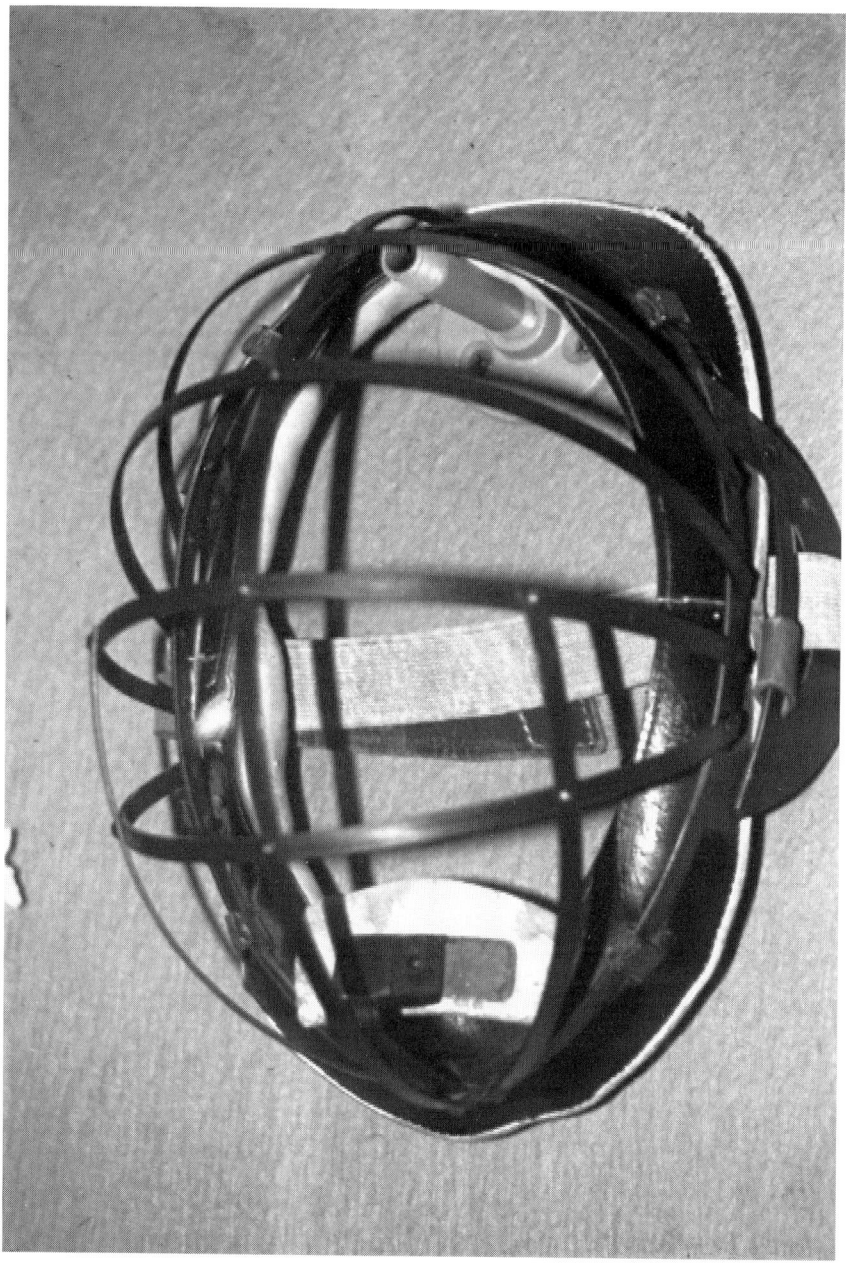

Figures 2.2 and 2.3 *The first catcher's masks used in the late 1800s. Note the vertical central bar that provided a distraction with visibility.*
(continued on next page)

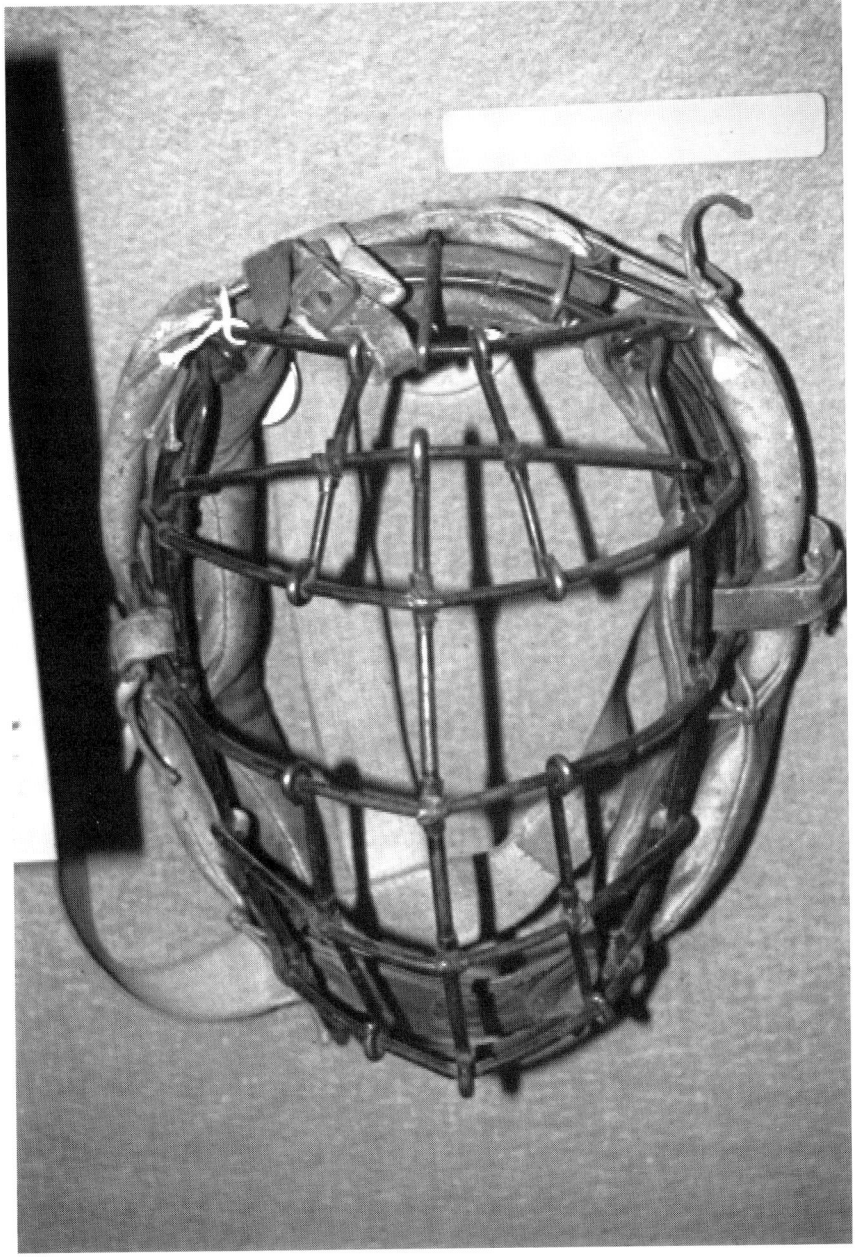

Figure 2.3 *Continued*

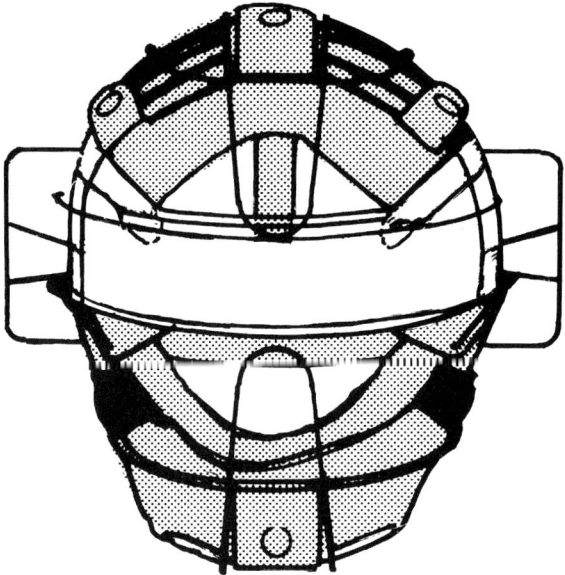

Figure 2.4 *The modern-day catcher's mask, made of steel wire frames and designed to give maximum facial protection and visibility.*

become more popular. This imposes a greater risk of an eye or facial injury to the sliding player from the base and/or the defensive player's lower extremity (e.g., knee, leg, foot). In the study by Zagelbaum et al (7) of major leaguers, one player stealing second base sustained blunt orbital trauma by colliding into the knee of the covering shortstop. This collision caused a malar fracture that required surgery, a lid contusion, and a subconjunctival hemorrhage.

When a player slides into a base, dirt is usually kicked up and thus there is a risk of sustaining a foreign body in the eye (Fig. 2.5). Finally, a sliding base runner may create a collision with the covering fielder, especially with catchers on close plays at home plate. On these types of plays, opposing catchers are usually blocking home plate with their bodies; thus the chance of a forceful collision is substantial.

The Umpire

At the Baseball Hall of Fame in Cooperstown, New York, there is one area on umpires that compares them to policemen: both wear blue uniforms, are respected in their professions, have complete authority when performing their duty, and are proud individuals dedicated to their work. However, that is where the analogy ends.

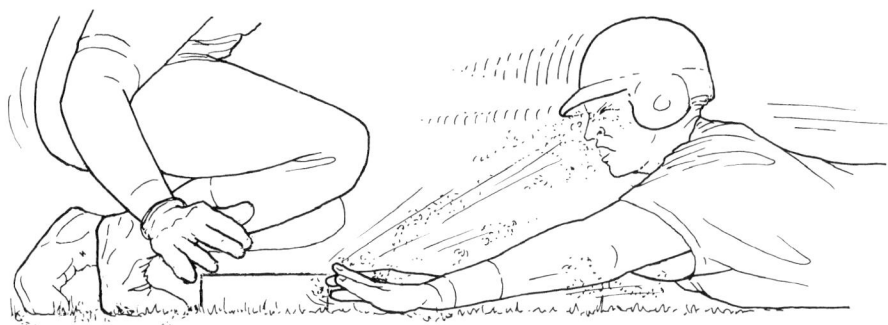

Figure 2.5 *Players sliding headfirst into the base have a greater chance of sustaining an eye injury from either the dirt kicking up or collision with the covering defensive player.*

Whereas a policeman can expect some kind of a reward for a job well done, the umpire toils in relative obscurity receiving no decorations, applause, or even a simple thank-you. Often, the better they are, the less conspicuous they become. Only mistakes bring attention and notoriety. Yet without the umpire's integrity, there could be no baseball.

Although umpires are stationed on the playing field, one umpire stands behind the catcher. His job is to follow the pitched ball as it crosses home plate and, if it is not hit, to call it a ball or strike. Just a few feet in front of the umpire is the batter, taking a swing at the pitched ball. Should the batter graze the ball with the bat, a "foul tip" may be sent back at tremendous velocity and may easily strike the umpire. Although umpires can hide most of their bodies behind the catcher, their entire face is exposed. Fortunately, umpires wear protective face guards.

The Spectator

Those fans who come out to view a baseball game sit in the stands and cheer for their team. They sit back and relax while enjoying the game. Throughout the game, many high velocity batted balls are projected into the stands. Infrequently, a bat may slip out of a batter's hands into the stands.

During a professional game, where as many as 50,000 spectators are seen, the chance that a spectator will need medical attention is significant. During a previous season, a fan sitting in the stands behind third base was struck in the eye by a foul ball, resulting in a ruptured globe that required surgery (Olander K, personal communication). In a separate incident, one player's wife was hospitalized after being struck by a foul ball (11).

Tools of the Game

Bat and Ball

Although major league players are restricted to using bats made of wood, others (e.g., college players, youth leagues) may use bats made of aluminum. It has been postulated that a batted ball coming off an aluminum bat is hit harder and travels faster than if wood was used. In 1884, the first Louisville Slugger bat was produced for Pete Browning. It was 37 inches long and weighed nearly 48 ounces. Today, 31 to 33 ounce bats are common. There is no restriction on the weight of a bat; however, no reinforcement (i.e., cork) may be used in its construction. Incidentally, the reason a player would want to "cork the bat" is that the lighter bat provides quicker bat speed. The faster the swing, the further the baseball travels. A bigger bat, on the other hand, provides a larger hitting surface.

Baseball standards in the major leagues have not changed significantly in 50 years. Major league baseballs must conform to a weight of 5 to 5.25 ounces and a circumference of 9 to 9.25 inches. There is always a cork rubber center, 369 yards of wool and cotton yarn, a rubber cement coating, and a two-piece cowhide cover that is stitched together. Many youth league baseballs are filled with synthetic yarns or molded plastics (12). The relatively large size of an official baseball compared with a squash ball makes it less likely to fit into the orbit and directly strike the globe (Fig. 2.6). Both the bat and ball have undergone few changes compared with other baseball equipment over the years.

Modifications in the hardness and compressibility of baseballs have been developed with the intent of reducing the force of impact while maintaining performance characteristics (1). These softer baseballs have been referred to as reduced injury factor (RIF) balls. The core of these RIF balls compresses over a larger area and for a longer time to reduce the severity of impact. Although it is feasible that these softer baseballs may reduce death or serious injury, no studies have been performed on their impact regarding the incidence or severity of eye injuries.

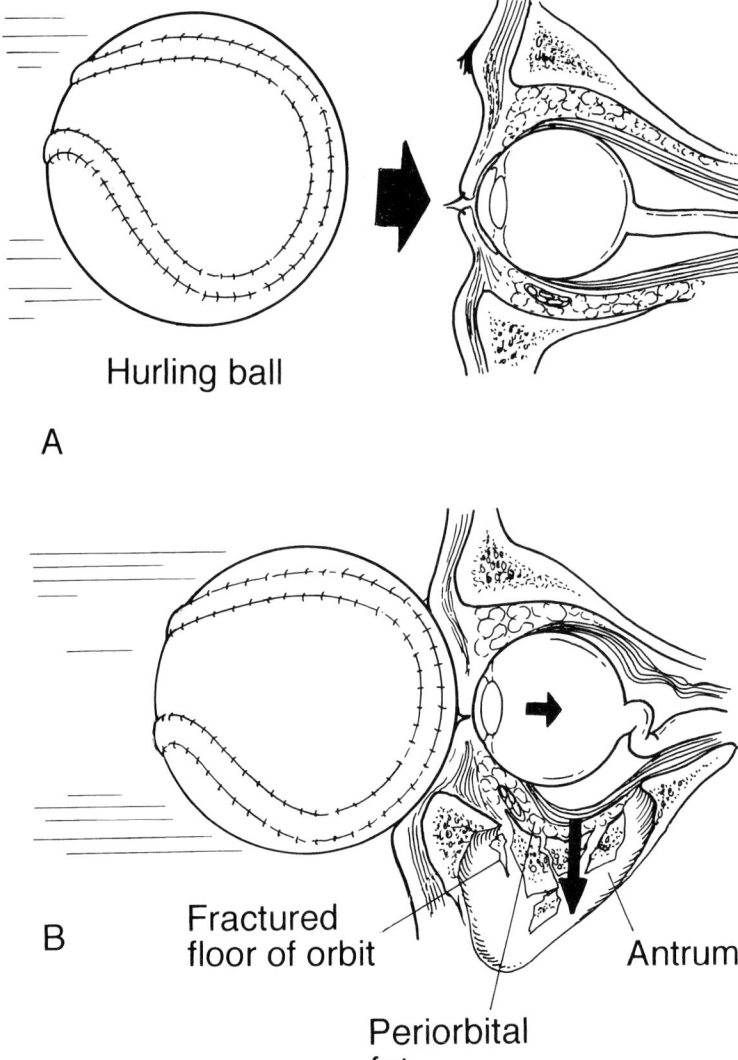

Figure 2.6 *The relatively large size of an official baseball makes it difficult to enter the orbit and directly strike the globe. (A) Just before impact. (B) After impact, the baseball creates a posterior volume displacement which may cause a floor fracture (longer arrow).*

Batting Helmet

The batting helmet was a Branch Rickey innovation. In 1952, the American Baseball Cap Company was born to manufacture the helmet (which was to replace the cap liner then worn by some players), and Charles Muse, Joseph O'Toole, and Edward Crick collaborated on developing the concept (Fig. 2.7). In 1953, the Pirates were the first organization to use batting helmets. The National League made the helmet mandatory for the 1956 season, and the American League followed 2 years later. The helmet ear flap was introduced in the minor leagues in the early 1970s and in the majors for rookies in 1983.

The helmet is made of a polycarbonate shell with foam liners that absorb the energy produced by ball contact. The fit of the helmet must be snug to prevent it from becoming dislodged while swinging the bat or running the bases. Helmets are constructed and tested for different aged players and head sizes. What may be considered safe for a 10-year-old may be unsafe for a 12-year-old. Helmets that are cracked or deformed should not be used. In addition, the foam must be in good condition. The National Operating Committee for Standards in Athletic Equipment (NOCSAE) stamp inside the helmet shows that the helmet has been properly tested. NOCSAE is an independent testing lab.

Little League Baseball

There are 2.7 million children that participate in Little League Baseball. According to Creighton Hale, president and chief executive officer of Little League Baseball, 5.2% of injuries within the league involve the eye (personal communication). Eighty-eight percent of these eye injuries are incurred in positions other than batter. Most injuries occur from contact with the ball, whereas only 5% of eye injuries occur from actions other than a batted, thrown, or pitched ball. According to Hale, there have been no injuries causing permanent loss of vision from 1989 through 1993.

In the early years of Little League Baseball, a wraparound helmet was used by batters, base runners, and coaches in the on-deck circle. The current helmet used today was introduced in 1959, and the catcher's helmet was introduced in 1972. Catcher's and umpire's masks were mandated since the league was first organized in 1939. Although batting helmets, catcher's masks, and umpire's masks are mandated, face guards on batting helmets are approved but not mandated. Similarly, the softer type baseballs are approved but not mandated.

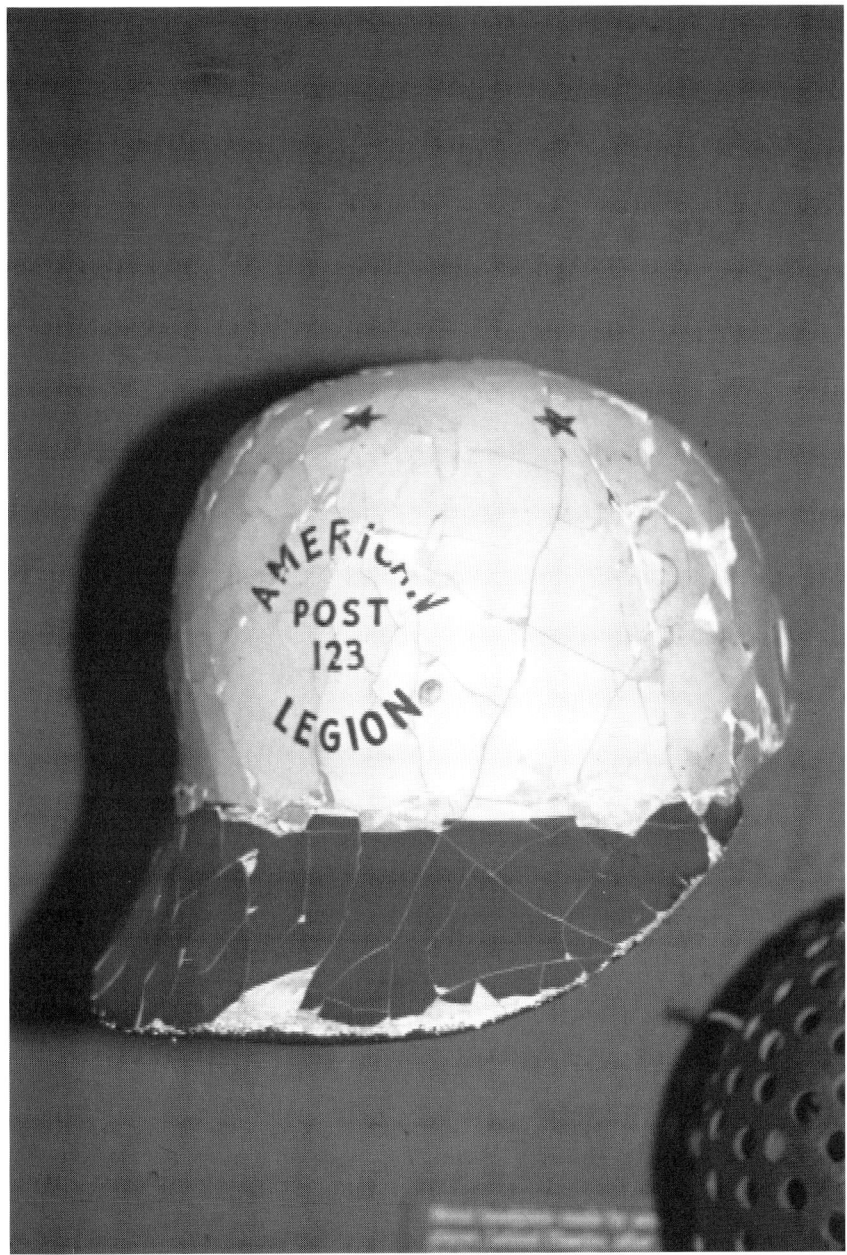

Figure 2.7 *The American Legion helmet was the very first helmet. Plaster was poured over the crown of a standard cloth cap.*

Little League Rulebook

The following are taken from the Little League Rulebook:

- ✗ *Little League Rule 1.11 h:* Shoes with metal spikes are not permitted. Shoes with molded cleats are permissible.
- ✗ *Little League Rule 1.08:* The league shall furnish player's benches, one each for the home and visiting teams. Such benches should not be less than twenty-five feet from the base lines. They shall be protected by fencing of wire.
- ✗ *Little League Rule 2.00 (bench):* Players and substitutes shall sit on their team's bench or in the dugout unless participating in the game or preparing to enter the game. No one except eligible players in uniform, manager and coach shall occupy the bench or dugout. When batters or base runners are retired, they must return to the bench or dugout at once. Batboys and/or batgirls are not permitted. The on-deck circle is adjacent to the dugout, but behind the protective fence in order to protect the player who is preparing to enter the game as the next batter.

Dixie Youth Baseball

The Dixie Youth baseball league has more than 400,000 players in 11 southern states. Players are children 12 years old or younger. For years, Dixie Youth Baseball has recommended facial protection, and on January 1, 1995, face guards were mandated to be worn by batters, base runners, and coaches on the first and third base lines. The league believes that if one child is spared an injury by wearing the face guard, it is well worth it. Dixie is the first youth baseball organization to require this facial protection; it is hoped that other programs will follow.

According to Nick Senter, executive director, Dixie Youth Baseball has led the safety movement over the years, being the first to move dugouts to a point out of range of foul balls, require all players warming up pitchers to wear facemasks, and prohibit shoes with any metal in soles, thus avoiding injuries from protruding cleats or metal pieces.

Major League (Professional) Baseball

On May 7, 1957, pitcher Herb Score of the Cleveland Indians was struck by a line drive off the bat of Yankee Gil McDougal (14). The ball, traveling at 120 mph, hit him squarely in the eye, causing a large hematoma and swelling (10,13). His vision was lacking light perception on initial examination because of retinal damage.

On August 18, 1967, at Fenway Park in Boston, Tony Conigliaro, a bright young baseball star, was struck in the head by a pitch (14). The impact fractured his left cheekbone, dislocated his jaw, and damaged his left retina. Conigliaro returned to the Red Sox in 1969 and played for approximately two more seasons before retiring. It was believed that since the initial injury, he was never quite the same.

On April 8, 1984, a major league player was hit by a pitch above the left eye (15). An all-star shortstop in 1983, he missed all of the 1984 season on the disabled list. For years, he had visual difficulties with impaired depth perception; however, he was able to resume playing baseball (16).

There have been other documented serious eye injuries that have been sustained by major league (professional) players. Whether a beginner, novice, or professional, all players, especially children, are at risk.

Eyeglasses and Baseball

Perhaps the secret of Babe Ruth's batting was that his eyes and ears functioned more rapidly than those of other players and that his brain recorded sensations more quickly and transmitted its orders to the muscles much faster than that of the average man. Babe Ruth's eyes were approximately 12% faster than those of the average human (17).

Years ago it was believed that baseball was responsible for causing eye strain (18). Glare, sweat in the eyes, and steady watching of the ball all contributed; it was especially noticeable in catchers, pitchers, and those sunny areas. Players were afraid their managers would discover that they should be wearing glasses; therefore, they refused to wear them, even off the field. George Torporcer was the first infielder who ever tried to play with glasses. His glasses were broken five times by bouncing balls. Today, most players requiring prescription eyewear wear contact lenses, although some use spectacles. Recently, a few professional players have worn protective sports goggles.

Face Guards

Over the past few years, two players who sustained facial or ocular injuries used a face guard made of an injection-molded polycarbonate during their rehabilitation. Unfortunately, this is usually the case, where the protective device is used after the injury has been sustained; it would be more important to prevent the injury from ever happening.

The face guard, if properly attached to the front of an appropriate NOCSAE-approved helmet, affords protection to the eyes, head, and face (Fig. 2.8, A and B). According to one company that manufactures the product, there has never been a reported eye or facial injury to any player wearing their device. As of January 1, 1995, face guards have been mandated for use by Dixie Youth Baseball. Little League Baseball approves of the guard but has yet to make it mandatory. The Franklin County Dixie Youth League of Virginia actually made face guards mandatory in 1981 (19). After two seasons of use, this league reported that no facial injuries had occurred while the guard was used. League officials spoke about children who were spared serious injury when baseballs bounced harmlessly off their face guards. By taking the fear out of being hit by a pitched ball, children are more comfortable and have more confidence while at bat. It is also comforting for parents. The face guard should also be used by base runners; however, it is important that they slide only feet first. Headfirst slides should not be permitted with the helmet and face guard because it can put undo pressure on the neck. Face guards provide full eye and facial protection. They are lightweight and do not interfere with visibility.

The American Society for Testing and Materials (ASTM) has a standard specification (F910-86) for face guards in youth baseball for batters and base runners (20). ASTM believes that in baseball, where the force of a pitched, hit, or deflected ball can cause facial injury, there is a need for head, facial, eye, and teeth protection. The impact test in this standard is designed to approximate the impact of a direct perpendicular blow from a baseball traveling at 31 m/s (70 mph). Any contact between a ball traveling at this speed with the test headform is considered a product failure.

C-Flap

Developed by a plastic surgeon, the C-flap is made of polycarbonate with an adherent inner foam patch that diffuses the force of an impact (Fig. 2.9). The C-flap was initially created to protect the cheek and jaw. To date, approximately 10 major league players have worn this device after sustaining an injury (Crow R, personal communication). Although this device seems to offer more facial than eye

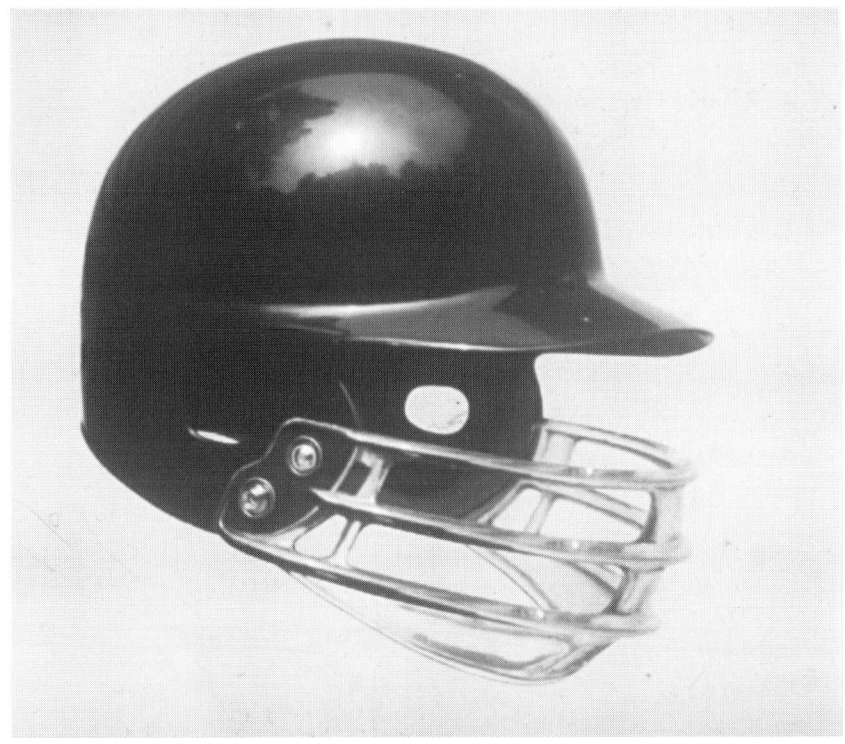

A

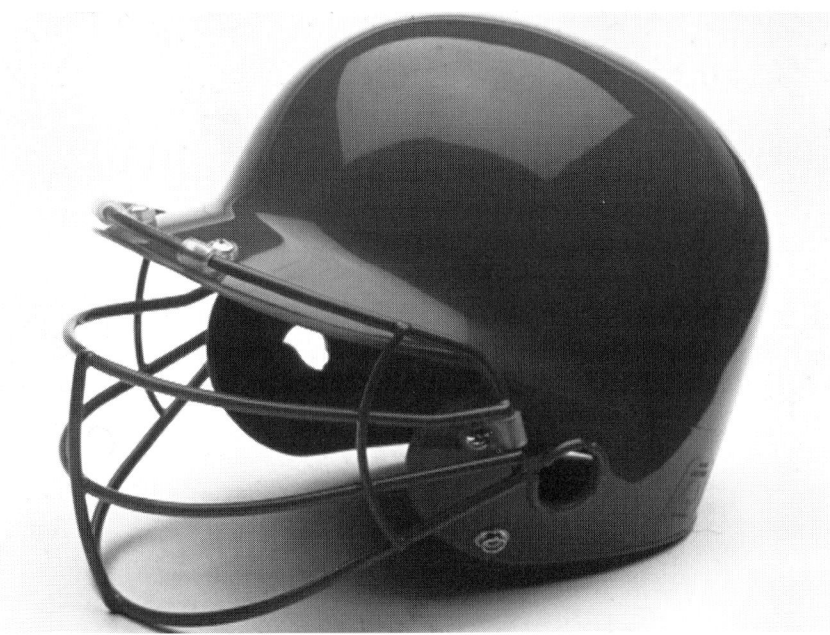

B

Figure 2.8 *The face guard affords protection to the eyes and face. Both types attach to the front of a NOCSAE-approved helmet. (A) Injection-molded polycarbonate design.* (Courtesy of Home Safe Face Guards.) *(B) Welded steel wire design.* (Courtesy of Schutt Sports Group.)

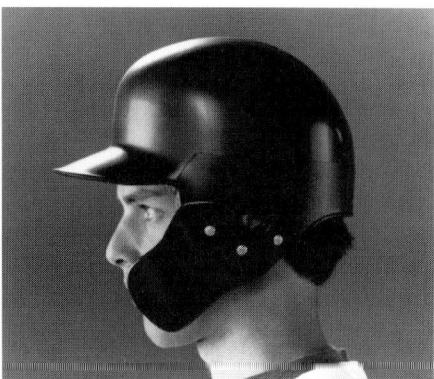

Figure 2.9 *The C-flap is made of polycarbonate and attaches to the front side of a NOCSAE-approved helmet.* (Courtesy of C-Flap, Inc.)

protection, it was designed so that the polycarbonate flap falls beneath the line of vision so that no visual interference occurs with its use.

Sunglasses

Almost anyone can recall seeing a professional baseball player losing a ball in the sun or stadium lights. Some of these balls have struck the fielding player. Sunglasses have been used by baseball players on sunny days for many years. Capable of flipping up or down by a hinge, they come with a strap that fits snugly around the back of the head. When used, they are usually kept in the up position until the fielder has to look at a ball in the sky. With the use of a finger, the player then flips the sunglasses down. Two major league players have sustained serious eye injuries when their flip-down sunglasses shattered on impact with the ball (14). Since 1986, Vision Master, Inc., the manufacturer of flip-down sunglasses, has switched to polycarbonate lenses, and no reported cases of shattered lenses have occurred (14).

Contact Lenses

Fourteen percent of major league baseball players wear contact lenses while playing (Zagelbaum BM, unpublished data). Of the 21 injuries sustained by major league players from July 1991 through July 1992, six (29%) had on contact lenses. All contact lens–related eye injuries were due to either a foreign body or eye rubbing; none was caused by a batted or thrown ball. A corneal abrasion was sustained in five of the six players; one player had bilateral corneal abrasions.

Naturally, achieving the best possible vision is important in any sport. This is especially true for baseball, where visual demands require picking up the flight of a baseball. With the use of contact lenses, there is a risk of eye injury from wind and swirling dirt, causing foreign bodies to strike the ocular surface and to lodge under a contact lens. A player sliding into a base may also create a cloud of dust. Contact lenses do not afford any protection against ocular injury, and protective eyewear is still recommended in addition to the contact lenses.

For players who wear contact lenses, soft hydrophilic daily wear lenses are recommended. Replacement contact lenses as well as contact solutions should be kept on hand at all times. All players wearing contact lenses should have periodic eye examinations. Any player complaining of a foreign body sensation in the eye, irritation, decreased vision, or redness should have his or her contact lenses removed immediately and examined, so that particular attention can be paid to the corneal surface.

Conclusion

Baseball is the number one cause of sports-related eye injuries in youngsters, and devastating injuries continue to occur. Eye injuries in baseball can occur from direct contact with a batted, thrown, or pitched ball; collision with another player; and foreign bodies. Most of these injuries can be prevented with the use of protective devices (e.g., face guards while batting) which should be mandated.

References

1. Committee on Sports Medicine and Fitness. Risk of injury from baseball and softball in children 5 to 14 years of age. Pediatrics 1994;93:690–692.
2. Jones NP. Eye injury in sport. Sports Med 1989;7:163–181.
3. National Society to Prevent Blindness. 1993 Eye injuries associated with sports and recreational products. Schaumburg, IL: National Center for Sight, 1994.
4. Larrison WI, Hersh PS, Kunzweiler T, et al. Sports-related ocular trauma. Ophthalmology 1990;97:1265–1269.
5. Tauber G. Batter up: with eye guards. Sightsaving 1984;53:1–5.
6. Mills N. Sports eye injuries: dimming the stars. Sightsaving 1985;54:2–7.
7. Zagelbaum BM, Hersh PS, Donnenfeld ED, et al. Ocular trauma in major-league baseball players. N Engl J Med 1994;330:1021–1023.
8. Bahill AT, LaRitz T. Why can't batters keep their eyes on the ball? Am Sci 1984;72:249–253.

9. Solomon H, Zinn W, Vacroux A. Dynamic stereoacuity: a test for hitting a baseball? J Am Optom Assoc 1988;59:522–526.
10. Hale CJ. Protective equipment for baseball. Phys Sportsmed 1979;7:59–63.
11. DeBenedette V. Medical coverage of sports events: the fans need attention, too. Phys Sportsmed 1988;16:195–200.
12. Vinger PF. The eye and sports medicine. In: Tasman W, Jaeger EA, eds. Duane's clinical ophthalmology. vol. 5. Philadelphia: Lippincott, 1994:1–103.
13. Bock W. The trick is quick diagnosis. Phys Sportsmed 1974;1:65.
14. Roanoke Times & World-News. Jan. 10, 1982. pg C-12.
15. Hohlfeld N. Thon told to rest his eyes. The Sporting News. June 23, 1986.
16. Fimrite R. You can't keep a good man down. Sports Illustrated. April 16, 1990.
17. Fullerton C. Eye, ear, brain and muscle tests on Babe Ruth. Western Optical World 1925;13:160–161.
18. Abel O. Eyes and baseball. Western Optical World 1924;12:41–42.
19. Mills N. Face shields for youth baseball. Sightsaving 1986;55:1–4, 16.
20. American Society of Testing and Materials. Standard specification for face guards for youth baseball: F910-86. Philadelphia: American Society for Testing and Materials, 1986.

CHAPTER 3

Basketball

Chad Starkey
Bruce M. Zagelbaum

History

The modern game of basketball was developed in 1891 by Reverend James Naismith (who later became a physician) as a form of indoor winter recreation for his parishioners. Using rules and strategies derived from popular New England sports such as ice hockey, soccer, and football, the original game involved two teams of nine players attempting to "toss" a soccer ball into peach baskets mounted to walls at each end of a room.

Near the end of the 19th century, colleges adopted the game of basketball as an intercollegiate sport with five players on each team. The early rules of competitive basketball were structured to eliminate the injuries associated with other team sports and were based on the premise that, "if the offense did not have the opportunity to run with the ball, there would be no necessity for tackling and we would thus eliminate roughness" (1). After viewing how contemporary basketball is played, it is humorous to note that the early game had a penalty box where, similar to ice hockey, a player who made physical contact with an opponent would be removed from the contest until the next goal was scored.

Today, basketball is a fast-paced game that permits, if not encourages, physical contact. Men and women of all ages compete on a playing area ranging from 74 ft long and 42 ft wide to professional- and college-sized courts measuring 94 ft by 50 ft. Basketball has a unique characteristic for an American sport: each athlete is expected to possess the requisite skills of running, jumping, throwing, catching, dribbling, and shooting. The actual number of participants in basketball cannot be calculated due to the growing popularity of recreational "pick-up" leagues, outdoor "street ball," 3-on-3 leagues, and the ever-present "driveway" games.

Eye Injuries in Basketball

Despite the fast-paced physical nature of the game of basketball, there is no required protective equipment. These factors invite the potential for injury and account for basketball's being the sport with the highest frequency of athletic-related eye injuries in the United States (2,3). In a Massachusetts study, 28.7% of all sports-related eye injuries were related to playing basketball (4). Within the sport, exceptional speed, strength, skills, and stamina are required by those who play under organized conditions. Unintentional contact by another player's finger, hand, or elbow; intentional punches with a closed fist; and contact with the ball itself all can cause serious trauma to the eye and its orbit.

Unfortunately, the use of approved protective eyewear in basketball occurs primarily as an afterthought once a player has sustained a significant injury. Although protective goggles do not prevent all eye injuries, the frequency of injury is significantly less for players who wear them. Athletes at all levels of competition must be encouraged, if not required, to wear protective eyewear.

Rules Mandating the Use of Protective Equipment

Of the popular team sports (e.g., baseball, football, ice hockey), basketball players' bodies are the most exposed to potentially injurious forces. Neither game rules nor uniform requirements stipulate the use of any type of protective equipment (the lone exception to this rule are those individual leagues that require the use of a protective mouthpiece). The rules do, however, stipulate protective devices that the player *cannot* wear. The rules of the National Collegiate Athletic Association (NCAA) governing the use of special equipment are prototypical of this type of regulation:

> *Elbow, hand, finger, or forearm guards, casts, or braces made of plaster, metal, or any other nonpliable substance shall be prohibited. Pliable (soft) plastic may be used as protective covering*

for an injury.... Equipment that could cut or cause injury to another player is prohibited, without respect to whether the equipment is hard (5).

Although this rule is the bane of many athletic trainers and team physicians, its obvious intent is to prevent the arms and hands from becoming more of a weapon than they already are.

Prevalence of Basketball-Related Eye Injuries

Basketball has been implicated as the most frequent cause of eye trauma in organized and recreational sports (2–4,6,7). It has been estimated that each season 10% of all college basketball players will suffer a traumatic injury to the eye (8).

Statistics provided by the National Society to Prevent Blindness (NSPB) cite the game of basketball as being the leading cause of sports and recreational eye trauma resulting in hospital emergency room visits (2,3). Of the 89,221 athletic-related eye injuries reported to the NSPB during 1992 and 1993, 16,825 (18.9%) were attributable to participation in organized or recreational basketball. According to age groups, basketball injuries are the most common cause of eye injuries in the 15- to 24-year-old and 25- to 64-year-old age groups. In 5- to 14-year-olds, baseball injuries are the most frequent, with basketball injuries being a close second. These numbers depict only the frequency of injury without accounting for the actual rate of eye injuries (e.g., 16,825 eye injuries are much more significant if 100,000 people were participating as opposed to 1,000,000 participants).

The National Basketball Trainers' Association's Eye Injury Study

The National Basketball [Athletic] Trainers' Association (NBTA) maintains a database of all injuries and illnesses that cause time lost (practices and/or games missed) or result in the athlete's being seen by a physician. From 1988 through the 1992 season, 3.2% of all injuries in the National Basketball Association (NBA) involved the eye (Table 3.1). Eye injuries in the NBA occur at the rate of 1.4 per 1000 athlete exposures (AE) (AE is defined as the number of individuals exposed to the opportunity for injury; thus, 15 athletes who participate in a single game account for 15 AE), a rate that exceeds many of the injuries traditionally associated with basketball compe-

Table 3.1 Relative frequency of eye trauma in the National Basketball Association occurring during the 1988 through 1992 seasons

INJURY	TOTAL FREQUENCY	(%)	RATE PER 1000 GAME EXPOSURES
Ankle sprain	488	(13.2)	3.2
Patellar tendon inflammation	254	(6.8)	0.4
Lumbar pathology	226	(6.1)	0.8
Knee sprain	135	(3.6)	1.0
Knee inflammation	125	(3.4)	0.2
Eye and periorbital trauma	**120**	**(3.2)**	**1.4**
Quadriceps contusion	117	(3.2)	0.9
Finger sprain/dislocation	100	(2.7)	0.7
Thumb sprain	56	(1.5)	0.4
Meniscal tear	37	(1.0)	0.2

tition. Most injuries reported in the NBTA's study involved soft-tissue trauma to the periorbital area (i.e., periorbital lacerations and contusions) (Fig. 3.1). However, approximately one-quarter of these conditions could have potentially resulted in permanent dysfunction if the condition was not initially identified and managed correctly. No injury resulting in long-term sequelae has been reported in the 10 years of data collection.

In a 17-month prospective study of professional basketball players (NBA), Zagelbaum et al (6) found that 5.4% of all injuries involved the eye. Thirty-one percent of these injuries occurred while the player was in the act of rebounding and 27% while the player was on of-

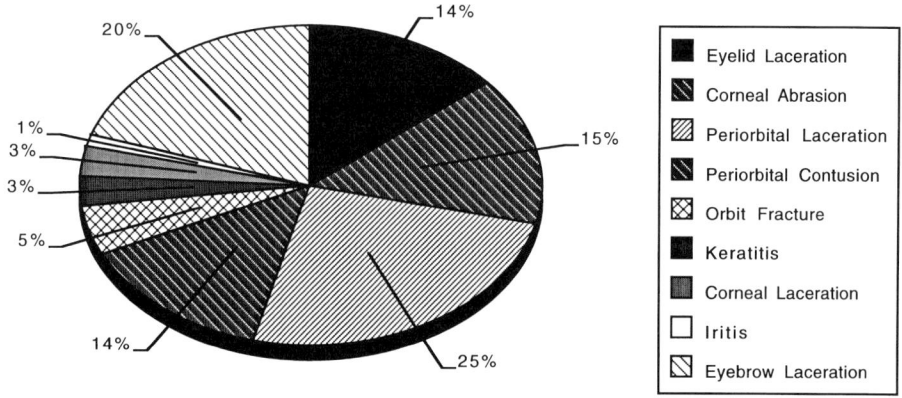

Figure 3.1 *Frequency of eye injuries in the National Basketball Association, 1988 through 1992 seasons.*

fense. The most common injuries seen were abrasions or lacerations of the eyelid (51%), contusions (edema and/or ecchymosis) of the eyelid (29%), corneal abrasions (12%), and traumatic iritis (12%). Five percent of all eye injuries were orbital fractures. Most injuries were caused by an opponent's finger (36%) or elbow (29%); 15% of all injured players missed subsequent games.

The distribution of eye injuries occurring in the NBA is most probably representative of those occurring at other levels of the game. Fortunately, in basketball the velocities of the fingers and ball are substantially less than those associated with baseball and racket sports. This allows for the body's reflexes to protect the globe from injury, albeit at the expense of the periorbital tissues.

Mechanisms of Injury

With the exception of dribbling, most of the psychomotor skills in basketball occur at a level above the waist. Skills such as shooting and rebounding occur above the athlete's head. The spatial relationship between the point in space to which the defender is reaching for the ball and the dynamic nature of the game makes inadvertent contact with the head, face, and eye all but unavoidable.

In the NBA, centers are the most predisposed to eye injury, suffering 1.94 injuries per 1000 exposures, followed by guards (1.41/1000 AE), and forwards (1.30/1000 AE). This statistic can be attributed to the center's traditional place close to the basket. The center's position on the court places this athlete in the middle of most of the activity occurring on the floor. Indeed, most of the player movement and ball passing occurs around an arc relative to the offensive center. On both the offensive and defensive ends of the court, centers are expected to "battle" for rebounds, set picks, shoot, and attempt to block shots.

Projectile Mechanisms

In athletics and recreational sports, most eye injuries occur as the result of a projectile striking the globe. However, during the course of normal basketball competition, the globe itself is rarely threatened by projectile-type injuries.

Basketballs are commonly made from leather or, in the case of outdoor or multipurpose balls, have a nylon covering, and weigh approximately 20 to 22 ounces. Their large circumference (regulation basketballs for men have a 30-inch circumference and for women a

Table 3.2 Mechanisms of eye injuries in the National Basketball Association between 1992 and 1993

MECHANISM	NUMBER	PERCENT
Finger	21	35.6
Elbow	17	28.8
Collision	8	13.6
Unspecified contact	6	10.1
Hand	2	3.4
Punched	1	1.7
Forearm	1	1.7
Ball	1	1.7
Unknown	1	1.7
Other	1	1.7

28.5-inch circumference) and relatively inelastic properties make a basketball unlikely to fit into the orbit and strike the globe directly; ball injuries usually affect the ocular adnexa over the orbital rim. During a 10-year analysis of injuries occurring to participants in the NBA, no injury to the globe has been caused by contact with the ball and only one injury to the periorbital region has resulted from the athlete's being hit with the ball (Starkey C, unpublished data, 1995).

Blunt Trauma

Most injuries in the game of basketball are caused by contact with the opponent's finger and elbow (Table 3.2) and occur while rebounding (Table 3.3). Typically when rebounding, two or more players leap for the ball with their arms and fingers extended (Fig. 3.2). Once the rebound is made, the rebounder traditionally clears space and moves the defensive players away by swinging the elbows while

Table 3.3 Athlete's activity at the time of injury

ACTIVITY	NUMBER	PERCENT
Rebounding (offense/defense)	18	30.5
Offense (general)	16	27.1
Defense (general)	11	18.6
Unknown	6	10.2
Loose ball	5	8.5
Transition	1	1.7
Stealing	1	1.7
Other	1	1.7

Basketball 49

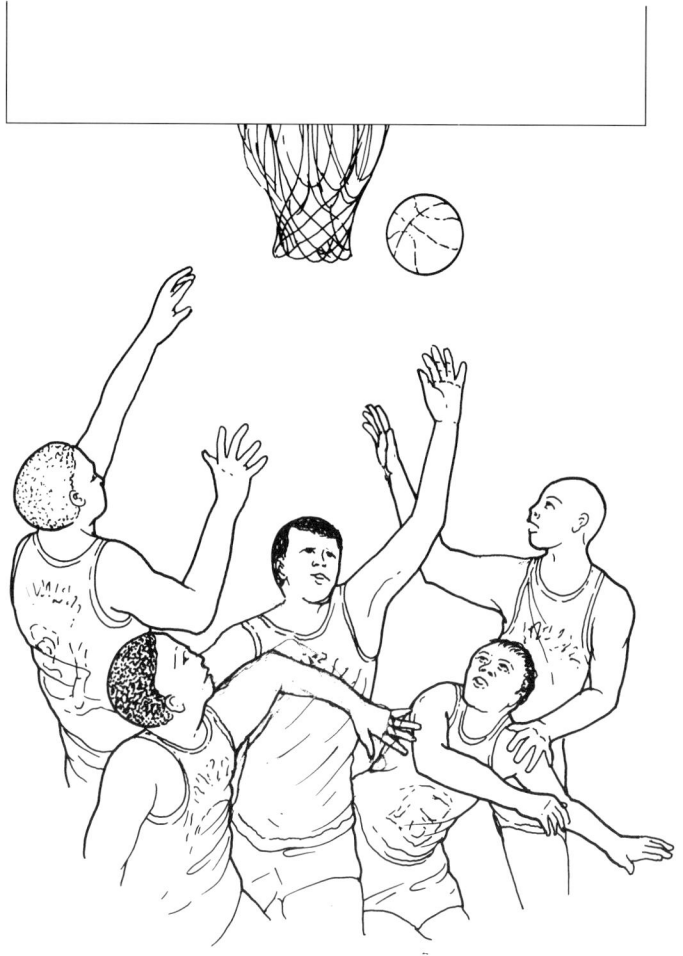

Figure 3.2 *While rebounding, players' arms and fingers are extended and go in all directions. Elbows are frequently seen hitting opponents.*

opposing players attempt to steal the ball. Direct blows from an elbow or fist may cause an orbital fracture.

On the offensive end, defensive players swipe at the ball in an attempt to steal it, and, when a shot is attempted, the defensive players attempt to block it with the hand (Fig. 3.3). Many injuries to guards occur while driving to the basket, only to encounter taller players, with their fingers extended, attempting to block the shot. Fingers and hands are usually going in all directions in an attempt to steal the ball, block the shot, and rebound. At times, a player on offense may use one hand to "ward off" the defender (Fig. 3.4).

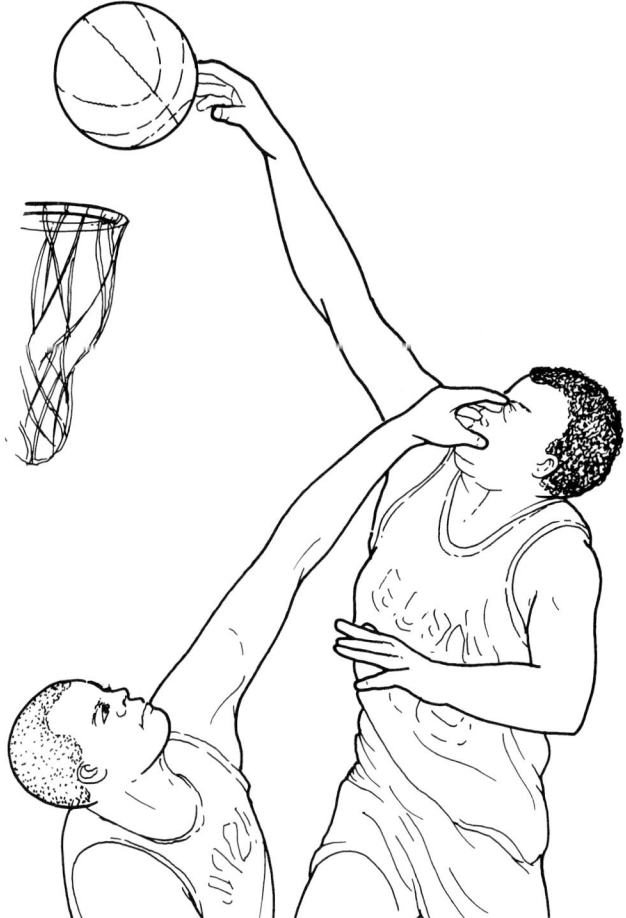

Figure 3.3 *The defensive player usually has arms and hands extended, looking to block the shot or steal the ball.*

Prevention

Chow et al (9) reported on an 18-year-old who was poked in his right eye by a finger while playing basketball and sustained an evulsion of the optic nerve with vision of no light perception. Park et al (10) reported on a 29-year-old male who had complete loss of vision (no light perception) after being poked in his eye while playing basketball. Despite the risk and potentially catastrophic consequences of basketball-related eye injuries, no major basketball sponsoring organization mandates or explicitly recommends the use of protective eyewear for basketball players. The NCAA 1994–1995 Sports Med-

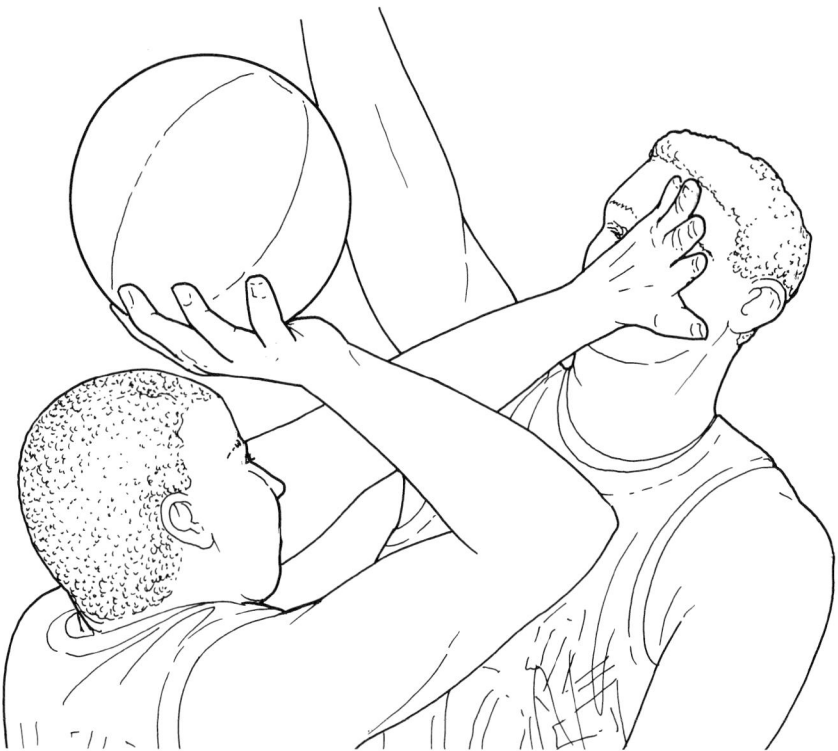

Figure 3.4 *This player on offensive is "warding off" the opponent with the use of his arm.*

icine Handbook does note that one-eyed participants "should" have eye protection (5). Other NCAA recommendations applicable to eye protection (although not specifically mandated) in basketball are listed in Table 3.4.

Most other team sports have ancillary methods of protecting the eye. Football and ice hockey players gain eye protection from the helmet and masks, as do Little League baseball players. Even higher level baseball players gain a degree of safeguard from the batting helmet, which can deflect many potentially injurious forces.

Anecdotally, it appears that the use of protective eyewear by basketball players is most often an afterthought. Most players begin wearing goggles only after a significant injury, but this is not always the case. During the 1993 season, one professional basketball player sustained four significant eye injuries over a 2-month period but at no time wore protective goggles. Yet other athletes wear protective

Table 3.4 NCAA Guideline 4B—Eye Safety in Sports. Excerpts applicable to basketball

- ✗ All participants in collision-contact sports [including men's and women's basketball] who use corrective lenses (including contact lenses) in their sports activity should have eye protection conforming to A through D [describing standards for eye protection].

- ✗ When external lenses (i.e., all other than contact lenses), either corrective or noncorrective, are used for eye protection, they should be of polycarbonate plastic or CR-39.

- ✗ All one-eyed participants [best corrected vision in their weaker eye is 20:80 or worse] in collision-contact sports should have eye protection conforming to definitions A through D.

lenses only while the injury heals and discontinue wearing them once the injury is resolved.

Protective Eyewear

Basketball players of all ages are susceptible to eye injuries. Ninety-seven percent of players in the NBA were not wearing any protective eyewear at the time of injury (6). Those who did had their eyewear dislodged, resulting in injury to the eyelid. The use of protective eyewear may prevent as many as 90% of all eye injuries (11). Protectors are readily available for the sport of basketball and prevent or minimize eye injuries by dissipating the force before it strikes the eye. Lenses should be constructed only of polycarbonate, a material much stronger (superior impact resistance) than standard plastic or glass. Standards for these protective devices (see Chapter 5) have been established and should be followed. Polycarbonate lenses can be custom-made to match the prescription of those athletes requiring glasses.

Regular streetwear glasses and contact lenses do not provide eye protection. To avoid ocular injury, we recommend approved sports goggles that are made of polycarbonate lenses (3 mm thick) and unbreakable frames. For those players who do not need prescription eyewear and those who wear contact lenses, molded polycarbonate sports frames with 3-mm polycarbonate plano lenses (no prescription required) are recommended (Fig. 3.5). Players who need corrective eyewear should use sports frames with 3-mm prescription polycar-

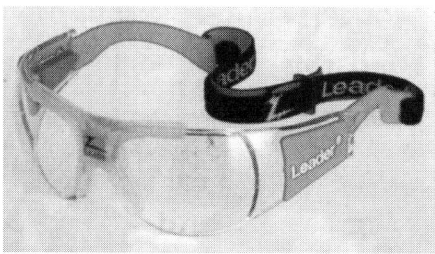

Figure 3.5 *Players who do not require prescription eyewear and those who wear contact lenses should wear approved polycarbonate goggles such as this model shown.* (Courtesy of Leader Sport Products, Inc.)

bonate lenses (Fig. 3.6). Proper fit is essential for optimal protection. Sports frames should fully cover the orbital region and should be properly fit, with contact at the bridge and both temples. In addition, they should contain safety bevels to prevent the lens from dislocating in (toward the eye).

Wearing protective eyewear does not guarantee elimination of eye injuries; however, it would dramatically decrease their incidence. Anecdotal reports describe instances in which the initial contact dislodges the player's goggles, thus exposing the eyes to trauma.

Perhaps the most iconographic statement for the use of protective goggles in basketball (perhaps for all athletic endeavors) is the image of Kareem Abdul-Jabbar (Plate 1). It was not until after his sixth corneal abrasion that he started wearing the now-famous goggles. Finding the proper pair of goggles was a trial-and-error process until he eventually found a pair that allowed him the necessary peripheral vision, did not fog during exercise, and were relatively comfortable to wear. In his book, *Kareem*, he notes, "eventually I found some [goggles] that worked, and every now and then I will feel the click of someone's nails on the lenses and know that it's been worth wearing all these years" (12). When asked if he planned on continuing to

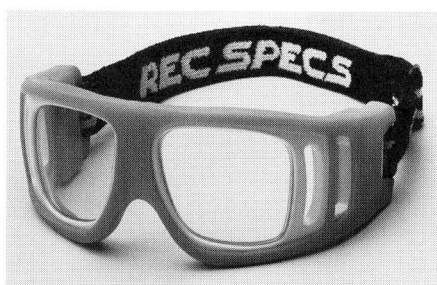

Figure 3.6 *Players who need prescription eyewear should use approved sports frames that can hold 3-mm polycarbonate lenses.* (Courtesy of Liberty Optical.)

wear his goggles, Kareem responded, "Of course! I'm down to my last pair of eyeballs!" (13).

Preparticipation Eye Examination

Keen visual acuity, perceptual vision, eye-hand coordination, and subsequent reaction time not only assist an athlete's playing ability but also decrease the likelihood of injury (14–17). The preseason physical examination of the basketball athlete should encompass a complete ophthalmologic examination. The goals of this examination are to measure existing visual acuity, to correct visual defects that may hinder performance, and, in conjunction with the coaching staff, to correlate visual skills with playing performance (18). The preparticipation eye examination can serve as a forum to promote and educate coaches and athletes alike on the need for protective eyewear.

The preparticipation eye examination should be supplemented by annual re-examinations at the start of subsequent seasons. The team's medical staff should be alerted to athletes who have conditions that further predispose them to injury, have a condition that may alter the evaluation of other medical conditions (e.g., anisocoria or nystagmus in an athlete suspected of suffering a concussion), or will need further evaluation or treatment for an existing eye condition.

Conclusions

Basketball accounts for the highest number of athletic-related eye injuries. Fortunately, most of these injuries are to the soft tissues surrounding the eye rather than to the globe itself. Injuries resulting in permanent disability are relatively rare when compared with racket sports. In the sport of basketball, centers are most predisposed to eye injuries, presumably because of their physical location on the court and their exposure to multiple injurious forces.

Commercially available eye protectors constructed of polycarbonate serve well in protecting the globe from injury. Unfortunately, there are no rules at any level of basketball competition requiring the use of such protective goggles. If young athletes were as concerned with what Kareem Abdul-Jabbar wore on his eyes (and why) as they are with what he wore on his feet, the prevalence of eye injuries would be markedly reduced.

References

1. Menke FG. The encyclopedia of sports. New York: A. S. Barnes and Company, 1953:160–161.
2. National Society to Prevent Blindness. 1993 Eye injuries associated with sports and recreational products. Schaumburg, IL: National Center for Sight 1994.
3. National Society to Prevent Blindness. 1992 Eye injuries associated with sports and recreational products. Schaumburg, IL: National Center for Sight 1993.
4. Larrison WI, Hersh PS, Kunzweiler T, et al. Sports-related ocular trauma. Ophthalmology 1990;97:1265–1269.
5. Benson MT. 1994–95 NCAA sports medicine handbook. Overland Park, KS: NCAA, Inc., 1994:59.
6. Zagelbaum BM, Starkey C, Hersh PS, et al. The National Basketball Association (NBA) eye injury study. Arch Ophthalmol 1995;113:749–752.
7. Zagelbaum BM. Sports-related eye trauma: managing common injuries. Phys Sportsmed 1993;21:25–42.
8. Vinger PF. The eye and sports medicine. In: Tasman W, Jaeger EA, eds. Duane's clinical ophthalmology. vol. 5. Philadelphia: Lippincott, 1994:1–103.
9. Chow AY, Golderg MF, Frenkel M. Evulsion of the optic nerve in association with basketball injuries. Ann Ophthalmol 1984;16:35–37.
10. Park JH, Frenkel M, Dobbie G, et al. Evulsion of the optic nerve. Am J Ophthalmol 1971:969–970.
11. Parver LM. Eye trauma: the neglected disorder. Arch Ophthalmol 1986;104:1452–1453. Editorial.
12. Abdul-Jabbar K, McCarthy M. Kareem. New York: Random House, 1990:112.
13. Putnam P. Return of old goggle eyes. Sports Illustrated 1974; Oct:22–25.
14. Beals RP, Mayyasi AM, Templeton AE, et al. The relationship between basketball shooting performance and certain visual attributes. Am J Optom Arch Am Acad Optom 1973;50:656–661.
15. Allard F, Graham S, Paarsalu ME. Perception in sport: basketball. J Sport Psychol 1980;2:14–21.
16. Stull RB. Study of hand and eye dominance and coordination of basketball players. J Am Optom Assoc 1960; Nov:293–298.
17. Applegate RA, Applegate RA. Set shot shooting performance and visual acuity in basketball. Optom Vision Sci 1992;69:765–768.
18. Scheller A, Rask B. A protocol for the health and fitness assessment of NBA players. In: Steingard PM, ed. Clinics in sports medicine. Philadelphia: WB Saunders, 1993:193.

CHAPTER 4

Hockey

Robert C. Pashby
Thomas J. Pashby

History

Although ice skating was introduced in Holland in the year 1400 (1), it was not until 1855 that ice hockey had its beginning. At that time, British soldiers cleared the snow on the harbor ice of Kingston, Canada, attached skates to their boots, and played a game with field hockey sticks and a lacrosse ball. Hockey derived its name from the old French word *hoquet*, which means a shepherd's staff.

The first recorded organized hockey game took place in Montreal in 1879, with 15 players on each side all playing at the same time. In 1890, the first hockey organization, the Ontario Hockey Association, was established in Toronto (2). Protective pads were not worn until well into the 1890s, because no one knew how to raise the puck. Incidentally, the hockey puck was developed from a lacrosse ball, both sides of which had been cut off. Once lifting the puck was introduced, goaltenders began to wear cricket pads, and skaters wrapped their shins in cardboard for protection. The goal consisted of two uprights that were dug into ice and frozen in place. The boards surrounding the playing surface were initially only 1 foot high.

During the late 1800s, hockey became popular in Canada and the United States. The winters were long and frozen ponds were plentiful. Leagues were formed and the competition began. The competition was so keen that Lord Stanley of Preston was prevailed upon to donate a cup; thus, the Stanley Cup was born in 1894.

In the United States, ice hockey made its appearance at Yale and Johns Hopkins universities during the 1890s. In 1903, Americans lay claim to the first professional hockey team, and in 1908, indoor rinks with artificial ice were established. The National Hockey League (NHL), born in 1917, consisted of five teams: the Montreal Canadiens, the Montreal Wanderers, the Ottawa Senators, the Quebec Bulldogs, and the Toronto Arenas. Today, the NHL is comprised of 26 teams. Hockey continues to grow in popularity.

Hockey Eye Injuries

Being one of the fastest and most aggressive team sports in the world, hockey is the leading cause of sports-related eye injuries in Canada and Sweden. The sport includes a high velocity projectile puck, a free-swinging stick, checking, fighting, and sharp skate blades; one can easily see why so many injuries result. There are impacts with a hard playing surface, rigid boards, and goal posts. Impacts range from the high velocity, low mass type (collision with a puck) to the low velocity, high mass type (collision with the boards or goal post).

The use of hockey helmets originated in Sweden and became mandatory in 1963 after a survey revealed approximately 100 closed-head injuries with one death, 22 concussions, and three facial fractures (3). All Canadian Amateur Hockey Association (CAHA) players were required to wear helmets by 1975.

Many years before injury statistics were gathered, two professional hockey players suffered career-ending eye injuries. In 1939, George Parsons was struck in the eye by a hockey stick, resulting in blindness. In 1952, Herb Dickenson was blinded in one eye when struck by a puck.

It was not until the early 1970s that the epidemiology of eye injuries in hockey was investigated. In 1973, Canadian ophthalmologists discussed the numerous hockey-related eye injuries they were treating, many destroying sight. The president of the Canadian Ophthalmological Society (COS) discussed this issue with Dr. Thomas Pashby and sought a solution. A retrospective study of eye injuries in Canadian hockey was then conducted by sending out questionnaire forms to 600 members of COS (4). These forms solicited information regarding hockey-related eye injuries that were treated during the 1972–1973 season. This study reported 287 injury reports that included 20 legally blind eyes; 74% of the eye injuries were stick induced (Table 4.1). A prospective study for the 1974–

Table 4.1 Mechanisms of eye injuries in hockey (Canada)

	1972–1973	1974–1975	1992–1993
Stick	74%	62%	41%
Puck	20%	31%	36%
Other	6%	7%	23%
Average age (yr)	14	16	26
Age of blind eyes			
Under 20 years old	61%	66%	0
Over 20 years old	39%	34%	100%

1975 season was then conducted and included 258 eye injuries, of which there were 43 blind eyes. Most of these injuries occurred in organized hockey in the 11- to 15-year-old age group. Sixty-two percent were caused by the hockey stick. Hospitalization for these injuries totaled almost 1000 days.

Statistics from the 1972–1973 and 1974–1975 seasons were presented to the CAHA and showed that most eye injuries were caused by hockey sticks. Therefore, new high stick rules were introduced for the 1975 season and sticks were not allowed to be brought over shoulder level (5).

In 1974, polycarbonate visors were attached to helmets, covering the eyes and extending down to the tip of the nose (Fig. 4.1). Wire mesh full face protectors, which were available, were considered unsuitable because a regulation hockey stick blade could penetrate them and strike the eye (Fig. 4.2). Before 1975, the CAHA rulebook stated that a player could wear facial protection only with a doctor's certificate and then only until the injury had healed.

In 1977, a Canadian Standards Association committee was set up and the preliminary standard, Z262.2-M1977, was established for eye and teeth protectors for hockey forwards and defensemen (6). There were three types of protectors: eye, teeth, and combination of both. These combination protectors were full face protectors and were either all wire or clear plastic above and wire below. No penetration of the protector was permitted by a 2 × .25-inch hockey stick blade. A full face polycarbonate protector was eventually developed (Fig. 4.3). In 1978, the standard was upgraded (Z262.2-M78) to include all players, including goaltenders, and to make it a face protector rather than an eye or teeth protector (7).

At the same time, in the United States, the American Society for

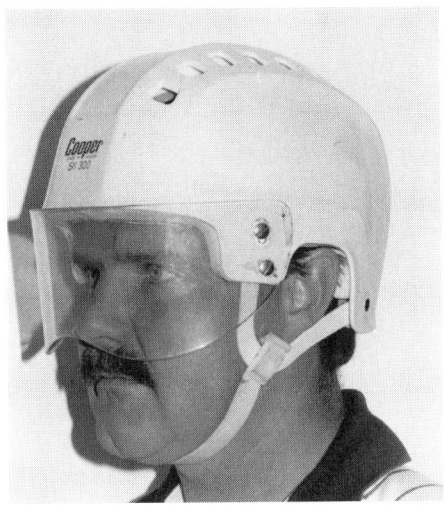

Figure 4.1 The original polycarbonate visor that was used in 1974.

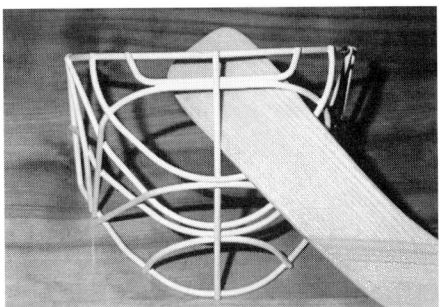

Figure 4.2 Full face wire mesh protector. Note that although the larger openings in the wire mask make them more acceptable to players, a hockey stick may penetrate the opening and strike the eye.

Testing and Materials (ASTM) established the standard F513-77 (8). This standard permitted a 1% probability of the hockey stick blade penetrating the mask, thus allowing for larger openings in the wire mask in attempts to make them more acceptable to players. Although this original ASTM standard did perform to the predicted 99% protection level, those injuries that did occur with the protectors in place were unacceptable. Therefore, the ASTM updated this standard (F513-80) to prevent any chance of penetration of the stick (Fig. 4.4) (9).

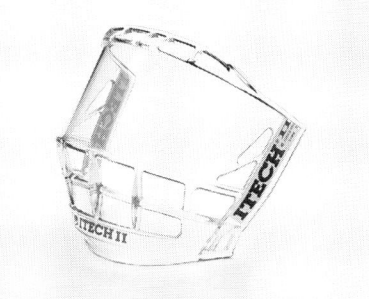

Figure 4.3 The modern full face polycarbonate protector attached to a helmet.

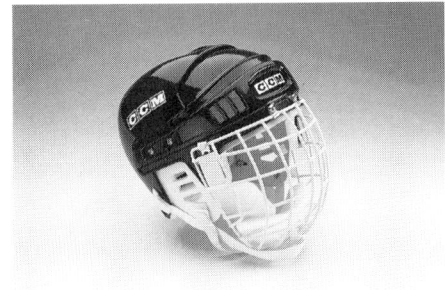

Figure 4.4 Updated wire mask that prevents any chance of stick penetration.

The Hockey Equipment Certification Council (HECC) was established in 1978 to set codes and standards for certifying equipment and facilities in the United States. The purpose of HECC is as follows:

> *To examine the needs and wishes of the various amateur hockey-governing bodies as they pertain to hockey equipment and safety. HECC seeks out and selects codes and standards, including test methods and other requirements for certifying playing equipment and facilities used in the sport of ice hockey. In addition, HECC promotes the use of certified products and monitors the effectiveness of its certification programs on the sport of ice prevention and/or reduction of ice hockey injuries. This is accomplished by studying playing rules, attitudes, playing surfaces, officiating, training, conditioning, and administration, among others (10).*

Meanwhile, the Canadian government insisted that CSA-certified protectors were to be the only ones that could be imported or sold in Canada. For the 1979–1980 season, CAHA ruled that all minor league hockey players (under 18 years of age) under their jurisdiction must wear a CSA-certified face protector that needed to be attached to a CSA-certified hockey helmet. Unfortunately, this was not made compulsory for junior and senior players. This standard was updated in 1983 and then again in 1990 to include visors.

In 1991, eight "old-timers" playing hockey suffered blinding eye injuries. Six were puck induced and two were caused by a stick. None of the injured players wore eye or face protection. At a meeting in 1993, CAHA finally ruled that all senior players under their jurisdiction must wear certified visors. Referees in Canadian amateur hockey must also wear a CSA-certified visor attached to a CSA-certified helmet.

The CSA face protector and visor standard lists four types: for skaters over 10 years of age, for skaters up to and including 10 years of age, for goaltenders, and for referees. The polycarbonate protectors must be tested optically for quality.

The benefits of masks may be seen by looking at the average age of injured players in the premask versus the postmask era. Before masks were introduced in 1975, the average age of an injured player was 14 years (see Table 4.1). Since masks were mandated for minor league hockey players, the average age of an injured player rose to 26 years. Again, note that where it is mandatory for players under age 18 to wear a CSA-certified face protector, juniors and seniors under CAHA jurisdiction have the option of wearing CSA-certified visors. Old-timers under Canadian Old Timers Hockey Association jurisdiction lose facial insurance coverage unless they wear at least a visor. Since protective masks have been introduced, there have been no blinding eye injuries for players under 20 years of age who have used a full-face protector.

Whereas the stick is becoming less of an injuring agent, the puck is becoming more frequently involved. The high velocity puck is made of rubber, weighs 6 ounces, has a diameter of 3 inches, and is 1 inch thick. Today, the puck is responsible for most blinding injuries. During the 1974–1975 season, 38% of blinding injuries were caused by a puck, whereas during the 1992–1993 season, 75% of blinding injuries were due to the puck. Of interest is that during the 1992–1993 season, one of the puck-related blinding injuries was to a 32-year-old who had previous radial keratotomy in the affected eye. Thirteen eye area injuries were reported during the 1992–1993 Canadian hockey season to players wearing visors. None of these injuries resulted in any visual loss.

Over a 21-year interval in Canada (1972–1993), 1790 hockey-related eye injuries have been recorded. Of these, 275 (15%) were blind eyes. Most of the injuries recorded were serious, as the data were recorded for players who required evaluation by an ophthalmologist (Table 4.2). Surprisingly, there were no serious eye injuries secondary to fighting. Over this 21-year period, most injuries seen were soft-tissue injuries and hyphemas. During the 1993–1994 season, two blinding eye injuries occurred to players wearing visors. The first was to a 35-year-old player who was struck in the eye by a stick. It was believed that the visor worn may have actually been displaced upward just before the injury. The second was to a 30-year-old player who was wearing a referee's visor (shorter model); an opponent swung his stick in the air to strike the puck and made contact with

Table 4.2 Types of eye injuries in hockey (Canada)

	1972–1973	1974–1975	1976–1992
Soft tissue	43%	31%	34%
Hyphema	24%	31%	27%
Other intraocular	21%	23%	23%
Cornea	7%	11%	9%
Orbital fracture	3%	3%	4%
Ruptured globe	2%	1%	3%
Total injuries	287	258	1214

his eye. During the 1994–1995 season, there were two junior players (ages 18 and 19) that sustained blinding eye injuries while wearing a CSA-certified visor. In both cases, the visor/helmet was displaced upward, exposing the eye to contact from a hockey stick.

From the gathering of data from this 21-year study, one can conclude that although visors may not afford as optimal protection as a full face protector, they offer substantially more protection than using nothing at all. It is unfortunate that most old-timers simply refuse to wear full face protectors. Amazingly, some will not even wear a helmet.

Other hockey-related injury studies have been published, giving data on ocular injuries. In a Montreal study, 33 (13.2%) of 250 retinal detachments due to a contusion of the globe were associated with hockey (11). Eighteen (54.5%) cases were caused by the stick and 14 (42.4%) cases were caused by the puck. In that series, 42.4% of the patients were legally blind in the injured eye even after successful repair of the retinal detachment. In 1974, a Minnesota study described 47 cases of eye trauma secondary to hockey (12). Also in 1974, another study looked at a three-season interval (234 games) of a Southern Hockey League team and found 233 injuries, including 4 fractured skulls (13). Two cases of traumatic iridoplegia were noted to result from direct blows to the periorbital area with a hockey stick. Finally, in a prospective study of a Swedish elite hockey team over a three-season period (1982–1985), 95 injuries were noted (14). There were 29 players with facial lacerations, of which only four had on a protective visor at the time of injury. The incidence of ocular injury was 1.4 per 1000 player-practice hours and 78.4 per 1000 player-game hours.

In the United States, USA Hockey is the governing body of amateur hockey, except for high schools and colleges. Collegiate hockey operates under the National Collegiate Athletic Association (NCAA). The NCAA mandates that all players, including goaltenders, wear full facemasks that meet HECC certification and the ASTM F513-89 standard. This standard requires that the full face is covered and the mask does not permit penetration of a hockey stick blade where it can strike the face. USA Hockey has more than 300,000 youth hockey players registered with 21,000 teams. Their guidelines (rule 304 d) state that all players, including goalkeepers, in the boys junior and under age groups (19 and under) and all girls/women/midget and under age groups (19 and under) are required to wear a full facemask certified by HECC to the ASTM F513-89 standard. All USA Hockey players who are playing in the junior and girls/women/midget age classifications, having reached the age of majority, shall be permitted to wear a HECC-approved half face shield. Junior A and junior B players who have reached the age of majority and who have signed a waiver shall be permitted to wear a facemask of their choice or no facemask at all. USA Hockey strongly recommends that all players and goalkeepers in all age classifications wear a HECC-approved full facemask for all games and practices.

The high school federation ice hockey rulebook requires that all players, including goalkeepers, wear full facemasks that meet the latest ASTM standard. When a new standard is established, high school players will have a 3-year grace period to comply with the new standard.

All players in the NCAA, high schools, and USA Hockey are required to wear ice hockey helmets. As of the 1995–1996 season, high school players are required to wear helmets certified by HECC to ASTM standard F1045-90a in all age classifications and to wear a HECC approved full facemask. Also, players under 13 years of age must use either a full facemask or a half facemask with an external mouthpiece. Players aged 13 to 16 years need a full facemask with an internal mouthpiece or half facemask with an internal/external mouthpiece.

Eye injuries in professional hockey are also a concern. Dr. Thomas Pashby knows of 28 professional players who have had career-ending eye injuries. In the NHL, suspensions have been handed out to players exhibiting unacceptable conduct (15). One player used his thumb to "gouge" the left eye of a rookie opponent during a brawl. The offender was suspended for 10 games for going to "extraordinary means in attempt to injure." Another player "whacked" an opponent in the eye area with his stick and received a 10-game suspension for using "excessive and careless tactics to check an opponent." As we know, there is a great deal of aggression and intimidation in professional hockey. There have been permanently disabling eye injuries in the NHL, such as the one suffered by Pierre Mondou of the Montreal Canadiens, who was forced into retirement in 1985 after getting poked in the eye (16).

Injuries can happen to anyone playing the game, as is evident by this story:

> *Every work day for the past 23 years, Tom Honsberger has gone to General Motors in St. Catharine's, Ontario, and put on safety glasses. It's mandatory. In nearby Grimsby, Honsberger played*

in a recreational old-timers league. Some players wear facial protection, Honsberger didn't. It's not mandatory. On February 13th, the 43-year-old supervisor of maintenance thrust his stick forward to block a slapshot and deflected the puck directly into his unprotected right eye. The impact split open his eyeball. Honsberger was off work for more than a month. Doctors tried to save his eye, then needed to replace it with a prosthetic eye. Now, he's back at G.M., but he will never get back the vision in his right eye (17).

The Rulebook

In the CAHA rulebook, there is a statement that CAHA does not approve of players or referees with only one eye, either playing or officiating. In the NHL rulebook, it states that if a player has one eye with a vision of 20/400 or less, that player is unfit to play.

In 1973, Greg Neeld, a promising 21-year-old junior hockey player in Toronto, was struck in his left eye by a hockey stick. Immediately after the injury, vision was lost in the affected eye. Twelve days later, the eye had to be removed. He was then drafted by the Buffalo Sabres of the NHL. Because of the rule in the NHL, he was considered unfit to play. In attempts to have Greg Neeld made eligible to play, he brought the case to court, believing that the NHL rule was a matter of "restriction of trade." He received a settlement of nearly $100,000. Greg and his father went on to develop a face protector (polycarbonate visor), the Neeld Shield, that would attach to a helmet. Greg also became a member of the CSA standards committee.

Goaltenders

In 1959, Jacques Plante, a goal tender for the Montreal Canadiens, was struck by a puck and suffered a severe facial laceration. At that time, Plante had designed a mask that he used during practice sessions only (Fig. 4.5). In those days, teams dressed only one goal tender and therefore Plante remained in the game. Plante insisted on using the mask to finish the game, which was against his coach's advice. This move became a tremendous influence on the future protection of all goal tenders.

Goaltenders in all leagues began to wear the Plante custom-molded masks (Fig. 4.6A). Certainly, protection was needed as the slapshot and curved hockey stick blades, which made the puck curve and

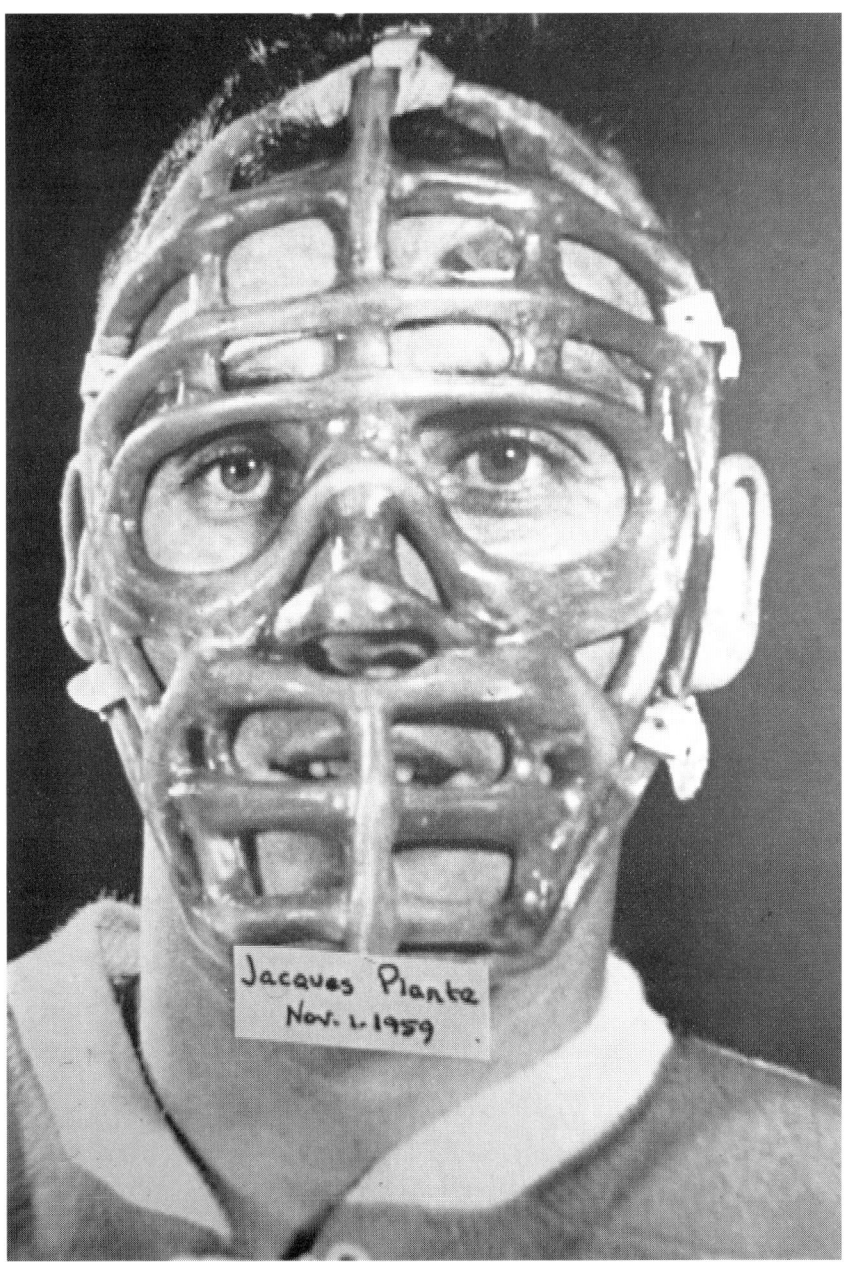

Figure 4.5 *The original goalie mask worn by Jacques Plante in 1959 after he was struck in the face by a puck.*

66 Sports Ophthalmology

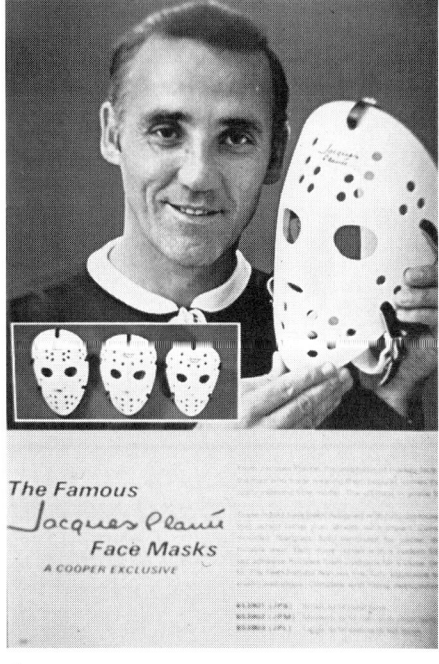 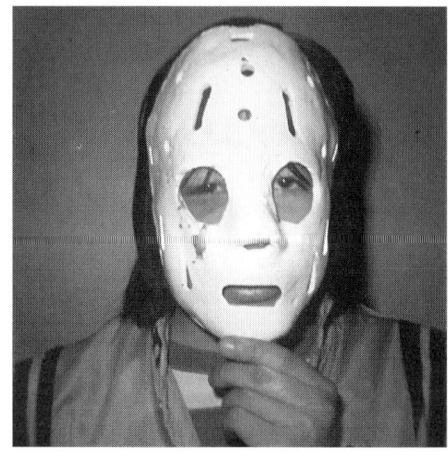

Figure 4.6 *(A) The Plante custom-molded mask. These were mass-produced and sold off dealers' shelves. (B) If a goal tender was having a poor game and allowing several goals, he tended to blame his mask and would enlarge the openings to improve visibility.*

drop, were introduced. To complicate matters, players began to crowd the area in front of the goal tender to obscure his view.

The Plante mask was mass-produced and sold off dealers' shelves. However, the fit was poor and allowed for uneven contact with the face. This resulted in injuries to amateur goalies when struck in the face with a high speed puck. Twelve amateur goal tenders suffered eye injuries while wearing the molded mask, five of whom sustained blinding injuries. At the same time, other molded masks for goal tenders became more popular and were now being custom-made to follow every contour of the face. This would allow any puck impact to transmit its forces evenly, resulting in fewer facial injuries.

The molded masks were not certified. Two NHL goal tenders, Bernie Parent and Gerry Desjardins, suffered career-ending eye injuries, whereas Mike Palmeteer sustained a serious eye injury, all while wearing custom-made molded masks. At times, if a goaltender was having a poor game and allowing several goals, he tended to blame the mask and would enlarge the eye openings to improve his view, resulting in decreased protection (Fig. 4.6B). In addition, molded masks offered no protection to the occipital area or temples.

Molded masks fell into disfavor, and the CSA-certified wire mesh masks were replacements (Fig. 4.7). The wire mesh protectors were either attached to a certified helmet or incorporated into a custom-made face protector and helmet unit. Some soft-tissue injuries still occur, often to the forehead and less frequently to the chin. However,

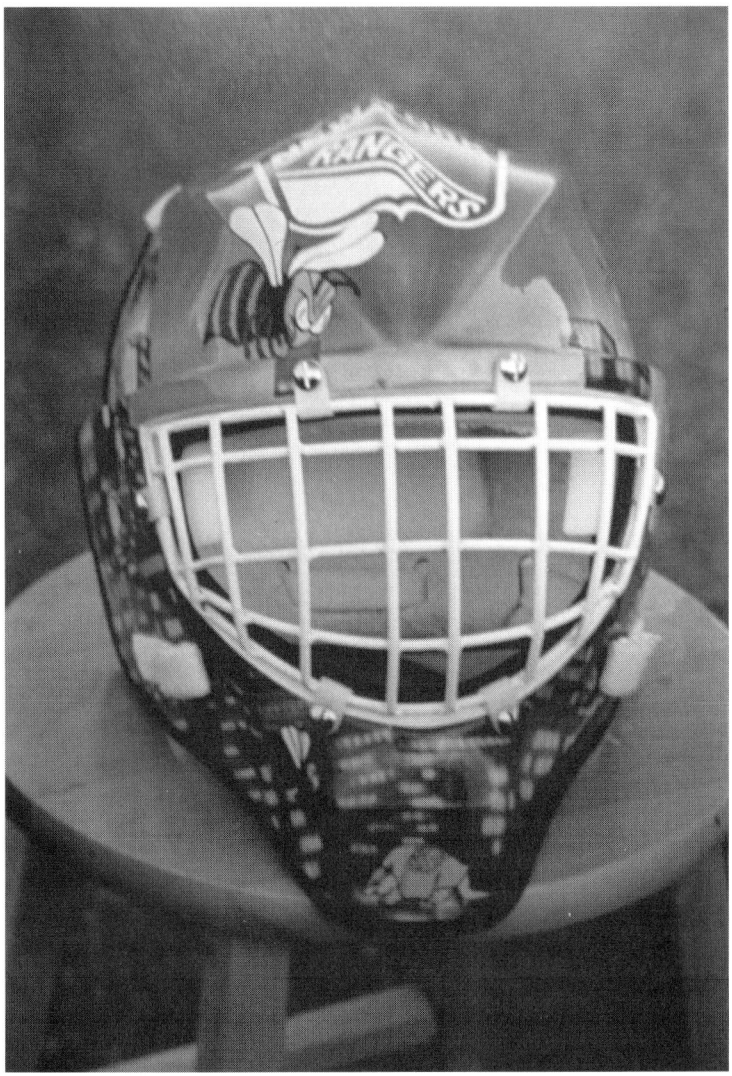

Figure 4.7 *Wire mesh protective mask worn by goalies.*

the wire mesh protector affords better protection, especially for the sides and back of the head. The force of energy impact is also dissipated throughout the helmet and padding. HECC no longer allows the use of form-fitting goalie masks. Currently, a standard for goal tender face and head protectors that will include puck impact is being drafted for both the United States (ASTM) and Canada (CSA).

International Organizations for Standardization

In 1979, the Amateur Hockey Association of the United States met in Lake Placid, New York. It was then decided that rather than have standards for safe hockey equipment produced in different hockey-playing countries, an International Standard Organization (ISO) committee should be established to set standards for hockey helmets and face protectors. As of 1980–1981, standards were already set for hockey equipment in the United States, Canada, and Sweden. The idea was to combine the best parts of these three standards and develop an ISO standard. It was not until 1987 that the first meeting of the ISO technical committee (TC83/SC5) took place, and annual meetings have occurred since then. The committee now includes all hockey equipment and facilities. We still await the final ISO standard for hockey helmets and face protectors (including visors).

Conclusions

In most countries today, eye protectors are worn in amateur hockey. In Canada, full face certified protectors must be worn by minors, whereas juniors and seniors must wear, at a minumum, certified visors. Available certified protective equipment is now available for hockey players that will prevent most eye injuries (Fig. 4.8, A–C).

The hockey face protector saves society $10 million a year by preventing approximately 70,000 ocular and facial injuries in 1.2 million protected players (18). In the NHL, during the 1992–1993 season, it was reported that 11% of players used visors.

Hockey is the fastest contact sport in the world. It is also one of the most aggressive team sports. The hockey stick is used like a golf club to shoot a hard rubber puck, all in a confined space averaging 85 × 185 feet. Some players today have the capability of shooting the puck well over 100 mph. The impact of a puck can reach more than 1200 pounds (19). The puck is often deflected away from its planned flight, making eye contact unavoidable at times. In addition,

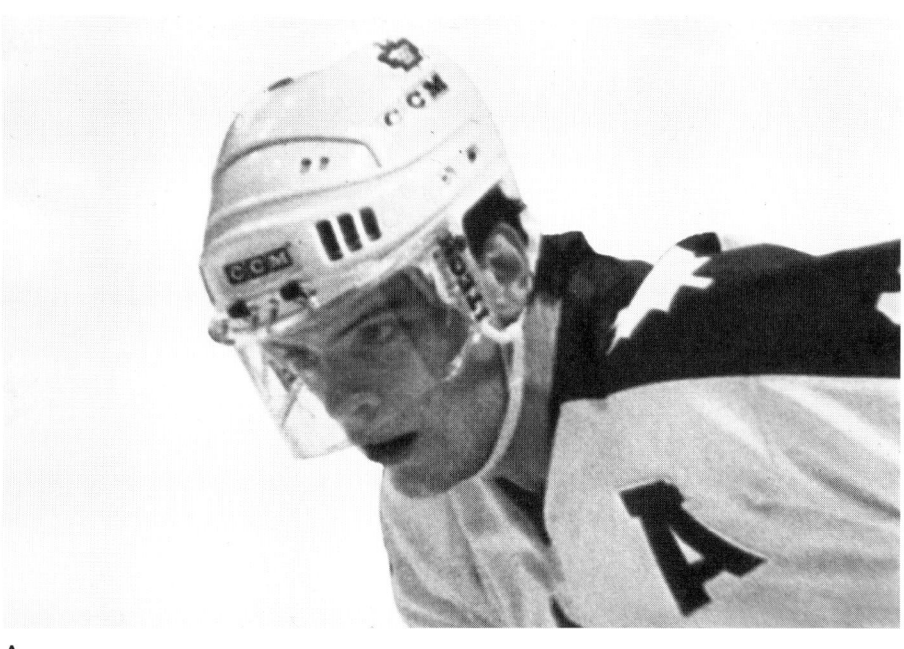

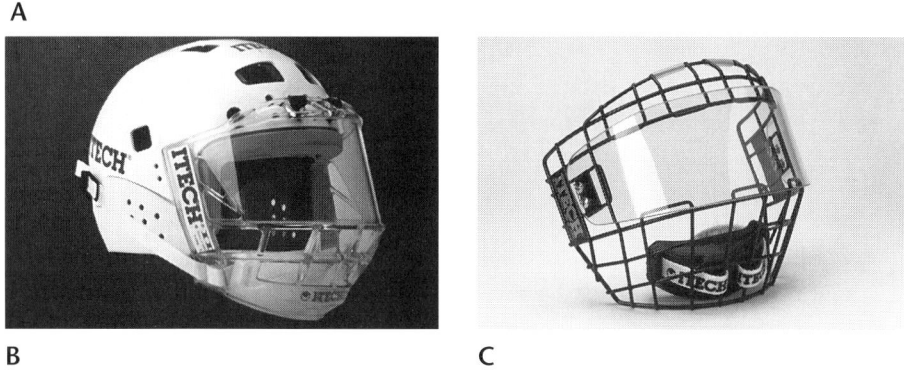

Figure 4.8 *(A–C) Available certified protective equipment that prevents most eye injuries.*

the occasional high stick is used. With these risk factors, it is no wonder serious eye injuries occur.

Over the years, the game has certainly changed. Once considered a recreational sport, professional hockey has now become a spectator sport televised worldwide. The players are bigger, stronger, and more skilled, which means they skate faster and collide harder. On the other hand, amateur hockey is usually played for fun and recreation, often before empty stands. Unfortunately, there are times when the amateur players try to emulate the professionals and play rough.

Changes and stricter enforcement of rules will help to reduce the number of injuries. Deliberate acts of intimidation, overly aggressive use of hockey sticks, and excessive body contact must be discouraged. The NHL has already made attempts to control fighting (20). Serious eye, face, and head injuries have been reduced since the helmet and face protector came into use.

Standards established concerning protective devices should hopefully eliminate the inferior products from the market. These standards provide a basis for continued investigation and the development of new products.

Professionals, amateurs, and recreational hockey players, especially the old-timers, must use the available equipment to protect their eyes. They must wear it properly and at all times, including practices, pick-up games, and organized games. In Canada, the war against hockey-related eye injuries, especially blinding ones, has finally been won. All other countries need to follow. Investigative studies regarding hockey eye trauma and the evaluation of products must continue. This information will provide the basis for what is needed by the sport and its players.

References

1. Pashby TJ. Eye injuries in hockey. In: Vinger PF, ed. International ophthalmology clinics. Boston: Little, Brown & Co., 1981:59–81.
2. Young S. One hundred years of dropping the puck: a history of the Ontario Hockey Association. Toronto: McCelland & Stewart, 1985.
3. Reynen PD, Clancy WG. Cervical spine injury, hockey helmets, and face masks. Am J Sports Med 1984;22:167–170.
4. Pashby TJ. Eye injuries in Canadian hockey: phase II. Can Med Assoc J 1977;117:671–678.
5. Canadian Amateur Hockey Association. Hockey Rules 1975–1976.
6. Canadian Standards Association. National Standard of Canada (Z262.2-M77): eye and teeth protectors for hockey forwards and defensemen. Rexdale, Ontario, Canadian Standards Association, 1977.
7. Canadian Standards Association. National Standard of Canada (CAN 3-Z262.2-M78): face protectors for ice hockey and box lacrosse players. Rexdale, Ontario, Canadian Standards Association, 1978.
8. American Society of Testing and Materials. Consumer safety specifications for eye and face protective equipment for hockey players (F513-77). Philadelphia: American Society of Testing and Materials, 1977.
9. American Society of Testing and Materials. Consumer safety specifications for eye and face protective equipment for hockey players (F513–80). Philadelphia: American Society of Testing and Materials, 1980.
10. Castaldi CR. Prevention of craniofacial injuries in ice hockey. In: Ranalli

DN, ed. Dental clinics of North America. Sports dentistry. Philadelphia: WB Saunders, 1991:647–666.
11. Antaki S, Labelle P, Dumas J. Retinal detachment following ice hockey injury. CMA J 1977;117:245–246.
12. Horns RC. Blinding hockey injuries. Minn Med 1976;255–258.
13. Rovere GD, Gristina AG, Nicastro JF. Medical problems of a professional hockey team: a three-season experience. Phys Sportsmed 1978;6:59–63.
14. Lorentzon R, Wedren H, Pietila T. Incidence, nature, and causes of ice hockey injuries: a three-year prospective study of a Swedish elite ice hockey team. Am J Sports Med 1988;16:392–396.
15. Swift EM. Blood and ice. Sports Illustrated. Dec. 5, 1988:57–60.
16. Duda M. Mandatory face shields in the NHL? Phys Sportsmed 1986;4:33.
17. Dryden S. Profile: the eyes have it. The Hockey News, Inside Hockey. June 25, 1990.
18. Vinger PF. The eye and sportsmedicine. In: Tasman W, Jaeger EA, eds. Duane's clinical ophthalmology. vol. 5. Philadelphia: Lippincott, 1994:1–103.
19. Sim FH, Simonet WT, Melton J, Lehn TA. Ice hockey injuries. Am J Sports Med 1987;15:30–40.
20. Moore M. Fighting NHL brawling with suspensions. Phys Sportsmed 1980;8:19.

CHAPTER 5

Racket and Court Sports

Michael Easterbrook

It is estimated that over 40 million Americans play racket sports (1). Every year, racket and court sports are responsible for approximately 8% of all sports-related eye injuries in the United States (2,3). According to Vinger (1), the risks of eye injuries for 100,000 playing sessions are as follows: squash, 5.2%; badminton, 3.6%; tennis, 1.3%; and table tennis, 0.1%. The risk of an unprotected squash player suffering significant eye injury after 24 years of playing 3 days a week is approximately 25%. The ocular injuries seen in racket and court sports are usually severe. Most result from being struck with either a high velocity projectile object (e.g., ball, shuttlecock) or a racket.

Badminton

The game of shuttlecock was played in Siam and China nearly 2000 years ago, yet it was not until 1872 that British officers introduced the game into England. The shuttlecock used in badminton is made of feathers and nylon. The length is anywhere from 2 1/4 to 2 3/4 inches, it weighs approximately 1 ounce, and fits perfectly into the orbit of the eye (Fig. 5.1).

Badminton is now an Olympic sport; therefore, there is a tremendous resurgence of interest internationally. Fifty percent of all badminton injuries involve some permanent loss of best corrected vision. In doubles play, shuttlecocks from both the partner and opponents hit the eye, yet racket impacts, which occur 14% of the time, are

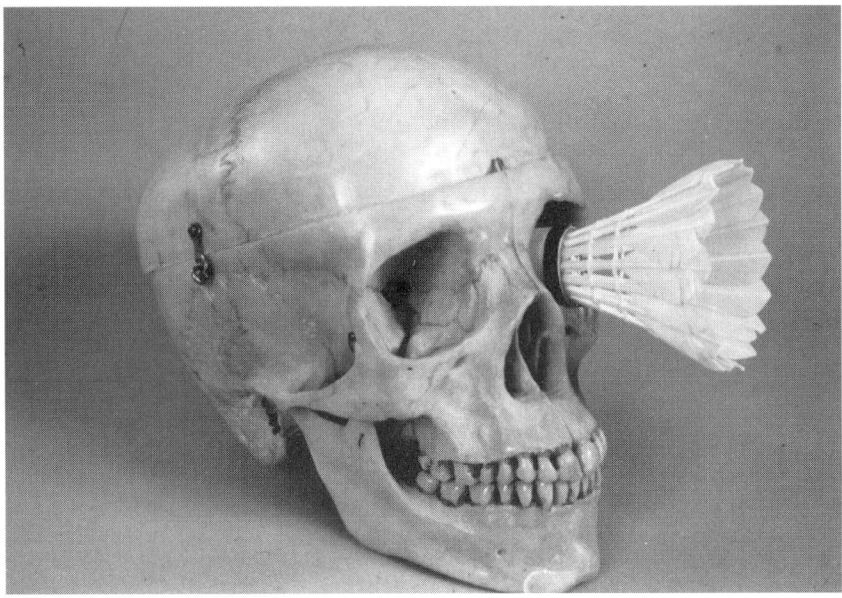

Figure 5.1 *The shuttlecock used in badminton, a perfect fit into the orbit.*

mostly caused by the doubles partner. Seventy percent of badminton eye injuries occur in doubles play. Badminton in Canada is now the most common cause of eye injuries in racket sports, replacing racquetball and squash (Table 5.1). No eye injuries to a player wearing an approved eye protector have ever been reported.

Tennis

In 1873, Major Walter Clopton Wingfield invented the game of tennis. It is debatable as to whether he actually modeled the game after an ancient Greek game or combined the games of court tennis and squash rackets. In the United States, the first game of tennis took place in 1874 in Staten Island, New York.

Tennis is one of the most popular sports in the United States, as it is played by people of all ages. Anyone visiting a recreational tennis center will see youngsters as well as old-timers engaged in matches. The tennis ball is made of rubber and is covered with wool. It is approximately 2 1/2 inches in diameter and weighs 2 ounces. Compared with a shuttlecock or squash ball, a tennis ball cannot enter the orbit as readily. However, the tennis ball is compressible, and because it can achieve speeds well over 100 mph, any direct eye contact could be devastating. Tennis players running to or close by

Table 5.1 Racket sports injuries (Canada)

YEAR	NO. INJURIES	RACQUETBALL/ SQUASH (%)	BADMINTON (%)	TENNIS (%)
1982*	90	73	13	14
1983	87	59	22	19
1984	115	58	16	26
1985	82	50	33	17
1986	83	39	33	28
1987	68	36	38	26
1988	46	39	46	15
1989	62	35	17	18
1990	40	35	55	10
1991	35	23	40	37
1992	33	24	52	24
1993	31	23	55	22
1994	27	26	56	18

* CSA standard published.

the net are at greater risk for sustaining an eye injury than those who remain in the backcourt. For those who wear regular street glasses, eye injuries have occurred when frames have collapsed, lenses dislocated through frames, or lenses shattered. Seelenfreund et al (4) described 10 patients who sustained eye injuries from a high speed tennis ball. Seven of the patients required either retinal surgery, laser, or both for retinal detachments and/or tears. All patients had vitreous hemorrhages.

Handball

Handball originated in Ireland nearly 1000 years ago and was brought to the United States in the 1880s. The soft rubber ball is 1 7/8 inches in diameter and weighs 2.3 ounces. The first protective racquetball eye guard, the lensless open guard composed of wire frame coated with rubber (Fig. 5.2), was first designed to prevent injuries in handball. Because lensless eye guards did not prevent eye injuries, the United States Handball Association in 1988 voted to require the use of one-piece lens polycarbonate protectors by all players participating in nationally sanctioned handball tournaments.

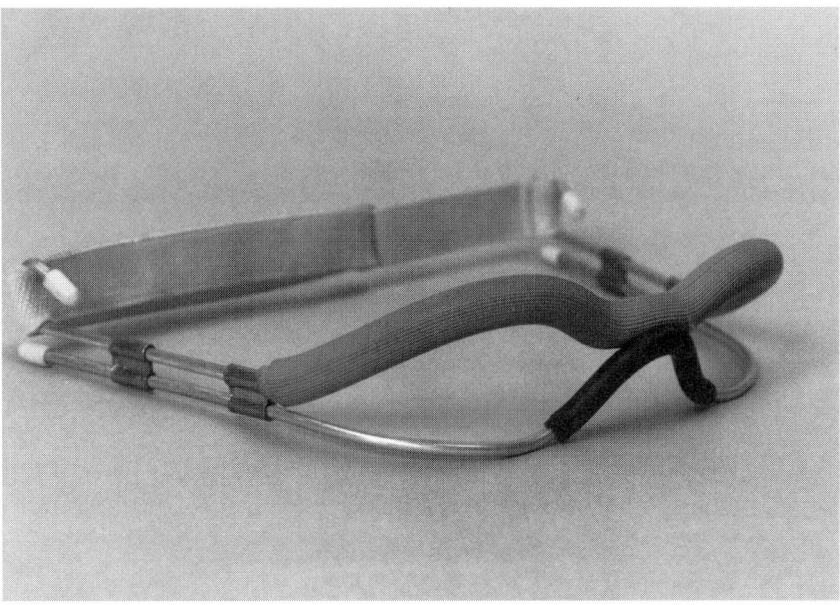

Figure 5.2 *First open eye guard, used in handball.*

Squash

The game of squash was first thought to have been played in the 1870s in England, and came to the United States in 1882. The squash ball, having a diameter of 1.75 inches, can travel at speeds up to 140 mph. The ball is capable of fitting within the orbit and directly striking the eye (globe) without deformation (Fig. 5.3) and thus is capable of causing enormous ocular damage. Like most other rackets, the squash racket may also strike the eye and adnexal region, creating damage to these areas (Fig. 5.4).

In 1976, Sabiston (5) reported on 25 squash-related eye injuries in New Zealand. Fifty percent of these injuries resulted in visual loss and two eyes required enucleation. Sabiston estimated that there were 100 squash-related eye injuries annually in New Zealand, with 50% of the injured losing useful vision. Ingram et al (6) examined 20 patients who sustained ocular injuries as a result of playing squash. This series included four ruptured globes, four hyphemas, and four cases of retinal pathology (e.g., detachment, edema). Other studies have also looked at squash-related eye injuries (7–23).

Within Canada, a preliminary standard was passed by the Canadian Standards Association (CSA) in 1982 (16). Squash balls are propelled at 90 mph toward the lens and hinge of the eye guard frame.

76 Sports Ophthalmology

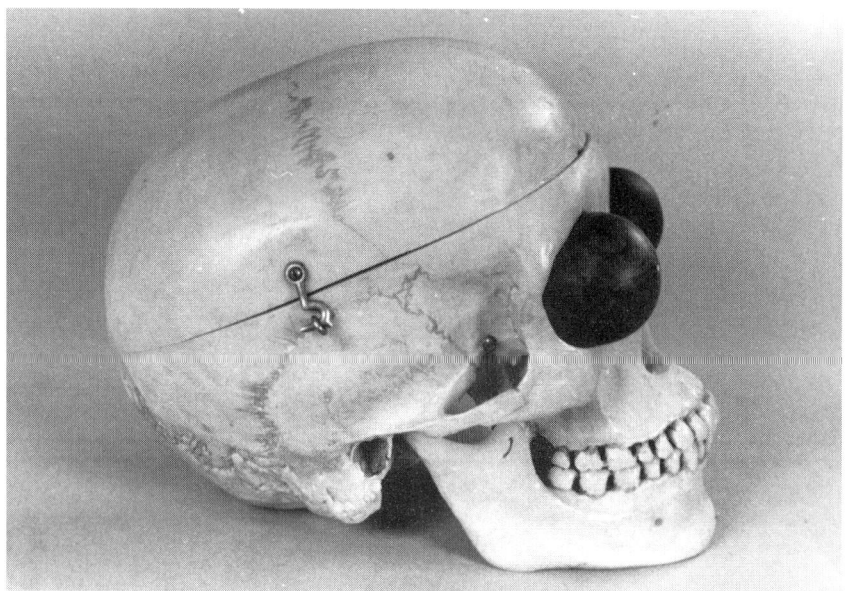

Figure 5.3 *A squash ball fits perfectly into the orbit.*

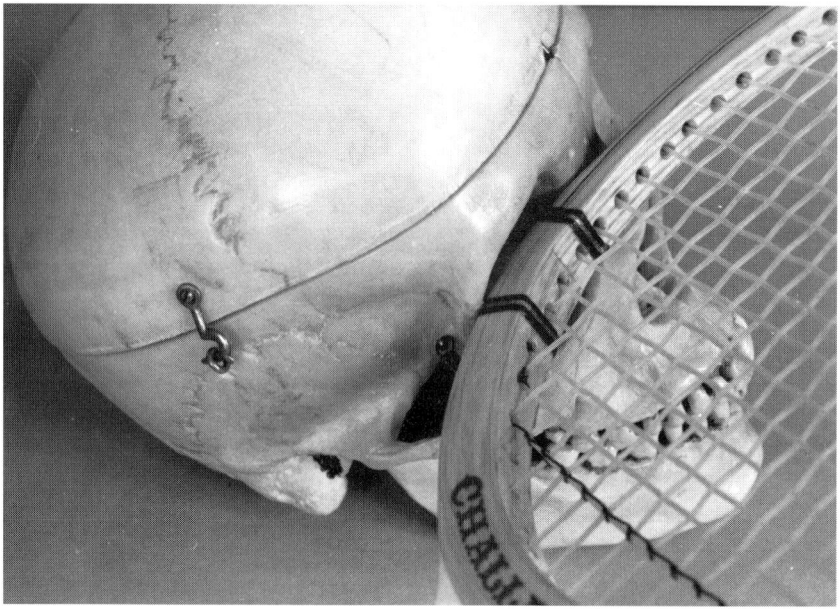

Figure 5.4 *Squash racket penetrating orbit.*

A failure results when any contact of the lens or frame with the headform occurs. Additional tests of field and optical clarity are also performed. In 1983, the American Society for Testing and Materials (ASTM) passed a similar standard (for performance, not design). Since 1986, eye protectors with lenses have been required for all United States Racquet Association (USRA) sanctioned tournaments. In 1987, the United States Racquetball association (USRA) incorporated eye guards into the rules of squash. In that same year, the American Amateur Racquetball Association (AARA) made polycarbonate-lens eyewear a rule of the sport:

> *AARA Rule 2.5 (Apparel):*
> *(a) Lensed Eyewear Required. Lensed eyewear designed for racket sports is required apparel for all players. The protective eyewear must be worn as designed and may not be altered. Players who require corrective eyewear also must wear lensed eyewear designed for racket sports. Failure to wear protective eyewear will result in a technical foul and the player will be charged with a timeout to secure eyewear. The second infraction in the same match will result in immediate forfeiture of the match. Effective Sept, 1995, the eyewear must be tested to meet or exceed ASTM F803 impact standards. The AARA recommends that players select eyewear with polycarbonate plastic lenses with 3 mm center thickness. Note: a list of approved eyewear is available by writing the AARA national office.*

It is well known that large numbers of participants at the "club level" do not wear any eye protection. Currently, the ASTM and CSA are trying to develop a North American standard, which hopefully will become a template for an international standard.

Racquetball

Racquetball was invented in 1949 on a Connecticut handball court by Joe Sobek. He designed the first short-strung paddle, devised rules combining the basics of handball and squash, and named it "paddle rackets." The sport quickly caught on and evolved into racquetball as we know it today. By the early 1970s, it was being played all over the United States and had a rapid and steady rise in popularity. In the 1970s and early 1980s, racquetball became one of the fastest growing sports in America. Today, approximately 7.5 million Americans play racquetball each year; it is played in 88 countries around the world.

78 Sports Ophthalmology

Racquetball-related eye injuries are very similar to those seen in squash. The ball velocities are similar; however, the racquetball is very compressible and readily penetrates the orbit (Fig. 5.5). Ninety percent of eye injuries in racquetball are caused by the ball, which can reach velocities as high as 140 mph. In 1978, the first series of racket sports–related eye injuries in Canada was reported in the *Canadian Medical Association Journal* (11). Since the late 1970s, ophthalmologists have been collecting data from players and physicians on mechanisms of injury, types of injury, and eye protectors, both adequate and inadequate. This experience has led to Canadian and American standards for better protection of recreational and professional racquetball players.

Data Collection

Since the late 1970s, questionnaires were sent out to racquetball and squash clubs and to all members of the Canadian Ophthalmological Society asking them to report on occurrence of an injury, mechanism of injury (ball vs. racket), level of player's experience, and eyewear used.

Table 5.1 summarizes the data from 1982 through 1994, dem-

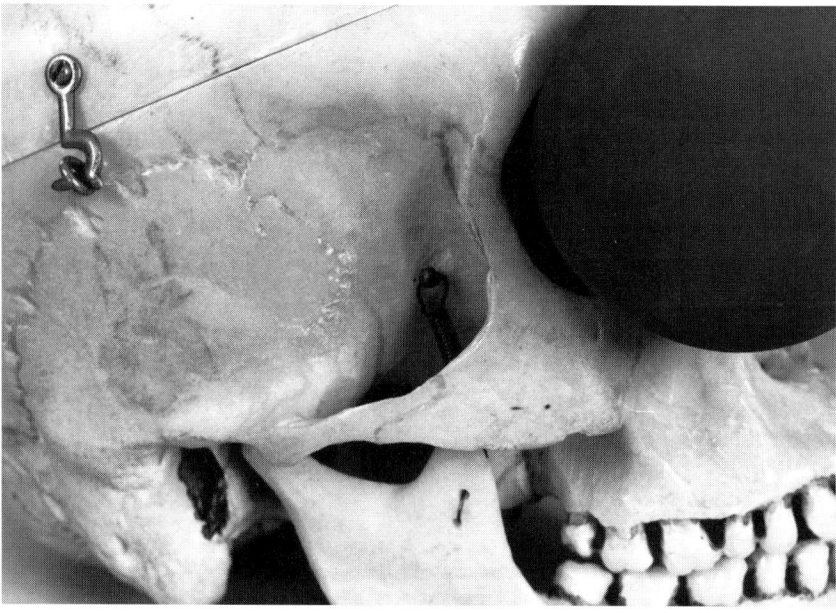

Figure 5.5 *Racquetball penetrating orbit.*

onstrating that with increasing use of protective eye guards by squash and racketball players, the relative incidence of eye injuries in badminton has increased.

Mechanism of Injury: Ball or Racket?

The data over the years suggest that in squash, 60% of ocular injuries are caused by the ball and 40% by the racket. In racquetball, 95% of ocular injuries are caused by the ball and only 5% by the racket. In badminton, most of the injuries are caused by the shuttlecock, not by the racket, and most injuries occur while playing doubles.

Ball and Racket Speeds

It is not surprising that in the confined space of a small court, ocular injury occurs. Table 5.2 illustrates the various velocities of the instruments used in racket and court sports. A novice 8-year-old squash/racquetball player has the ability to hit the ball 80 mph. A professional squash/racquetball player strikes the ball at 150+ mph. A professional badminton player was clocked with an overhead smash at 187.5 mph at the 1992 Olympic games.

Table 5.2 Ball and racket velocities

	AVERAGE SPEED (mph)
Racquetball	
Ball	85–110
Racket	85–90
Squash	
Ball	130–140
Racket	95–110
Tennis	
Ball	90–110
Handball	
Ball	60–70
Badminton	
Shuttlecock	130–135

Experience: Help or Hindrance?

There is a common misconception among racket sports players that the experienced player is more protected than the novice. However, our experience (11–22) along with that of others suggests that the experienced racket sports player is at a greater risk of injury. The novice squash player generally plays watching the front wall, not the ball. The experienced racket sports player never takes his or her eyes off the ball, so that the next shot may be anticipated. Players frequently look behind them while their opponent is about to strike the ball.

In a New Zealand prospective study, the highest incidence of facial injuries occurred in squash over a 1-year period in the top level of play (23). In our series, the mean playing experience of squash players that sustained ocular injury was nearly 6 years (20).

Streetwear Glasses: Increased or Decreased Risk?

Nearly 50% of the population wear glasses or contact lenses. In Canada, there have been 21 players who have sustained serious ocular injury when their prescription glasses with hard or plastic lenses shattered. Players who are myopic (nearsighted) wear lenses that are very thin in the center; these players are at a greater risk of sustaining an eye injury. There is a misconception that plastic streetwear glasses are protective; however, this is untrue. Lenses must be made of polycarbonate and used in an approved sports frame to be protective.

Polycarbonate Protective Lenses and Contacts

Polycarbonate is a very high impact resistant plastic initially used in jet canopies and riot police gear that will stop a 22-caliber bullet (24). This material is very strong and is available in almost all prescriptions for the recreational player. Players wearing contact lenses and those who do not require glasses for vision should wear polycarbonate lenses with no prescription in a protector designed for racket sports. These sports eye protectors have a posterior lip that should prevent the lens from traveling posteriorly (dislocating in toward the eye) if hit by a ball or racket (25).

Soft contact lenses neither hurt nor help a player in avoiding eye injury; however, hard gas permeable lenses may break on impact and cause a corneal laceration. Any player wearing contact lenses should wear a polycarbonate eye guard over the contact lenses.

Eye Guards

Open Eye Guards: Protective or Risky?

In the mid-1970s, lensless polycarbonate open eye guards (Fig. 5.6) were used, initially in handball and then in squash and racquetball, in an attempt to reduce the risk of ocular injury. These eye guards are still sold in Europe and Britain. It is apparent that the squash ball and racquetball readily penetrate the open eye guard (Fig. 5.7).

The open eye guard may actually contribute toward ocular injury, because it gives players a false sense of security, allowing them to follow the ball at all times. Moreover, it may expose them to the increased risk of being struck by a direct shot with penetration of the racquetball or squash ball through the eye guard, allowing it to strike the eye. One would argue that the open eye guard funnels the malleable squash ball and racquetball into the eye and may very well contribute toward ocular injury (Fig. 5.8).

In racquetball, where almost all injuries are caused by the ball, the open (lensless) eye guard is of no use and may contribute to injury. In squash, where 40% of injuries are caused by the racket, there may be some limited use of the eye guard against the racket. Some players have reported that their eyes were protected by the open eye guard

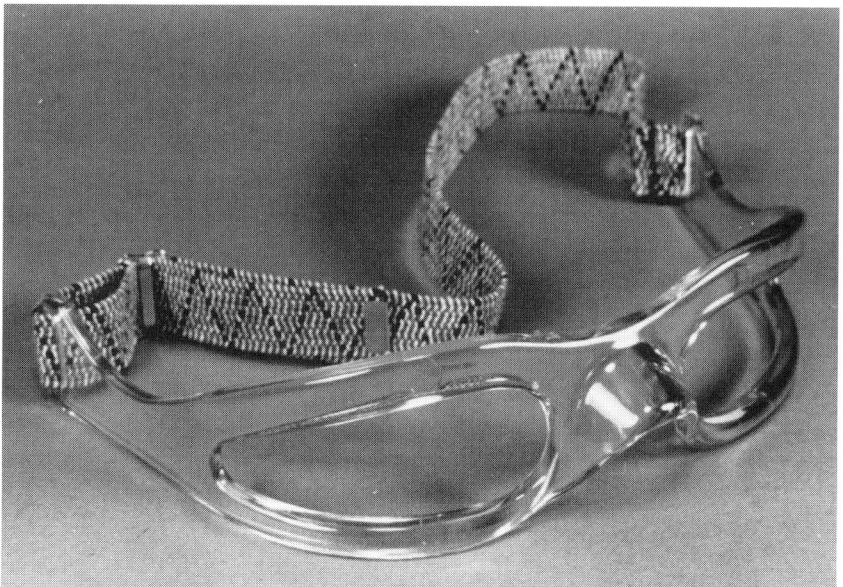

Figure 5.6 *Open (lensless) eye guard, no longer used in North America.*

82 Sports Ophthalmology

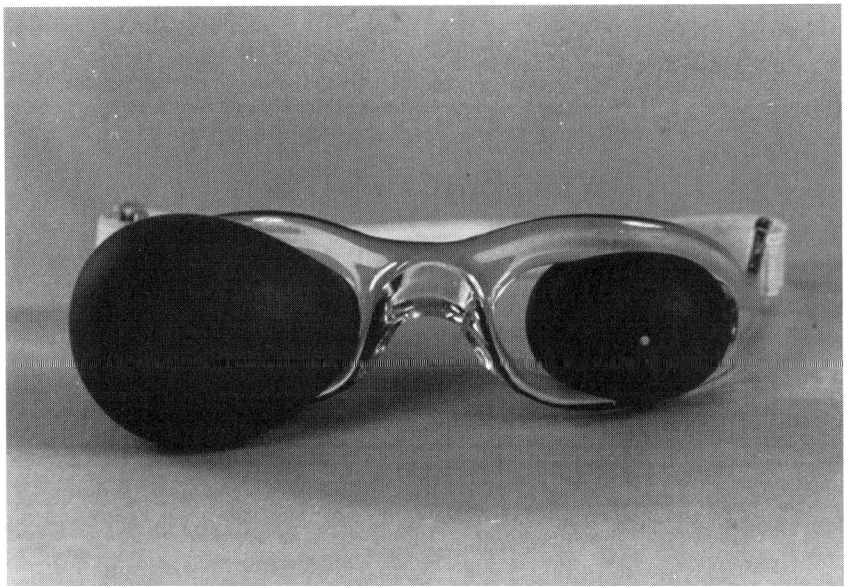

Figure 5.7 *Open eye guard permitting penetration by squash ball and racquetball.*

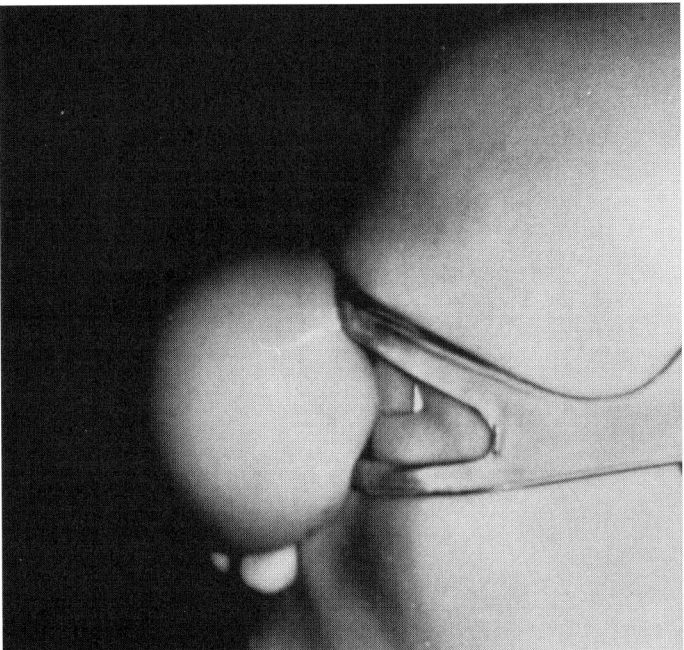

Figure 5.8 *Penetration of open eye guard by racquetball. Note the ball going through the open eye guard and striking the eye.*

when they were struck by a squash racket. In the late 1970s and early 1980s, many injuries occurred in players wearing open eye guards. By 1980, many ophthalmologists were publicly stating that open eye guards did not prevent ocular injury in squash or racquetball and might actually contribute to injury.

Table 5.3 demonstrates the first 80 ocular injuries sustained by players who wore an open eye guard. After speaking with each of these individuals: 69 (86%) believed that the ball penetrated the open eye guard they were wearing at the time of injury. The remaining 11 (14%) believed that the open eye guard was too narrow and displaced upward into the eye, thus contributing to their ocular injury. Pat Bishop was commissioned by the CSA to examine whether these eye guards were protective. With the use of high speed film, all open eye guards were demonstrated to allow penetration at speeds as low as 50 mph. These eye guards were placed on a headform (Fig. 5.9). Molding of the squash ball and racquetball on contact with the open eye guard permitted contact with the eye of the Alderson headform (see Fig. 5.8). The CSA has further refined the headform with reproducible measurements of the eye area. This headform is available in several different sizes from the CSA and is now the headform of choice when testing eye guards in racket sports.

Prescription and Nonprescription

The first generation of polycarbonate eye guards (Fig. 5.10) was popular with racket sports and basketball players. There are now many models of nonprescription polycarbonate eye guards available that meet CSA or ASTM impact standards (Figs. 5.11 and 5.12). For those players requiring a prescription, polycarbonate prescription lenses can be inserted in a sports frame designed for racket sports (a posterior lip prevents backward dislocation into the eye) (Figs. 5.13 and 5.14). Table 5.4 lists racket sports eye guards, which manufacturers indicate are tested to ASTM F803 or CSA standards.

Wearing Eye Guards

Those of us who wear streetwear glasses have little difficulty in adjusting to eye protection for racket sports. Players who do not wear glasses should wear eye guards around the house for a weekend until they become accustomed to the apparent restriction of peripheral vision. This is an apparent restriction because players who anticipate will never take their eye off the ball. They actually use their central vision and not peripheral vision to anticipate the next shot.

84 Sports Ophthalmology

Table 5.3 Injuries sustained by 80 athletes wearing open eye guards

	NUMBER
Injury	
Eyelid hemorrhage	11
Eyelid laceration	3
Corneal abrasion	10
Iritis	8
Hyphema	56
Mechanism of injury	
Ball	77
Racket	3
Ball penetrated eye guard	69
Ball displaced eye guard	11
Sport	
Squash	24
Racquetball	56

In the mid-1980s, eye guards with an antifog coating became available. It was also recommended that players wear a thick headband to prevent sweat from running onto the eye guard. Eye guards should be removed between games or when a player is resting or arguing about a shot, as rising body heat may contribute to fogging. Fogging in North America is rarely a problem; however, in very humid climates such as Hong Kong, squash players have had difficulty even with some of the antifog coating materials. Manufacturers are

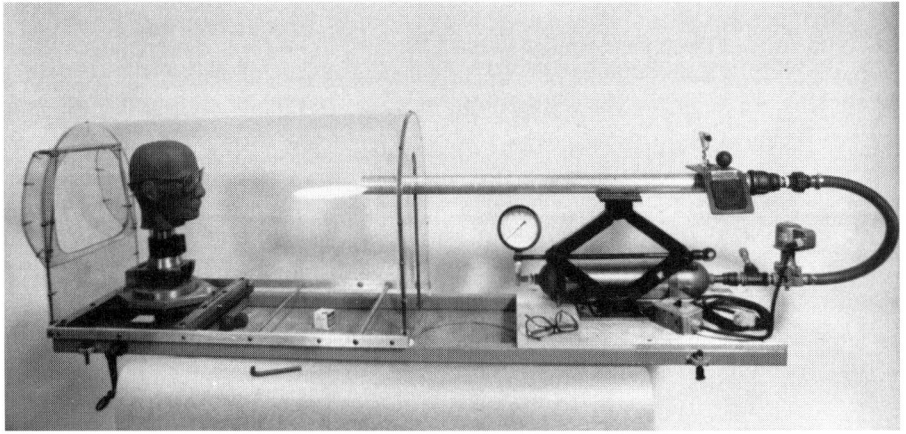

Figure 5.9 *Eye guard on Alderson headform.*

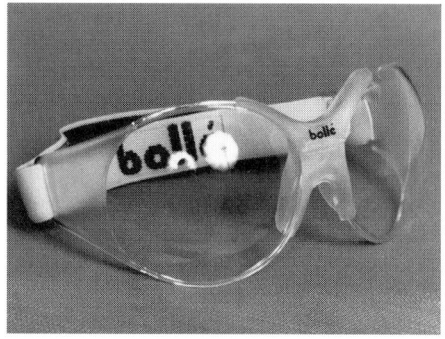

Figure 5.10 *Eye guard for nonprescription wearers.*

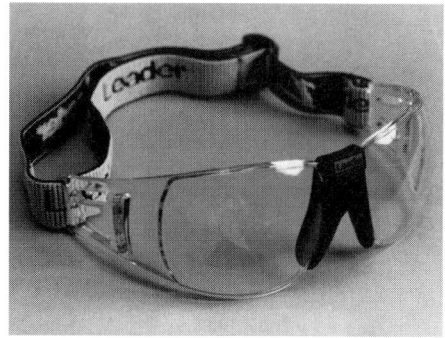

Figure 5.11 *Polycarbonate nonprescription eye guard.*

being asked to send samples to humid climates for testing, as antifog coatings are improving on a yearly basis.

Voluntary or Mandatory?

In 1985, before the approval of ASTM and CSA standard specifications, the USRA made the wearing of eye guards mandatory at all national championships for all levels of play. Subsequently, the USRA has made lensed eye guards mandatory. Eye guards are now an integral part of the game. The rules of doubles squash and 70+ squash make wearing of a closed lensed eye guard mandatory.

Certification and Standards for Eye Guards in Racket Sports

Sports-related eye injuries have been reported in many countries, including the United States, Australia, New Zealand, Canada, and Brit-

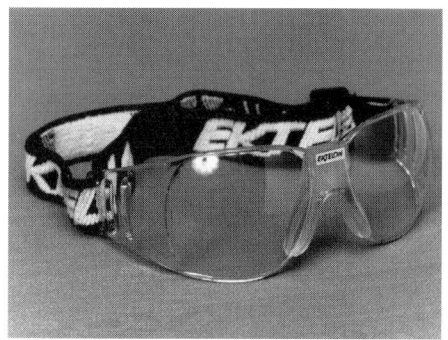

Figure 5.12 *Polycarbonate nonprescription eye guard with antifog coat.*

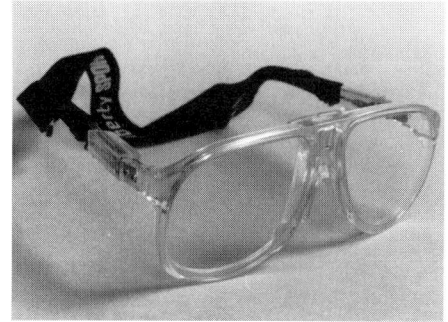

Figure 5.13 *Hinged protector with polycarbonate prescription or nonprescription lens: hinge will withstand ball at 90 mph.*

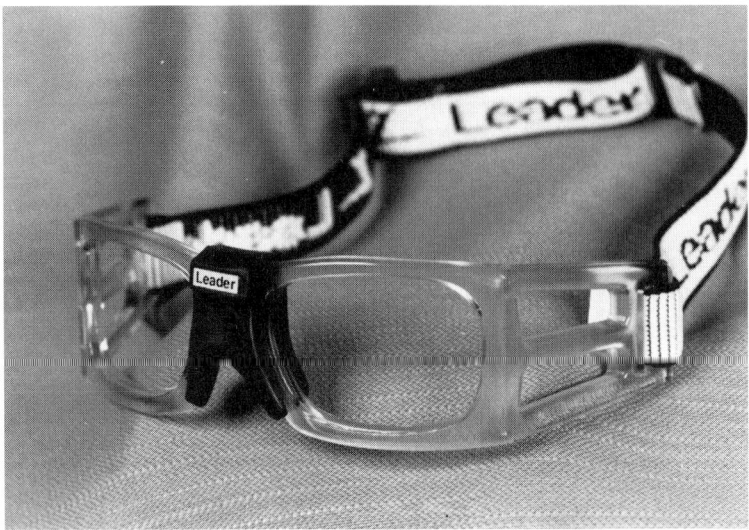

Figure 5.14 *Polycarbonate sports frame into which polycarbonate prescription lenses are fitted.*

ain. During one 6-month period in England, 339 players were injured while playing squash (23). Although some national organizations, particularly in Europe, believe the risk of injury in squash is small, this one series showed that ophthalmologists in most squash-playing countries are seeing squash eye injuries on a regular basis.

Impact studies were commissioned by the ASTM in the United States and the CSA in Canada. Pat Bishop in Canada and C. A. Morehouse and Michael Elman in the United States performed elegant experiments using high speed film and an Alderson headform, demonstrating that the open eye guard did not prevent injury with a squash ball or racket and readily allowed the penetration of the squash ball into the orbit. In 1980, a committee of the CSA, composed of manufacturers, opticians, ophthalmologists, optometrists, and representatives of consumer groups, was formed to write a standard for racket sports eye protection. In early 1982, the CSA passed a preliminary standard. In 1983, ASTM passed a similar standard for racket sports eye protectors that has been subsequently updated. These standards are not design standards; they are performance standards. Eye guards that pass these standards will prevent eye contact of a squash ball or racquetball at speeds of 90 mph when impacted from the front or the side. Hinges are tested at similar speeds. There are also standards of optical quality and field of vision.

Table 5.4 Sports eye protectors (eye guards)

Protectors into which a 3-mm prescription polycarbonate spectacle lens may be inserted
- Liberty Sport, Liberty Optical Company (Newark, NJ)
    - Junior Rec Specs, small — R,S,T,H
    - Junior Rec Specs, large — R,S,T,H
    - All Pro Rec Specs, small — R,S,T,H
    - All Pro Rec Specs, large — R,S,T,H
    - Sportgoggle 2 — R,S,T,H
    - Sport-Lok, small — R,S,T
    - Sport-Lok, large — R,S,T
    - Pro Guard Rec Specs — S,T,H
- Black Knight USA (San Jose, CA)
    - Action Eyes
- Eagle Eyewear, Inc. (Whitehouse, NJ)
    - REP 1, small
    - REP 1, large
    - REP 2
- REM (Los Angeles, CA)
    - Sports Goggle 1
    - Sports Goggle 2
    - Sports Goggle 3

Plano-molded protectors (for emmetropes or contact lens wearers)
- Black Knight USA
    - Sight Guards
- Leader Sports Products, Inc. (Plattsburg, NY)
    - New Yorker
    - Albany
    - Dallas
    - Optivue
    - Maxum

Plano goggle-type molded protector (may be worn over streetwear spectacles)
- Leader Sports Products, Inc.
    - Vizion II

Tested either by independent laboratory or by manufacturer to ASTM F803 or CSA racket sports eyewear standards. List may be incomplete and is subject to change. R, racquetball; S, squash; T, tennis; H, handball; no letter, specific racket sport not stated by manufacturer. (Data collected by Tom Woods, Michael Easterbrook, and Paul Vinger; tests not certified by authors.)

The American and Canadian standards are similar but not identical. A committee has been formed that hopefully will produce a common standard acceptable in Canada and the United States, as well as internationally.

In 1986, after 6 years of testing, six racket sports standards were certified by the CSA, who sets standards and tests eye guards. In the United States, the ASTM sets standards, but independent laboratories perform the testing.

Manufacturers, representatives, ophthalmologists, physicians, and racket sports organizations formed the Sports Certification Council under the auspices of the National Society to Prevent Blindness in an attempt to certify eye protectors for general use by squash and racquetball players in the United States. Manufacturers initially certified eye guards but found the cost of certification was expensive. In some certification areas, the manufacturers were responsible for two or three annual visits to the manufacturers' plant. Many manufacturers believed that their profit margins were too thin and could not afford this expense. Consequently, at the present time we have no certified eye protector in North America.

Manufacturers, however, can and do submit their eye guards to independent laboratories to determine whether they do meet the standard. Players should look for some notification on the package or eye guard suggesting that the eye guard has met ANSI F803.94 (a) or CSA impact standards before wearing such an eye guard.

Conclusion

Racket sports and court sports are played by millions of participants around the world. The speeds that these sports' projectile objects (e.g., ball, shuttlecock) reach are enormous; a professional badminton player was recorded hitting the shuttlecock at 187.5 mph. Eye injuries within these sports are devastating yet continue to occur. Preventing these injuries is possible with the use of approved protective eyewear.

References

1. Vinger PF. The eye and sports medicine. In: Tasman W, Jaeger EA, eds. Duane's clinical ophthalmology. Philadelphia: Lippincott, 1995;5:1–103.
2. National Society to Prevent Blindness. 1992 Eye injuries associated with

sports and recreational products. Schaumburg, IL: National Center for Sight, 1993.
3. National Society to Prevent Blindness. 1993 Eye injuries associated with sports and recreational products. Schaumburg, IL: National Center for Sight, 1994.
4. Seelenfreund MH, Freilich DB. Rushing the net and retinal detachment. JAMA 1976;235:2723–2726.
5. Sabiston D. Squash and eye injuries. NZ J Sports Med 1976;4:3–5.
6. Ingram DV, Lewkonia I. Ocular hazards of playing squash rackets. Br J Ophthalmol 1973;57:434–438.
7. North IM. Ocular hazards of squash. Med J Aust 1973;1:165–166.
8. Barrell GV, Cooper PJ, Ilkington AR, et al. Squash ball to eye ball. Br Med J 1981;283:893–895.
9. Blonstein JL. Eye injuries in sport with particular reference to squash rackets and badminton. Practitioner 1975;215:208–209.
10. Genovese MT, Lenzo NP, Lim RK, et al. Eye injuries among pennant squash players and their attitudes towards wearing protective eyewear. Med J Aust 1990;153:655–658.
11. Easterbrook WM. Eye injuries in squash: a preventable disease. Can Med Assoc J 1978;118:298–305.
12. Easterbrook WM. Eye injuries in racquet sports: a continuing problem. Can Med Assoc J 1980;123:268.
13. Easterbrook WM. Eye injuries in racquet sports. Int Ophthalmol Clin 1981; 21:87–119.
14. Easterbrook WM. Eye injuries in squash and racquetball players. Phys Sportsmed 1982;10:47–56.
15. Easterbrook M, Cameron J. Injuries in racquet sports. In: Schneider R, et al, eds.: Sports injuries: mechanisms, prevention and treatment. Baltimore: Williams and Wilkins, 1985:553–564.
16. Easterbrook M. Ocular injuries in racquet sports. Int Ophthalmol Clin 1988;28:232–237.
17. Easterbrook M. Assessing ocular trauma in athletes. Can J Diagn 1988; 43–49.
18. Easterbrook M. Keeping an eye on sports—retinal injuries. Curr Ther 1989;2:21, 33.
19. Easterbrook M. Eye protectors in racquet sports. In: Torg J, Welsh RP, Shepherd RJ, eds. Current therapy in sports. vol. 2. Philadelphia: B. C. Decker, 1990:356–362.
20. Easterbrook M. Standards for protective eye guards. In: Hermans GPH, Mostend WL, eds. Sports, medicine and health. Amsterdam: Excerpta Medica, 1990:1101–1106.
21. Easterbrook M. Prevention of eye injury in badminton. In: Hermans GPH, Mostend WL, eds. Sports, medicine and health. Amsterdam: Excerpta Medica, 1990:1107–1110.
22. Easterbrook M. Eye injuries in sports. Protection and care. Can J Diagn 1993;77–89.
23. Clemett RS, Fairhurst SM. Head injuries from squash: a prospective study. NZ Med J 1980;92:1–3.
24. Davis JK. Perspectives on impact resistance and polycarbonate lenses. Int Ophthalmol Clin 1988;215–218.
25. A ball in the eye. Br Med J 1973;195–196. Editorial.

CHAPTER 6

Boxing

Vincent J. Giovinazzo

Boxing causes more damage to the eye than any other sport. Although traumatic injuries that potentially damage vision can occur in noncontact sports, such as badminton, and full contact sports, such as football, boxing is the only sport in which winning is predicated on causing intentional ocular injuries. Boxers are trained to "target" areas of previous scarring over the eyebrows of their opponents in an attempt to cause hemorrhages and decrease vision (Fig. 6.1). Inadvertent gouging of the eye by a thumb, although reason for suspension of a bout, occurs frequently in the ring and produces perhaps the most damaging trauma to an eye (Fig. 6.2). Referees are trained to stop bouts if excessive swelling of an eyelid or hemorrhage from cuts over the eyebrow causes impaired vision in one eye of a boxer. Traditionally, if a boxer is deemed to be functionally monocular by a referee or doctor, a bout is stopped.

The eye has always been a prime target in the ring and as such is subject to more trauma in a boxer's career than it would be in any other sport. Given the long tradition of organized professional and amateur boxing, it is surprising that larger numbers of reports on the ocular injuries that can be sustained in the ring have not been published. For years, the ophthalmic literature was conspicuously devoid of studies that accurately determined the frequency and severity of ocular injuries from boxing. In fact, reports on the frequency of ocular injuries incurred from boxing have been surprisingly low. In 1955, Doggart (1) suggested that ruptures of Descemet's membrane, hyphema, glaucoma, iridodialysis, cataracts, retinal de-

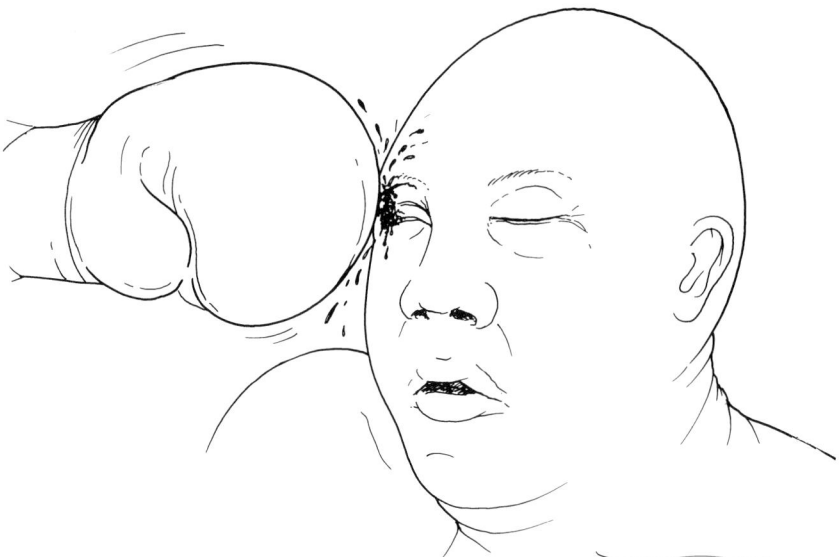

Figure 6.1 *Boxers take aim at their opponent, looking for susceptible areas that may hemorrhage and obscure vision.*

tachments, vitreous hemorrhage, maculopathies, and choroidal ruptures were potential ocular complications from boxing, but reported no data. Palmer et al (2) studied a group of 55 former boxers and reported a prevalence of 8.2% angle recessions. They also reported seeing cataracts and retinal detachments in this group, which had an average age of 59 years. No patient with angle recession had glaucoma. In 1981, Whiteson (3) stated that retinal detachments were uncommon in boxing. However, Maguire et al (4) retrospectively found eight retinal detachments in boxers over a period of 2 years at the Wills Eye Hospital. Enzenauer et al (5) found that ocular injuries occurred in 5% of soldiers hospitalized for boxing-related trauma from 1980 through 1985 in the United States Army. In recent years, more scientific examination of the prevalence and incidence of ocular injuries in boxers has been undertaken. In 1987, Giovinazzo et al (6) reported on a prospective randomized control study of active asymptomatic professional boxers over a 2-year period in cooperation with the New York State Athletic Commission. They found that over 66% of boxers had at least one pathologic change in either the anterior or posterior segment. A total of 58% of boxers suffered what they termed "vision threatening injuries." The percentage of injuries was confirmed in a study of amateur boxers in Austria by Wedrich et al in 1993 (7).

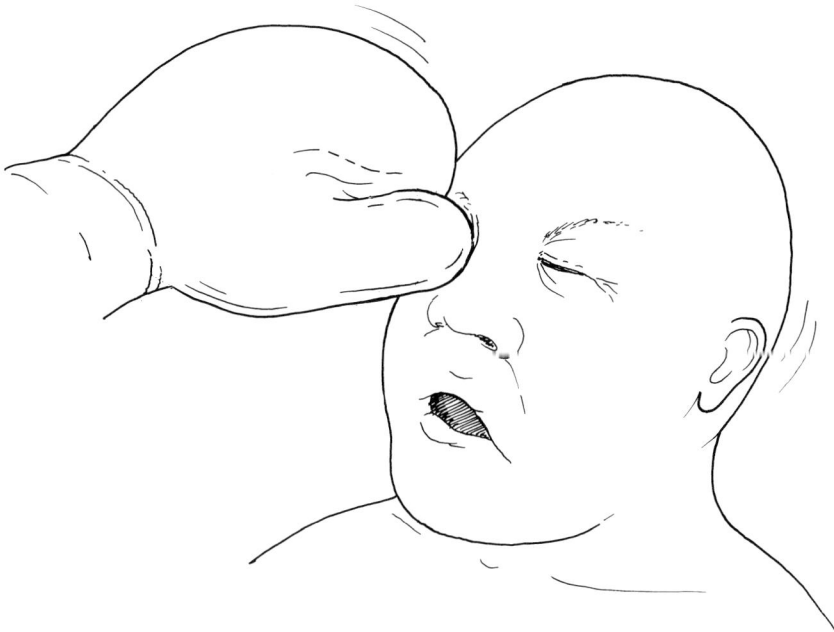

Figure 6.2 *Gouging of the eye by the thumb may create enormous ocular damage.*

Knowledge of the impact that boxing has on the visual system must first include an understanding of the mechanisms underlying the type of injury, the specific types of structural damage found in boxers, and timely and appropriate diagnosis and treatment. Special consideration must be provided to those boxers with specific visual problems, including those with myopia who use contact lenses and those postsurgical boxers after cataract and retinal detachment surgery. Finally, a better understanding is needed of the currently available means of prevention of injuries and the institutional reforms necessary to keep a boxer's eyes safer during his career in the ring.

Mechanisms of Injury

Three mechanisms have been described to explain the ocular complications of blunt trauma: coup, contrecoup, and equatorial expansion (8). The concepts of coup and contrecoup injuries were first described to explain the types of injuries seen in the brain after blunt trauma to the skull. These theories were applied by Walter (9) to explain ocular injuries occurring after blunt trauma.

Coup

Coup injury is caused by a direct blow that produces local damage (Fig. 6.3). Coup forces that have an impact on the outer surface of the globe can directly injure the lids and cornea. A direct inferior temporal blow that strikes the globe where it is unprotected by the orbital rim causes a coup-type damage to the sclera, underlying ciliary body, and retinal tissue. The types of structural damage that are seen from direct blows secondary to blunt trauma can produce cutaneous lacerations, especially over hard structures such as the superior orbital rim. Corneal abrasions are not commonly seen, but subconjunctival hemorrhages and cutaneous ecchymoses are common. The type of structural damage created by a coup injury can create focal areas of necrosis in underlying tissues, and this may partly account for the frequency of retinal holes secondary to coup-type ocular damage.

Contrecoup

The concept of contrecoup was refined by Courville (10) to account for the brain damage that occurs away from the area of impact in

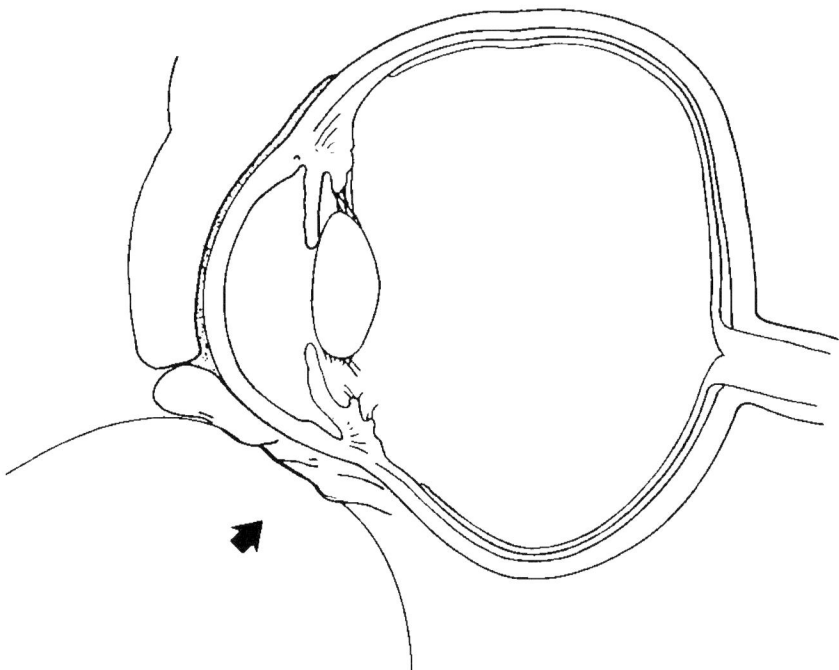

Figure 6.3 *Local damage to the eyelids occurs from a coup-type injury. Note that the direct blow to the eye (arrow) produces the local damage.*

cases of blunt head trauma. A direct blow produces a line of force traversing the skull. Damage is found to be localized at interfaces or those structures that are borders between tissues of differing densities (Fig. 6.4). This theory of damage occurring along a line of force at interfaces has been used to explain certain eye injuries such as anterior subcapsular cataracts, posterior subcapsular cataracts, traumatic retinal pigment epitheliopathies at the macula, and macular hole formation (9).

Equatorial Expansion

Equatorial expansion is the third mechanism that has been proposed specifically to explain peripheral retinal damage from blunt trauma (11). As the globe is compressed along the anterior-posterior axis, the circumference of the equator increases (Fig. 6.5). As the sclera at the equator expands, the underlying retina and pars plana are suddenly pulled from their attachment to the vitreous base. This traumatic separation can result in an avulsion of the vitreous base, tears in the retina and the ciliary epithelium of the pars plana, and retinal dialysis. This sudden ocular compression is with the indentation of the cornea; acute forcing of aqueous tissue into the angle may also account for the rupture of ciliary body tissue and the production of angle recession.

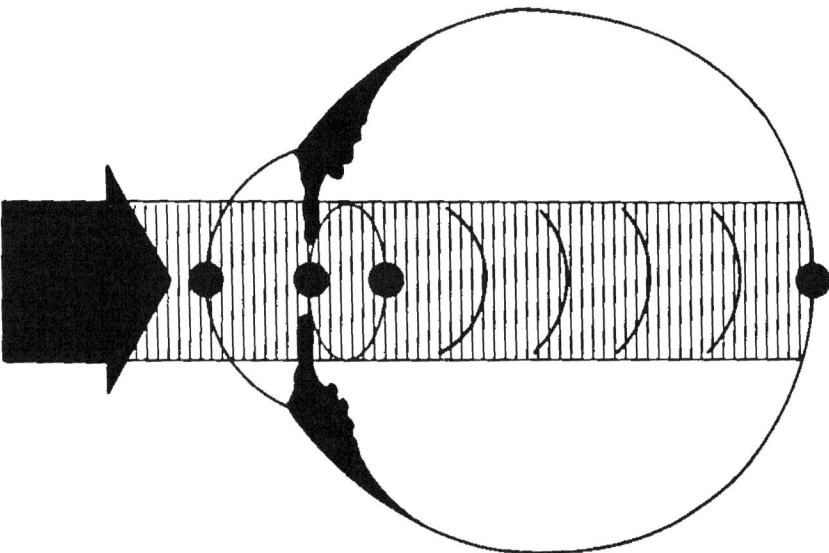

Figure 6.4 *Contrecoup lesions occur at interfaces between tissues of different densities.*

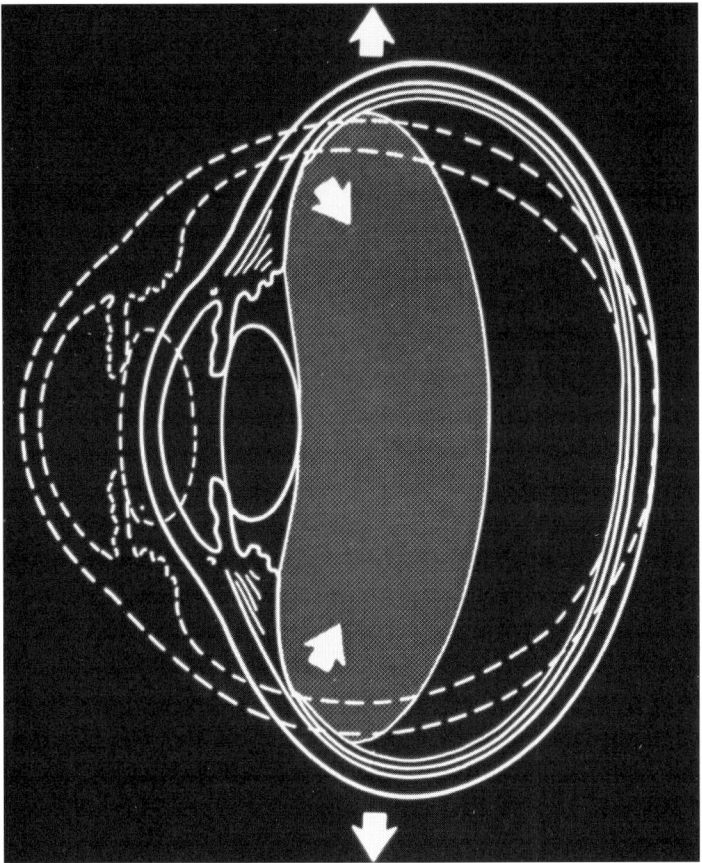

Figure 6.5 *Equatorial expansion. As the globe is compressed along the anterior-posterior axis, the circumference of the equator increases.*

Type of Injury

Vision-Threatening Injuries

The best available data on the prevalence of injuries in boxers are from *The Ocular Complications of Boxing* (6), a prospective study of active asymptomatic boxers that found over half (52%) of all eyes and two-thirds (66%) of the boxers examined had pathologic changes (Table 6.1). Fortunately, many of the injuries recorded were not vision threatening in nature. Small corneal opacities, cutaneous scarring, and iris abnormalities such as sphincter tears are examples. A large number of injuries, however, were of the type that might be vision threatening, either acutely or insidiously. These "vision-

Table 6.1 Type and frequency of injuries

INJURIES	PERCENT OF BOXERS
External	
Ptosis	4
Motility	5
Decreased sensation	1
Scars	1
Iris	
Sphincter tears	9
Rubeosis iridis	1
Angle	
Recession	9
Anterior synechiae	4
Pigment dispersion	5
Lens-cataract	
Posterior subcapsular	14
Anterior subcapsular	3
Nuclear sclerosis	3
Macula	
Hole	1
Cyst	3
RPE degeneration	4
Peripheral retina	
Atrophic hole	4
Opercular tear	8
Horseshoe tear	16
Detachment	3

RPE, retinal pigment epithelium.

threatening injuries" were defined as significant damage to the angle, lens, macula, or peripheral retina. When only vision-threatening injuries were selected in the examined boxers, 58% of boxers had at least one vision-threatening injury.

Injuries to the Angle

There is a high frequency of angle abnormalities in boxers ranging from recession and tears in the ciliary body to peripheral anterior synechiae and increased angle pigmentation. Although no patients had an elevated intraocular pressure, glaucomatous disk changes, or visual field defects, the potential for glaucoma exists in these boxers. Palmer et al (2) examined 55 former boxers and similarly found a high degree of angle abnormalities, with no incidence of glaucoma.

The reported prevalence of chronic glaucoma after a traumatic angle recession ranges from 7% to 9% (12–14). The onset of glaucoma may not occur until 10 or more years after injury. Most patients who have glaucoma secondary to trauma have an angle recession of at least 180 degrees (15) and perhaps an underlying tendency toward the development of chronic open angle glaucoma (13). A long-term longitudinal study of former boxers would be helpful to establish the frequency of late onset glaucoma in eyes with angle injuries.

Injuries to the Lens

The overall prevalence of cataracts is 19%. This is an extremely high frequency of cataracts in a population of active boxers with a mean age of 25. No cataracts were present in a control population of college varsity athletes of the same age. Over 70% of cataracts in boxers are posterior subcapsular. The mechanism of the lens changes can be accounted for in the contrecoup theory, especially the anterior and posterior subcapsular cataracts in which the interface between the lens and the vitreous may account for damage occurring at this site. In active asymptomatic boxers, the visual decrease secondary to cataract formation is small. Only one cataract in this series of boxers was severe enough to produce a visual decline to 20/40. However, given the progressive nature of posterior subcapsular changes, as boxers continue their careers, these cataracts may become more significant. Many boxers have had their careers ended by significant cataract formation. Once visual acuity reduces to the level of 20/60, a boxer is at a significant disadvantage within the ring. The ability to see fists and incoming blows from his opponent is diminished. The bright lights under which most boxers perform also contribute to the glare and the significant visual disability boxers with cataracts have. Although anabolic steroid use is not common among boxers, its presence should be questioned if cataracts are diagnosed.

Injuries to the Macula

Several different traumatic manifestations in the macula are noted, including macular cysts, macular holes, and hyperplastic-atrophic pigment epitheliopathy. Traumatic changes in the retinal pigment epithelium were the most commonly seen and presumably occur from a mechanism of either equatorial expansion at the macula or a contrecoup mechanism. Boxers can historically report the exact blow that produced a macular hole. Choroidal ruptures are also seen in boxers and can be one of the more common causes of severe vision loss if it occurs in the macula. Although no long-term longitudinal study on boxers has been performed, these macular abnormalities may place boxers at a greater long-term risk for changes of macular degeneration.

Injuries to the Peripheral Retina

A finding of considerable significance is the extremely high number of retinal tears seen in asymptomatic boxers. Peripheral retinal tears were found in 24% of boxers (6,7). There were no retinal tears found in a control population of college varsity athletes. The finding of traumatic retinal tears in boxers suggests that they are at high risk for the development of retinal detachments. An attempt to identify those risk factors that might be predictive for ocular injury was performed. Variables examined included age, weight division, right- or left-handedness, total number of bouts, and total number of losses, and total number of years in boxing (Table 6.2).

Univariate and multivariate statistical analyses were important in identification of risk factors predictive of ocular complications. It had been suggested that right- or left-handedness would be a significant factor in determining right versus left eye injury. The typical right-handed boxer fights with his left hand held high, close to his left eye and his right hand held lower, below his right eye. This stance might leave his right eye relatively vulnerable to injury. One right-handed boxer with an unorthodox stance held his right hand very low. He had no retinal tears in his left eye but five retinal tears in his right eye. Multivariate analysis, however, showed no significant difference between handedness and prevalence of right and left eye injuries in boxers. Statistically significant correlations were found, however, between the total number of bouts and the total number of losses and

Table 6.2 Risk factors predictive of retinal tears in boxers

RISK FACTORS	PERIPHERAL TEARS
Age	NS
Weight division	NS
Total bouts	$p < 0.01$
Total losses	$p < 0.03$
Handedness	NS
No. of years boxing	NS

NS, not significant.

the presence of retinal tears. As seen in Table 6.2, the relationship is almost linear between losses and retinal tears, with a 20% prevalence of retinal tears after five losses. After 75 bouts, the prevalence of retinal tears in the boxers studied was well over 90%. It is reasonable to presume that the number of punches a boxer has suffered in his career, which is perhaps measured by the number of losses and the total number of bouts, is the causative factor in the development of retinal tears.

The natural history of these traumatic tears is characterized by a relatively asymptomatic, slowly progressive detachment with multiple demarcation lines. This fact mandates a dilated retinal examination in the evaluation of every boxer. Retinal tears in boxers are more commonly found anterior to the equator with dialysis at the ora serrata, one of the more common types of tears seen in boxers. Only a dilated retinal examination with scleral depression will identify this very significant ocular pathology.

Given the larger number of retinal tears seen, there were surprisingly few retinal detachments. Reasons for the paucity of detachments noted may be the young age of boxers with their correspondingly formed vitreous, the lack of a longitudinal follow-up and the slowly progressive natural history of traumatic tears, and the nature of this particular study selection, which involved asymptomatic boxers.

The knowledge that retinal detachments are not uncommonly found in boxers, coupled with the high frequency of retinal tears, presents an opportunity to the examining ophthalmologist to diagnose and prevent further damage with appropriate treatment.

Diagnosis and Treatment

Frequent complete ocular examinations are vital during a boxer's career. A complete dilated eye examination should be performed before initiating either an amateur or a professional career and at intervals during a boxer's career when injuries are most likely to be detected. This would be best predicated on the available data that significant injuries such as retinal tears can be detected after six bouts or two losses. Professional boxers in New York State have a complete dilated eye examination every year upon renewing their license. If a ringside physician detects an ocular injury or the gouging of an eye with a thumb, an eye examination should be mandated and performed within several days of the bout. The study of one boxer best illustrates the importance of a dilated examination. This asymptomatic boxer was found to have a visual acuity of 20/25 in the right eye and 20/20 in the left eye. During a dilated examination, a large supranasal retinal detachment was identified in the right eye with a localized detachment (Plate 2). It is important to note that the macula was not involved in this detachment. This boxer was scheduled to fight 4 days after this examination. The fight was canceled, and the boxer's retina was successfully repaired. An examination limited to visual acuity testing and an undilated view of the fundus would not have detected this serious vision-threatening injury.

Ocular Examination

The ocular examination should include visual acuity with and without refraction, for both distance and near vision. A complete visual field should be obtained. Specific notation should be made of any cutaneous scarring. Examination of the cornea, conjunctiva, anterior chamber, and iris with gonioscopy should always be performed noting any degree of angle recession present. A dilated examination of the lens is important as peripheral opacities may be identified, especially posterior subcapsular changes. The vitreous is a common source of pathology, as avulsions of the vitreous base or pigmentary debris in the vitreous are frequently seen. These may also be a clue to the presence of retinal tears or detachments. A full, dilated examination of the fundus with scleral depression is mandatory in boxers.

Diagnosis

It is important to identify all ocular injuries in boxers, specifically those that are vision threatening. Many vision-threatening injuries can be treated if they are detected early. Early treatment of retinal tears can prevent their progression to a clinically significant retinal detachment. Identification of reduced vision in a boxer may be cause for appropriate suspension or termination of their career.

No one can participate in the sport of boxing if they are monocular. A "one-eyed athlete" is defined as any person with less than 20/40 vision with the other eye being normal visual acuity in one eye less than 20/50. This should be the standard used in deciding whether a boxer can continue his career once an ocular injury is suffered. Whether the cause of decreased vision is a maculopathy, retinal detachment, or cataract, visual acuity less than 20/40 is not acceptable in a boxer for two reasons. Any serious injury to the other eye would leave a vision of less than 20/40 in the remaining functioning eye, which would preclude obtaining a driver's license in most states. Second, with visual acuity reduced to this level in one eye, it is unlikely that sufficient visual acuity over an appropriate field could enable defense in the ring.

Treatment

Advances in treatment of ocular diseases have provided an opportunity for injured boxers to return to the ring and continue their careers. There is no cross-sectional or longitudinal data on postsurgical boxers and their continued careers. There have been many empiric observations and many stories of treated boxers successfully competing. However, all cases must be considered on an individual basis, with the full knowledge that boxing is an extremely high risk sport for damage to the eye.

Treatment of Retinal Tears

The most common and the most significant injury identified in the ocular examination of boxers is traumatic retinal tears. Traditional therapy for retinal tears involves either laser photocoagulation or cryotherapy. These treatments produce an adhesion from the retina to the underlying retinal pigment epithelium. It has been extremely successful in reducing the progression of retinal tears to clinically significant retinal detachments in the general population. Special consideration must be given to boxers because they will continue to suffer from repetitive trauma to their eyes after laser photocoagulation or cryotherapy. There is a potential that after treatment they may be susceptible to new complications because of the repeated blows to their eyes. There is currently no data on this issue, but this potential must be understood by boxers and their physicians.

Treatment of Cutaneous Lacerations

Plastic closure of any lacerations is important in boxers. The production of hypertrophic scars is not uncommon because of the repetitive trauma to the areas around the orbital rim. The more successful the repair, the more tensile strength the eye has, and accordingly there is a reduced risk for recurrent lacerations produced by repeated blows in the ring. Primary plastic closure soon after each bout is recommended.

Special Situations in Boxing

Contact Lenses

The use of contact lenses is now permitted by the U.S. Olympic Committee's Amateur Boxing Association. Although boxing is a sport that takes place in close quarters, opponents are usually never more than 5 feet apart; boxers who are myopic may need contact lenses to perform successfully.

The likelihood of damage from contact lenses in the ring is small. It is more likely that a contact lens will be lost from the eye during a severe blow. If contact lenses are to be used in the ring, provision must be made to stop the bout if a boxer loses a contact lens; the boxer may not know whether the lens is lost or whether vision has been decreased by a sustained ocular injury. No attempt should be made to retrieve and replace the lost contact lens, but spare contact lenses should be kept in the corner and both the corner men and the referee should be trained in contact lens insertion.

Only soft contact lenses should be used, preferably of a large diameter to help reduce the risk of displacement during a bout. The use of contact lenses in the ring may enable more myopic boxers to participate in the sport. Eyes with high myopia are at a higher risk for retinal detachment. Putting highly myopic boxers in the ring may potentiate the risk for a retinal detachment. Both doctor and patient must be aware of the potential for this increased risk, and more frequent examinations of myopic boxers may be necessary.

Postretinal Detachment Surgery

An increasing number of boxers are returning to the ring after retinal detachment surgery and resuming their careers with an uneventful postsurgical ocular history. Although this is true with many boxers who have had a successfully repaired retinal detachment, there are many boxers who should not return to the ring after retinal detachment. Plate 3 illustrates a redetachment in a boxer who returned to the ring after an initially successful repair of a retinal detachment. The large temporal retinal tears, produced after a return to the ring, should preclude any further participation in the sport of boxing.

Each boxer must be evaluated on an individual basis. The more successful both the structural and visual rehabilitation of the eye postoperatively, the greater the chance a boxer can successfully return to his career. However, even poorly treated retinal tears may predispose a fighter to further retinal injuries. In boxers with successfully treated retinal tears, there should be frequent follow-up but no contraindication to a return to their careers.

Postcataract Surgery

Recent developments in cataract surgery, such as small incision surgery with foldable implant lenses, have made it possible for boxers to return to the ring after cataract surgery. Larger incisions are a potential source of weakness and possible scleral rupture. This type of incision would preclude a return to a boxing career. The presence of a polymethylmethacrylate (PMMA) implant lens has the potential for more intraocular damage with the repeated blunt ocular trauma sustained in the ring. Small incision surgery performed through a scleral tunnel with implantation of a foldable soft silicone implant lens appears to reduce the risk of damage to a boxer's eye. Boxers have successfully competed after this operation but must be followed closely. One major risk is dislocation of the implant lens from repeated blows.

Any boxer who has undergone treatment for an injury sustained in the ring must be followed more closely than the boxer who has not sustained an injury. Boxers with developing cataracts must again be followed more closely, and when they cross the visual threshold of 20/50 visual acuity or less than 20/40, they should be suspended from fighting. There is no substitute for a careful and complete ocular examination including refraction. A boxer is being placed at risk of further damage to the eye by participating in the sport when an undetected vision-threatening injury may be present. No one should enter the boxing ring and be unable to defend oneself because of inadequate vision from either eye.

Prevention and Reform

Gloves

The thumb of the standard boxing glove is of sufficient size to effectively fit within the orbital rim and gouge the eye. The recent changes in glove design have been important in preventing this gouging from occurring. Most amateur boxers and some professionals use a thumbless glove. The thumbless glove (Fig. 6.6), by suturing the thumb entirely to the mit of the glove, prevents gouging of the eye.

The thumb-locked glove (Fig. 6.7) has a small leather tether from

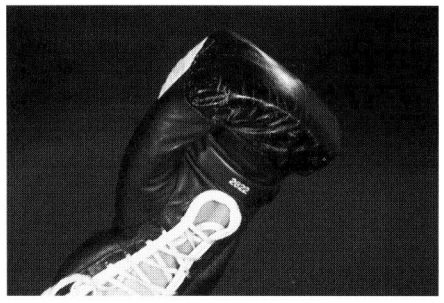 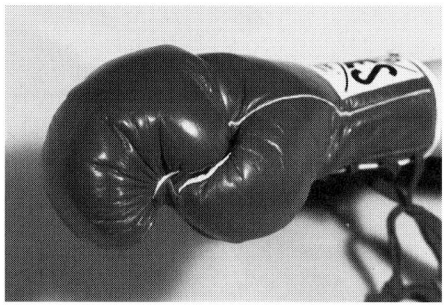

Figure 6.6 *The thumbless glove has the thumb permanently sutured to the hand.*

Figure 6.7 *The thumb-locked glove has the thumb tethered to the hand by a piece of leather.*

the tip of the thumb to the mit. By the end of a bout, this tether can become weak and stretched, and possibly break. Although the thumbless glove is preferable, the thumb-locked glove is acceptable and is now the standard in most professional bouts.

Guidelines

Specific recommendations for both the examination and treatment of boxers have been made by the American Academy of Ophthalmology. These reforms include the following.

Examination of Boxers

1. There should be specific requirements regarding ocular examination of boxers as follows:

   a. An initial complete eye examination should be required before licensure for either amateur or professional boxing. This initial examination should include visual acuity, visual field, slit-lamp biomicroscopy, intraocular pressure measurement, gonioscopy, and a dilated vitreoretinal examination including indirect ophthalmoscopy with scleral depression by an ophthalmologist.

   b. A repeat complete eye examination should be performed after 1 year, six bouts, two losses, the stopping of a fight after an eye injury, or at the discretion of the ringside physician.

2. A mandatory temporary suspension from sparring or boxing should be required for specific ocular pathology. When a retinal tear is identified and treated, a minimum 30-day suspension from the ring should be enforced. When a retinal detachment is treated and a ca-

reer is to be resumed, a minimum of 60 days' mandatory suspension should be enforced. Suspensions may be individualized in consultation with the medical advisory board of each state athletic commission.

3. The minimal visual requirements for boxing should be as follows:
   a. A corrected visual acuity better than 20/50 in each eye.
   b. A full central visual field of not less than 30 degrees in each eye.

4. An ophthalmologist should serve on each state and medical boxing advisory board to advise on a boxer's eligibility for licensure.

Safety Equipment

5. There should be adopted by state and local licensing agencies adequate safety equipment to minimize ocular injuries. The thumb of most regulation boxing gloves is small enough to penetrate the orbital rim. It is an important cause of blunt ocular trauma sustained in the boxing ring. This injury can be eliminated by the use of the thumbless or thumb-locked boxing glove. The use of the thumbless or thumb-locked boxing glove should be mandatory not only in all amateur and professional bouts but also in all sparring matches.

Regulations

6. There should be established in the United States a "National Registry of Boxers" for all amateur and professional boxers, including sparring mates. A computer-based central registry of this kind would be effective in recording licensed bouts and specifically noting knockouts and significant ocular injuries. When a bout is stopped because of ocular injury, proper records and documentation should ensure adequate examinations of injured boxers.

7. There should be a program of training and recertification of ringside physicians in the proper identification of serious eye injuries sustained in the ring. The diagnosis of serious eye injuries and specific criteria for suspension of a bout should be planned and conducted in cooperation with the American Association of Ringside Physicians and the American Academy of Ophthalmology.

8. There should be adopted by state and local licensing agencies a uniform code of safety requiring that a boxing match shall be stopped upon the occurrence of specified ocular symptoms or injuries

such as visual field loss and blood in the anterior or posterior segment of the eye.

It is quite clear that participation in boxing results in a large number of ocular injuries. The effects of these injuries can be quite variable and are best exemplified with the story of two United States Olympic gold medal winners, the two Sugar Rays. Sugar Ray Leonard, an Olympic gold medal winner in 1976, turned professional and became the welterweight champion. He suffered a retinal detachment, underwent surgery, and resumed his career. He subsequently won several championship belts and earned millions of dollars by the age of 30. Sugar Ray Seals, an Olympic gold medal winner in 1972, suffered bilateral retinal detachments. After more than 400 bouts and seven vitreoretinal surgeries, he is now bilaterally blind. These two individuals illustrate the wide range and potentially devastating effects of ocular injuries in boxing. Although a high incidence of ocular injuries occurs in boxers, many of these injuries are treatable if detected early. A complete dilated eye examination by an ophthalmologist is necessary to diagnose ocular injuries before they cause vision loss. Uniform regulations enacted on a nationwide basis mandating required eye examinations and safety equipment will reduce the frequency and severity of ocular injuries in boxing.

References

1. Doggart JH. The impact of boxing on the visual apparatus. Arch Ophthalmol 1955;54:161–169.
2. Palmer E, Leberman TW, Burns S. Contusion angle deformity in prizefighters. Arch Ophthalmol 1976;94:225–228.
3. Whiteson AL. Injuries in professional boxing: their treatment and prevention. Practitioner 1981;225:1053–1057.
4. Maguire JI, Benson WE. Retinal injury and detachment in boxers. JAMA 1986;255:2451–2453.
5. Enzenauer RW, Mauldin WM. Boxing-related ocular injuries in the United States Boxing Army, 1980 to 1985. Southern Med J 1989;82:547–549.
6. Giovinazzo VJ, Yannuzzi LA, Sorenson JA, et al. The ocular complications of boxing. Ophthalmology 1987:587–596.
7. Wedrich A, Velikay M, Binder S, et al. Ocular findings in asymptomatic boxers. Retina 1993;3:114–119.
8. Benson WE, Shakin J, Sarin LK. Blunt trauma. In: Duane TD, ed. Clinical ophthalmology. vol. 3. Philadelphia: Harper & Row Publishers Inc., 1985:1–13.
9. Walter JR. Coup-contrecoup mechanism of ocular injuries. Am J Ophthalmol 1963;56:786–796.

10. Courville CB. Coup-contrecoup mechanism of craniocerebral injuries. Some observations. Arch Surg 1942;45:19–42.
11. Weidenthal DT, Schepens CL. Peripheral fundus changes associated with ocular contusion. Am J Ophthalmol 1966;62:465–477.
12. Blanton FM. Anterior chamber angle recession and secondary glaucoma. A study of the after effects of traumatic hyphemas. Arch Ophthalmol 1964; 72:39–43.
13. Mooney D. Angle recession and secondary glaucoma. Br J Ophthalmol 1973;57:608–612.
14. Kaufman JH, Tolpin DS. Glaucoma after traumatic angle recession: a ten year prospective study. Am J Ophthalmol 1974;78:648–654.
15. Tesluk G, Spaeth GL. The occurrence of primary open-angle glaucoma in the fellow eye of patients with unilateral angle-clearage glaucoma. Ophthalmology 1985;92:904–911.

CHAPTER 7

Football

John B. Jeffers

Over 1 million youngsters participate in organized football programs (1). The contact sport of football is played at various levels, from youngsters to professionals. Like most athletes, football players continue to get bigger, stronger, and faster every year. Many efforts have been made in providing protective equipment to prevent injuries; however, football is responsible for approximately 432,000 injuries per year in the United States (2). A 2-year prospective study of collegiate athletes playing football showed the overall injury rate was 6.32 per 1000 athletic exposures or 45.27 per 100 athletes (3).

In 1993, football accounted for 5% of all sports-related eye injuries (4). Despite the improvements in helmets and faceguards, ocular and facial injuries continue to occur. One study looked at ocular trauma in college varsity sports at Michigan State University and found that football was responsible for 4.1% of all eye injuries (5).

History

Historians claim that we can thank the Chinese for being the first to introduce a form of football in 2000 B.C. Although the use of an inflated ball took place in 500 A.D., it was not until the Middle Ages that the ball was made from a cow's bladder (the modern "pigskin"). In the United States, the first intercollegiate game was played in 1869 between Princeton and Rutgers.

From 1888 through 1906, American football was considered a "deadly game" in which brute force was involved. Various lineups such as the "V formation" and "flying wedge" resulted in a large number of serious injuries as well as some fatalities. These lineups were eventually outlawed, and in the 1920s football had begun to grow in popularity.

Visual Performance in Football

Football is a contact sport that requires a specific degree of visual function depending on the position and level at which it is played. Whether football is played under unorganized or organized conditions, from playground roughtouch, through high school and college, and ultimately to the professional level, adequate visual acuity and depth perception along with hand-eye coordination and timing are important to the position played.

The players that require optimum visual performance are designated as the skill positions. The quarterback, wide receiver, tight end, running back, defensive back, linebacker, and kickoff and punt return specialist are all considered skill players. Centers may also be included because of their role in long snaps for punts, point after touchdowns, and field goals. The nonskill (a definite misnomer) positions refer to linemen whose strength and quickness are more important than optimal visual acuity.

The visual requirements of the quarterback include precise distance visual acuity to interpret the hand signals quickly and accurately from the sidelines and then before the "snap" to instantaneously "read" the defensive alignment. A full field of vision is needed while dropping back to pass to survey the defensive deployment and predict exactly where the intended receiver will be open. The quarterback then passes the ball in anticipation of "hitting" the receiver in stride at a precise spot.

The defensive backs, on the other hand, must possess excellent visual acuity and a wide field of vision to "pick up" the potential offensive receivers, while tracking the flight of the ball. It is necessary for the defender to keep pace with the receiver while anticipating the pass.

The kickoff and punt return specialists are receiving a ball that is coming directly toward them at a high trajectory. This requires exceptional visual acuity and depth perception. The potential exists for adverse factors such as the wind changing the flight of the ball or the sun making it difficult to see; the player, therefore, must make adjustments accordingly.

The need for increasingly precise visual performance will be dependent on the skill level of the game and relative athletic maturity. The skills of the young player differ greatly from the more sophisticated high school, college, or professional player. Visual acuity, depth perception, and reaction time may be an absolute necessity at the higher levels of organized football.

Football Eye Injuries

Eye injuries in football can occur in all positions played. The defensive lineman may be seen with hands going under an offensive player's faceguard (cage) while attempting to block or penetrate the line (Fig. 7.1); a running back or quarterback may be seen giving an opponent the "straight arm" to his face to ward him off (Fig. 7.2); and a defensive player may grab an opponent's faceguard in an attempt to tackle and inadvertently have fingers penetrate it (Fig. 7.3).

A study of North Carolina high school players found that of 4,287 football injuries, 52 (1.2%) were to the eye (6). Helveston (7) discussed two professional football players who sustained eye injuries; the two injuries were caused by the same defensive player in a similar manner. Remarkably, both injuries occurred on the same play, and a

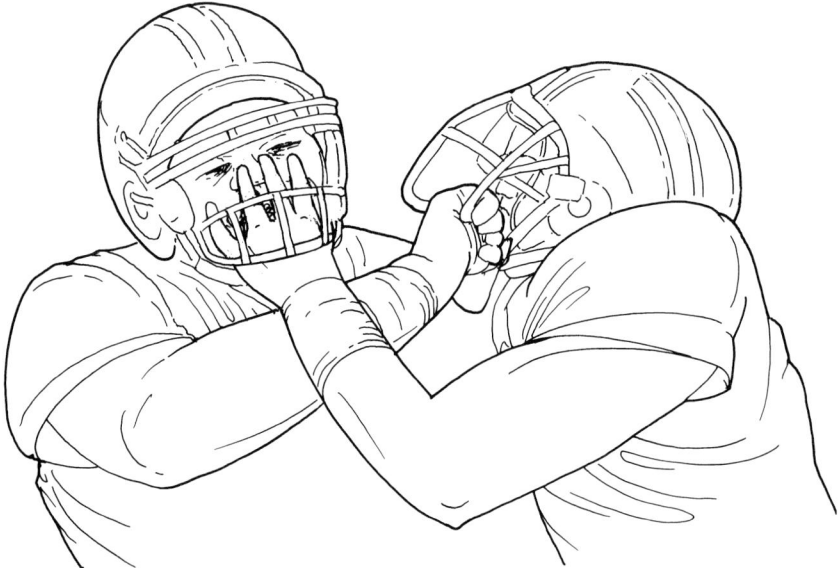

Figure 7.1 *Hands may be seen sliding under an opponent's faceguard, especially while blocking on the line of scrimmage.*

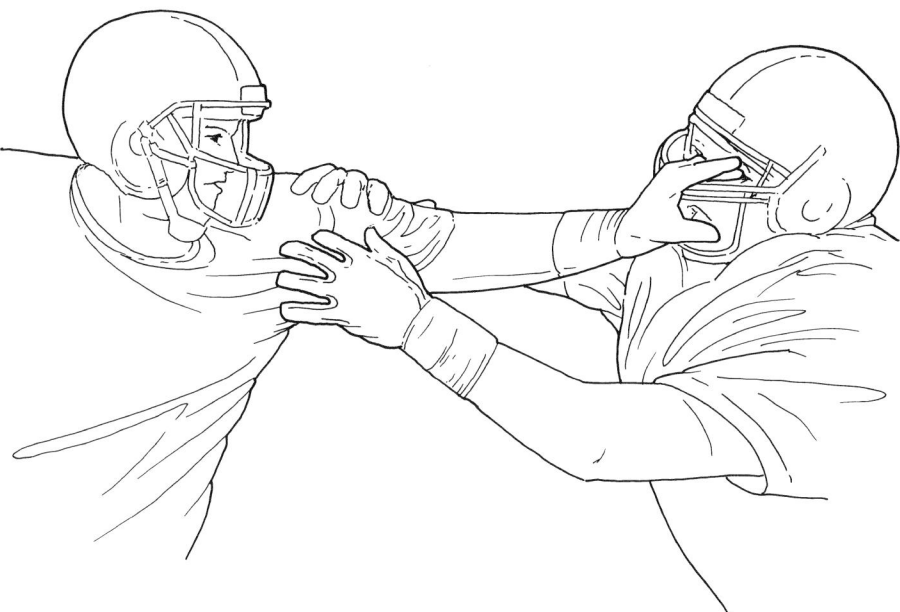

Figure 7.2 *The offensive quarterback or running back may give an opponent the "straight arm," in which fingers may penetrate the faceguard.*

fingernail was the offending agent. Heinrichs et al (8) reported on a 19-year-old collegiate varsity defensive tackle who sustained a giant retinal tear, retinal detachment, vitreous hemorrhage, and eyelid laceration when an opponent's thumb went through the facemask. This player went on to have major ophthalmic surgery and had an excellent visual recovery. Inadvertent fingers and hands are capable of penetrating all football faceguards. One university team doctor saw three injuries occur in this manner over a 1-year period (9).

Mechanisms of Injury

Blunt trauma is the most common cause of eye injuries in football. Fingers are the usual etiology of an injury because they directly penetrate the opening of the faceguard. When rule changes allow for an increased use of the hands, the hands may slide up under the faceguard and impact the eye.

The most common types of ocular injuries occurring in football are foreign bodies on the cornea and conjunctiva, periorbital contusions in the form of ecchymosis and edema of the lids ("black

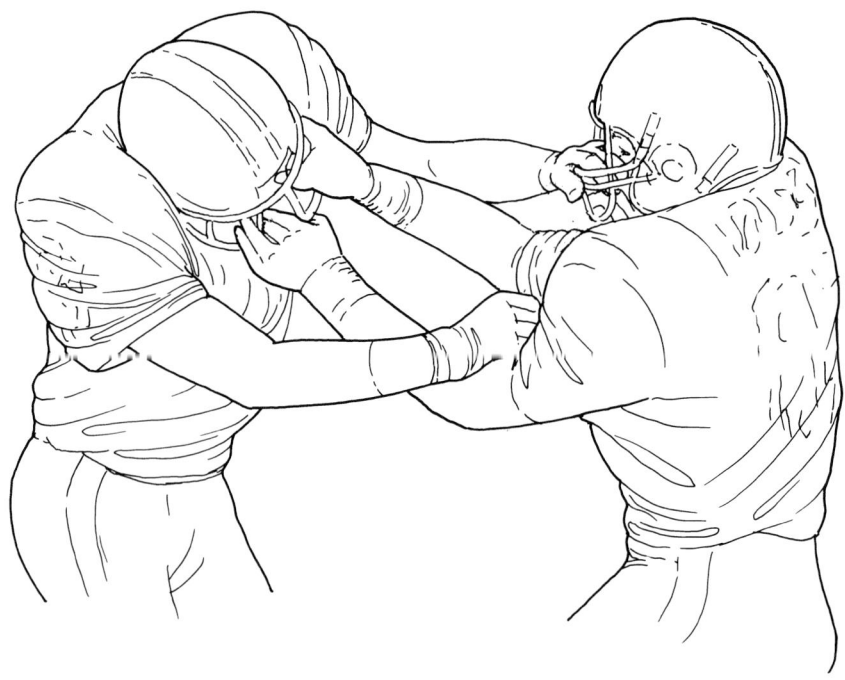

Figure 7.3 *This defensive player is shown grabbing the facemask, his fingers penetrating it.*

eye"), corneal abrasions, and traumatic iritis (see Chapter 11). Less common injuries involve orbital bone fractures, lacerations of the lid or conjunctiva (usually by a fingernail), traumatic hyphema, and commotio retinae.

During a National Football League (NFL) professional game, an offensive lineman was intentionally "poked" in the eye through the faceguard by the finger of a defensive lineman. The injury resulted in 80% of the corneal epithelium being torn off along with a contusion of the medial rectus muscle, resulting in transient double vision. At the time of examination, an avulsed optic nerve and/or orbital fracture was suspected. These were ruled out by CT scan. Since the injury, that player has developed a recurrent erosion (the surface epithelium of the cornea, as it is healing, does not adhere to the basement membrane sufficiently and is repeatedly torn off either by light eye rubbing or opening of the eyelid after sleep).

When football is played on a grass field, there is the ever-present possibility of a conjunctival and/or corneal foreign body getting into the eye. In games played on artificial turf, there is the potential of "carpet dust" getting in the eye. Both types of playing surfaces have field markings and thus there is also a danger of sustaining a chemical injury to the eye (Fig. 7.4).

During one professional game, the kicker, while running down after a kickoff, was literally jabbed in the eye by the opposing player. The injured kicker described a feeling of "actually being lifted off the ground." The injury resulted in a conjunctival laceration with retinal edema and hemorrhage opposite the point of external impact. The recommendation for temporary protective eyewear was accepted by the player but overruled by the coach after a subsequent missed field goal with the goggles in place. The player informed the ophthalmologist, "Doc, I just blew it—it wasn't the goggles."

During a college game, a traumatic hyphema occurred in a tight end who was attempting to block an opposing player. The opposing player's hand slid up under the faceguard, impacted the eye, and produced the bleeding.

Prevention and Protection

Football Helmet

According to the American Plastics Council, in the early 1900s a padded leather "head harness" was developed as a means of protecting football players from traumatic blows to the head. After World War II, manufacturers began to use plastic. Today, the football helmet's outer shell is polycarbonate and is lined with several layers of material: a vinyl-and-rubber foam to absorb the shock of a jarring collision, polyurethane foam to increase comfort, and a sheet of vinyl to protect the foam inside the helmet from hair and body oils. Specialized custom helmets may contain inflatable vinyl cells that can be pumped with air to provide more of a cushion.

Although the first faceguard was made in the mid-1930s, it was not until the mid-1950s that the use of faceguards became common. The faceguard is composed of steel and coated with two ultrathin layers of plastic. It is mounted on the helmet with brackets and comes in many different configurations.

The modern football helmet with the attached faceguard is constructed so that the occurrence of severe ocular injuries is at a minimum. The football helmet and faceguard have been instrumental in protecting players and have resulted in an 80% to 90% reduction in facial injuries (10,11). The football helmet with attached faceguard offers excellent facial protection; however, its effect on reducing the

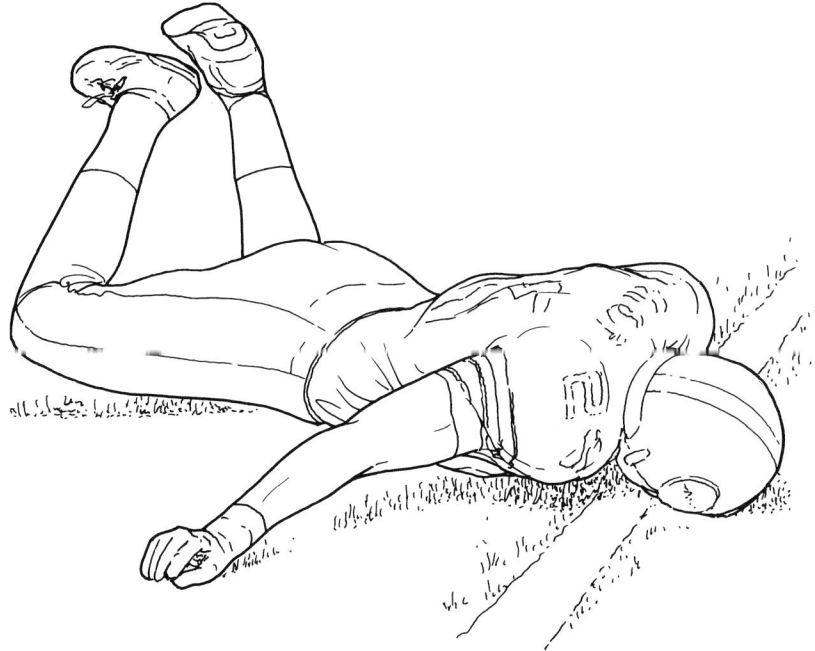

Figure 7.4 *An eye injury may result from either a foreign body or chemical coming off the turf. This player can be seen facedown on the line markings, which should consist of an inert nontoxic component.*

number of eye injuries is not impressive. All faceguards today will allow an opponent's finger to penetrate it or a hand to slide up underneath the faceguard and strike the eye from below. The faceguard itself comes in many styles, each having varying sizes of openings.

The structure of faceguards may vary in the number of horizontal and vertical bars, and the position played will dictate the player's choice. A kicker, for instance, may choose one that has a single horizontal bar with a large opening so it does not impair the vision (Fig. 7.5), whereas a lineman's faceguard with numerous bars may closely resemble a "cage" (Fig. 7.6). Skill position players usually prefer no central vertical bar that might interfere with a full field of vision.

Polycarbonate Shield

In 1974, Frank Pupello developed the first football shield visor from an automobile racing helmet (12). He constructed it for a University of Tampa player who had been poked in the eye by a finger. In 1984, Pupello, then the equipment manager for the Tampa Bay Buccaneers, made a more advanced model for linebacker Hugh Green. Other

Football 115

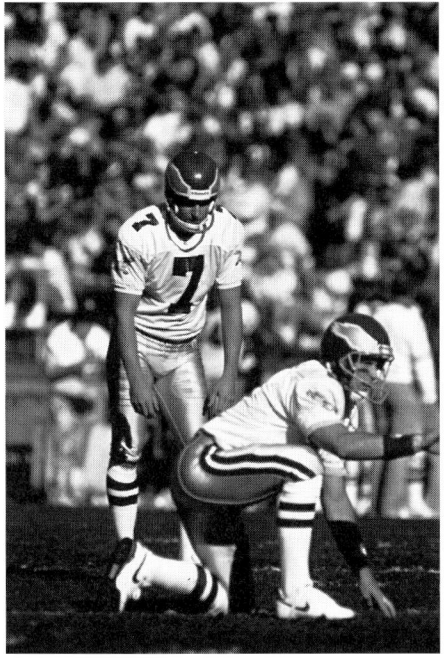

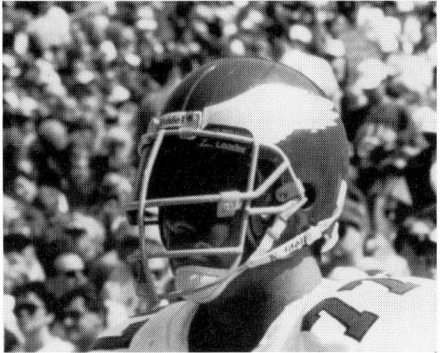

Figure 7.6 *This lineman wears a "cage-like" mask in addition to a polycarbonate tinted visor. Note the vertical bar running through the center.* (Courtesy of the Philadelphia Eagles.)

Figure 7.5 *The placekicker usually has a large opening in the facemask to improve visibility.* (Courtesy of the Philadelphia Eagles.)

players in the league became interested in the shield, and soon manufacturers began producing it. One problem with the shield was that it would occasionally fog up. In addition, in adverse weather conditions such as rain, snow, or a muddy field, the visor would have to be wiped off.

For a player to wear a polycarbonate shield, the NFL now requires a prescription to be on file in their office indicating the need. Some state high school athletic associations will not allow the players to wear the shield without a prescription or letter from their ophthalmologist.

The polycarbonate shield, attached to the faceguard, offers protection from direct blows through the faceguard but not from underneath (Fig. 7.7). Appropriate well-fitted polycarbonate sports goggles are the only means to give almost complete protection from the hands of the opposing players (Fig. 7.8).

Many professional players are reluctant to wear protective eyewear because they believe the goggles interfere with their peripheral

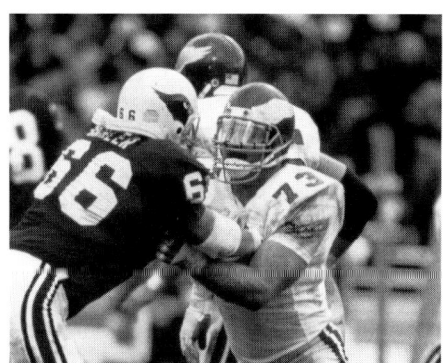

Figure 7.7 *The polycarbonate visor comes in different shades. Although this type of facial/eye protection is recommended, an opponent's hands are capable of sliding up underneath the mask.* (Courtesy of the Philadelphia Eagles.)

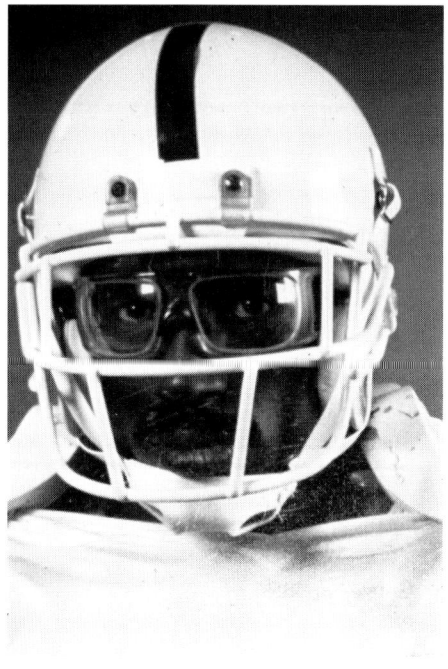

Figure 7.8 *These Helmet Specs differ from other protective frames in that they are better designed to fit under a helmet and contain a strap to go around the top of the head.* (Courtesy of Liberty Optical.)

vision: "it's not macho, it's not my style, it ruins my game." Some team owners may also have negative opinions about players' wearing eye protection (which they believe adversely affects the players' game). However, if indicated, the medical staff has to be emphatic about the recommendation.

By agreeing to wear polycarbonate sports goggles while an injured eye is healing, a player may be allowed to return to action sooner. Professional athletes are more apt to accept wearing eye protection for a short period while the eye is healing.

Functionally One-Eyed Player

The functionally one-eyed player is one with 20/40 or better, best corrected vision in one eye and worse than 20/40 best corrected vision in the other eye. To play football, this player must be required to wear the polycarbonate shield as well as polycarbonate sports goggles under the helmet for maximum protection. It is important to understand that regular streetwear glasses or contact lenses do not afford adequate eye protection.

If a player has lived with amblyopia all through life, there are usually minimal problems with gross depth perception because monocular clues are used to adjust. Wesley Walker, former all-pro wide receiver with the New York Jets, was functionally one-eyed secondary to amblyopia related to a monocular cataract, yet he was able to perform at a very high level and had an extremely successful career.

If the athlete is past the amblyopic age (approximately 9 years old), has had binocular vision, and then acutely becomes a functionally one-eyed person (most often as a result of injury), it is extremely difficult to adjust and perform athletically at the same optimal level.

Visual Training and Visual Enhancement

There are no controlled scientific studies to prove the efficacy of visual training or visual enhancement (see Chapter 14). In football, it seems that extra time on the practice field would accomplish more in improving quality of play than spending time trying to improve the player's visual function in front of a board that, among other things, is used to measure and improve reaction time (i.e., eye-hand speed).

My own personal experience suggests that the younger, more athletically immature football players (grade school and junior high school age) may benefit from these vision enhancement exercises by increasing their awareness of their potential visual acuity and visual field. However, the young athlete must then bring this increased awareness to the field and put it into "action."

References

1. Goldberg B, Rosenthal PP, Nicholas JA. Injuries in youth football. Phys Sportsmed 1984;12:122–130.
2. Jones N. Eye injury in sport. Sports Med 1989;7:163–181.
3. Zemper ED. Injury rates in a national sample of college football teams: a 2-year prospective study. Phys Sportsmed 1989;17:100–113.
4. National Society to Prevent Blindness. 1993 Eye injuries associated with

sports and recreational products. Schaumburg, IL: National Center for Sight, 1994.
5. Marton K, Wilson D, McKeag D. Ocular trauma in college varsity sports. Med Sci Sports Exerc 1987;19(suppl):S53.
6. Blyth CS, Mueller FO. An epidemiologic study of high school football injuries in North Carolina 1968–1972. Washington, DC: US Product Safety Commission, 1974.
7. Helveston EM. Football. In: Pizzarello LD, Haik BG, eds. Sports ophthalmology. Springfield: Charles C Thomas, 1987.
8. Heinrichs EH, Willcockson JR. Catastrophic eye injury in a football player. Phys Sportsmed 1982;10:71–72.
9. Sherwood DJ. Eye injuries to football players. N Engl J Med 1989.
10. Vinger PF. The eye in sports medicine. In: Tasman W, Jaeger EA, eds. Duane's clinical ophthalmology. vol. 5. Philadelphia: Lippincott, 1994:1–103.
11. Schneider RC, Antine BE. Visual-field impairment related to football headgear and face guards. JAMA 1965;192:120–123.
12. Craig Neff, ed. The Darth Vader look. Sports Illustrated Dec. 5, 1988, pp. 21–22.

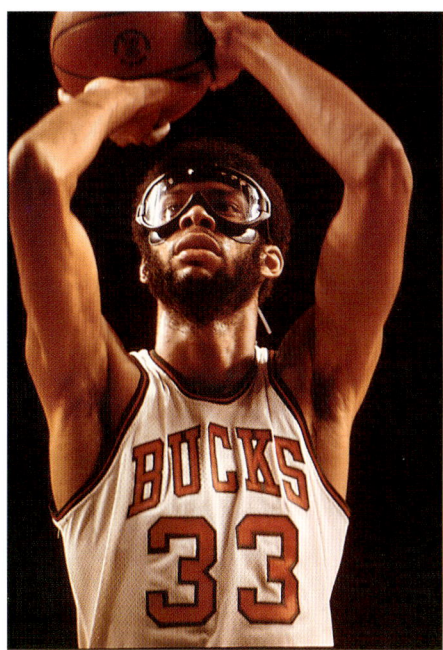

Plate 1 Many basketball players begin wearing protective eye goggles post injury. Perhaps the most famous instance of this is Kareem Abdul-Jabbar who began wearing protective eye wear, shown here in his vintage aviator's goggles, following his sixth corneal abrasion. Although these goggles were short lived, his polycarbonate goggles soon became an icon in professional basketball. (Reprinted with permission from John Jaconol Sports Illustrated.)

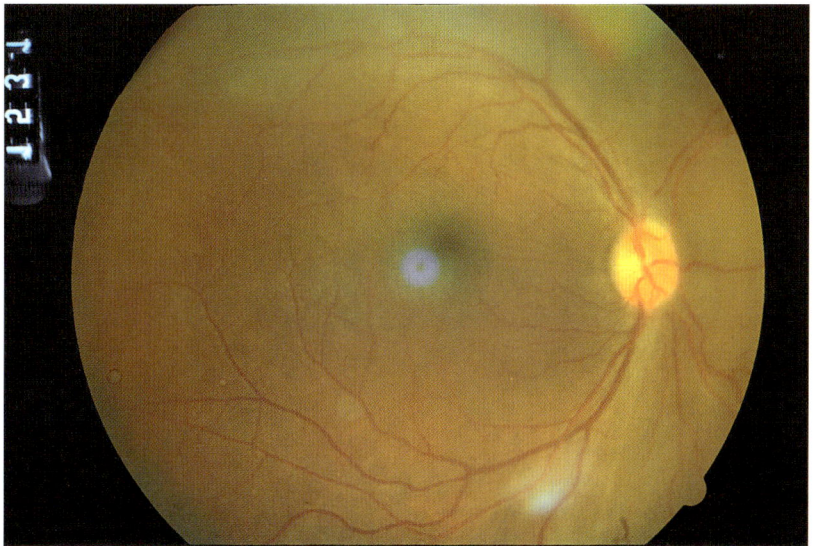

Plate 2 The macula is attached and this boxer has excellent visual acuity. However, a dilated fundus examination reveals a quadrantic retinal detachment with a giant retinal tear.

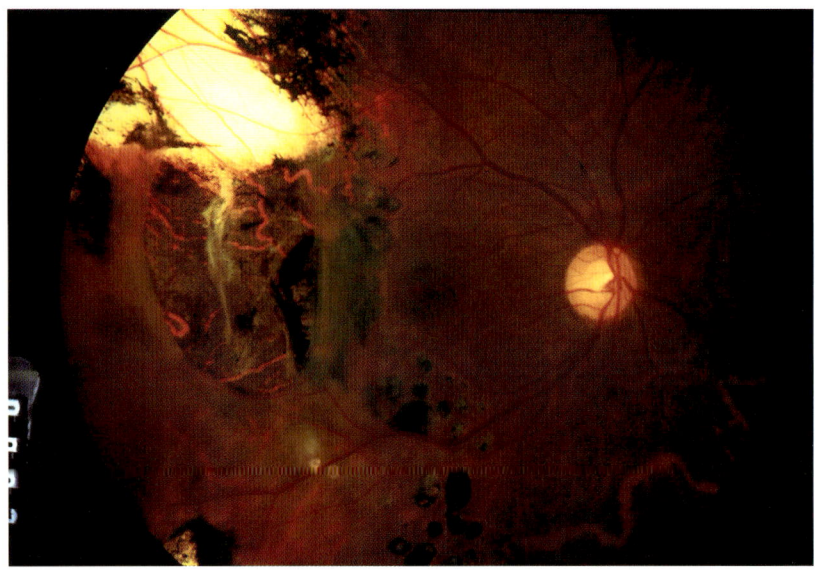

Plate 3 *The visual acuity of this boxer is 20/30, yet significant peripheral retinal pathology precludes a safe return to a career in boxing.*

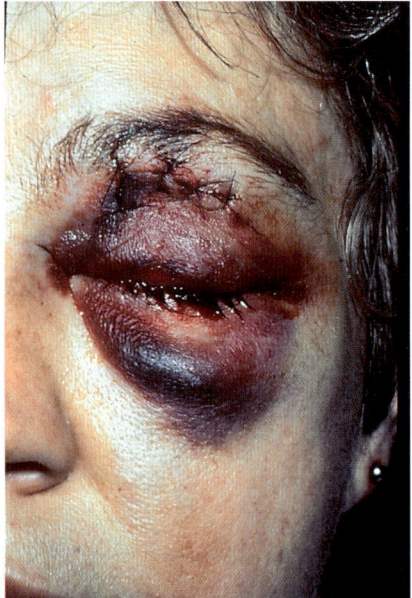

Plate 4 *This individual was struck with a high velocity golf ball. External evaluation reveals an eyelid laceration (sutured) as well as periorbital edema and ecchymosis. A ruptured globe was present.*

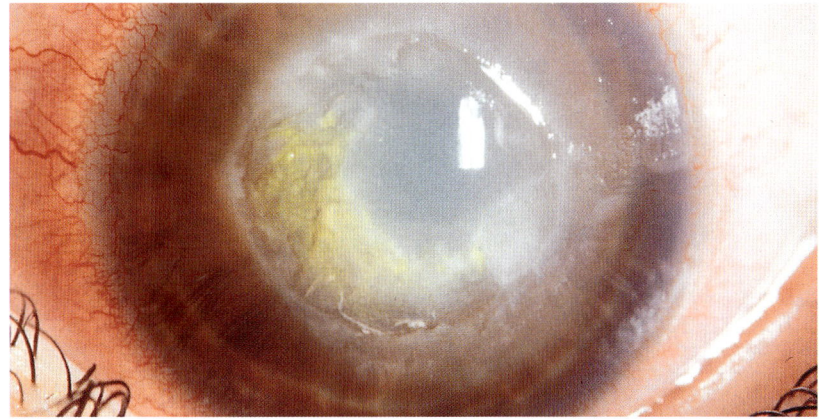

Plate 5 *This painful ring-like corneal infection proved to be Acanthamoeba. The patient was a contact lens wearer.*

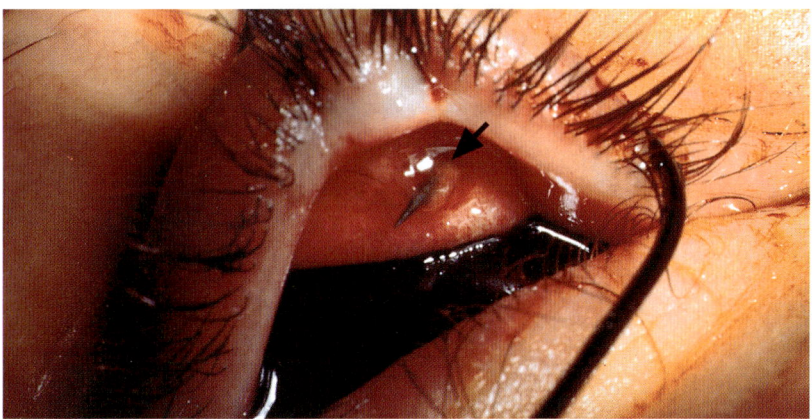

Plate 6 *This fish-hook penetrated the upper eyelid.*

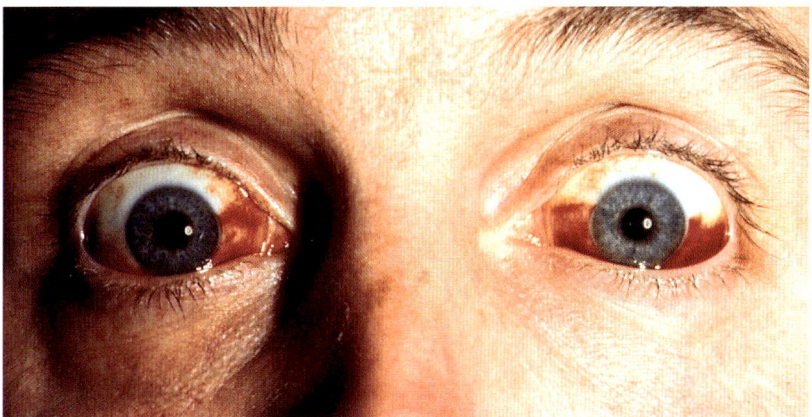

Plate 7 *Ocular squeeze as seen here may result in bilateral subconjunctival hemorrhages.*

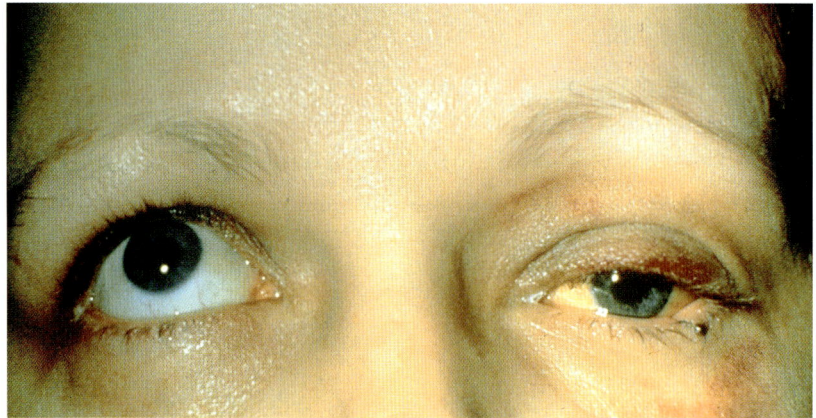

Plate 8 On upgaze, this patient's left eye was unable to look up. A left orbital floor fracture was present with entrapment of the inferior rectus muscle.

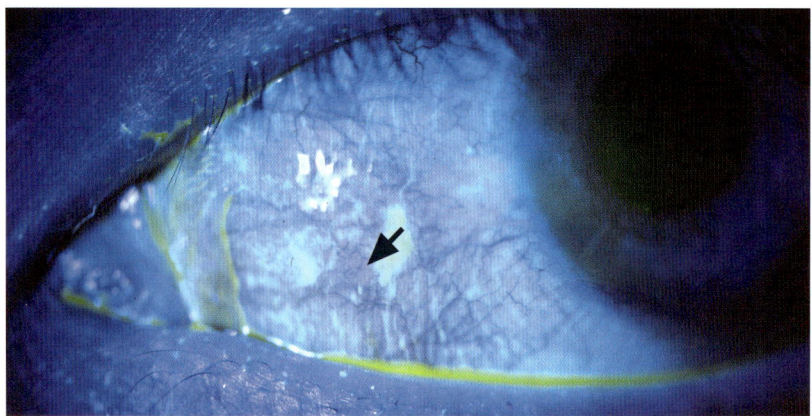

Plate 9 This conjunctival abrasion (arrow) shows bright green fluorescein uptake. The patient was poked in the eye while playing basketball.

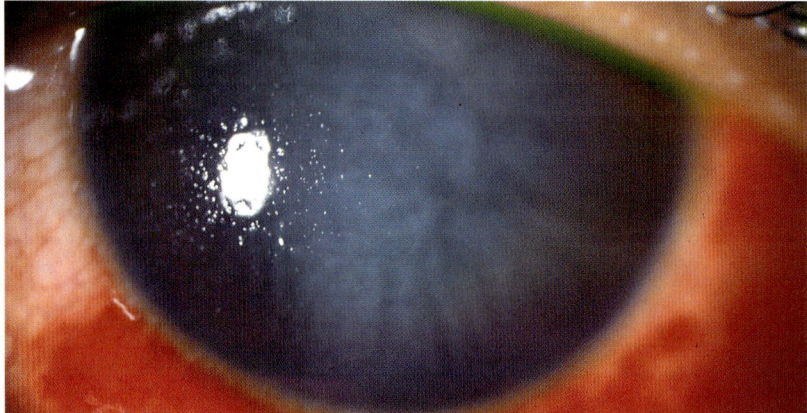

Plate 10 The corneal clouding (white area) present is corneal edema.

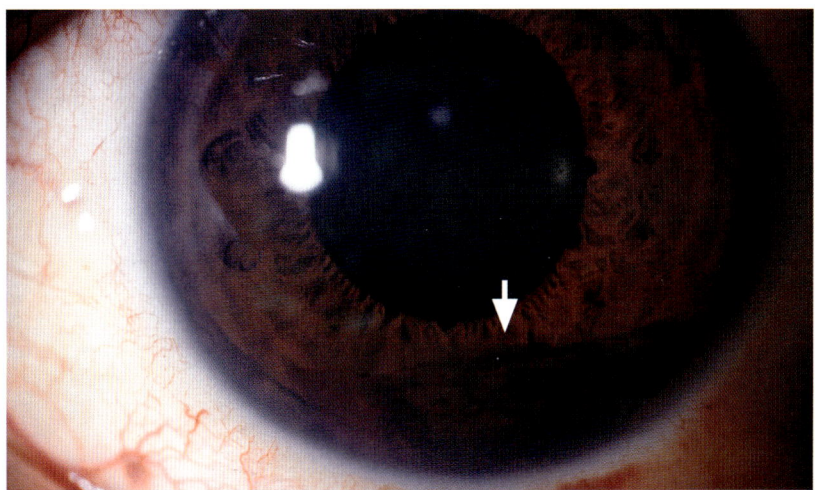

Plate 11 Blood in the anterior chamber is known as a hyphema. In this case, the hyphema is layered (arrow).

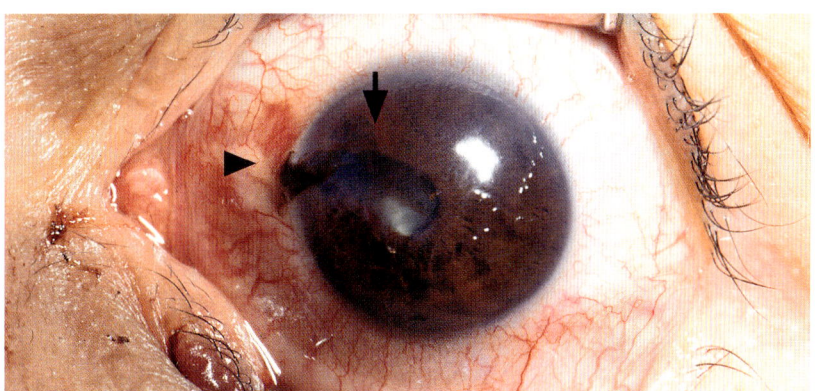

Plate 12 A peaked (irregular) pupil (arrow) is recognized in a patient with a ruptured globe. Note the prolapsed iris through the corneal laceration (arrowhead). A traumatic cataract is present.

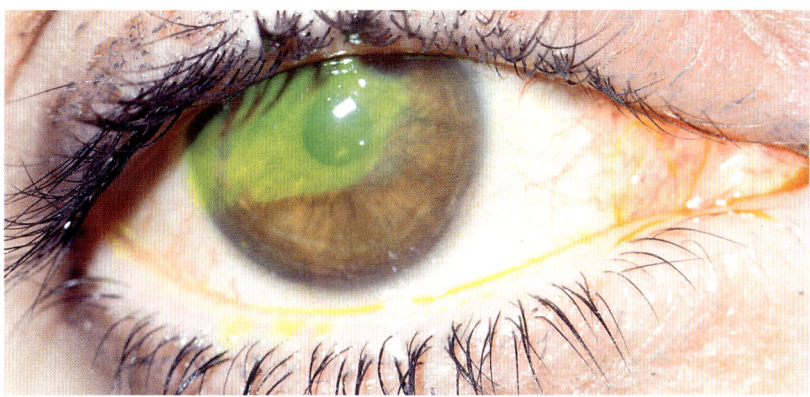

Plate 13 Bright green staining on this patients' cornea using fluorescein dye confirms the diagnosis of corneal abrasion.

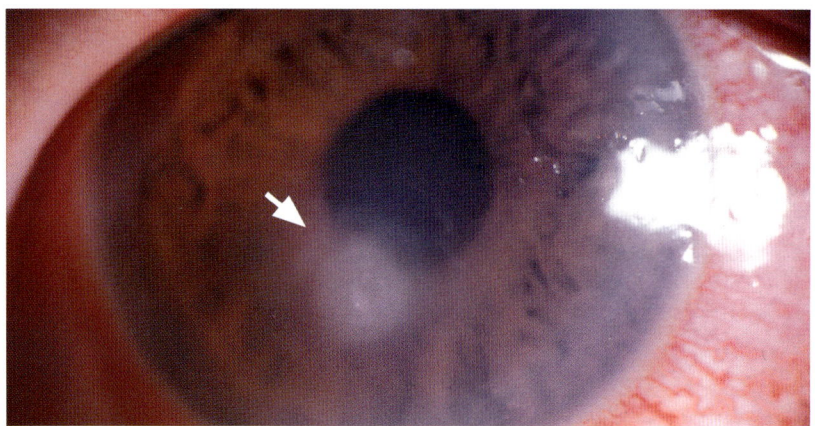

Plate 14 *An infectious corneal ulcer is seen as a white lesion on the cornea (arrow).*

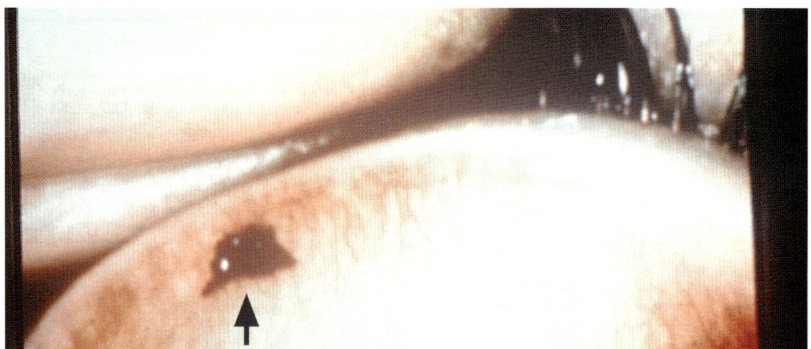

Plate 15 *In this case, a foreign body (arrow) is found embedded on the inner surface of the eyelid (tarsal conjunctiva).*

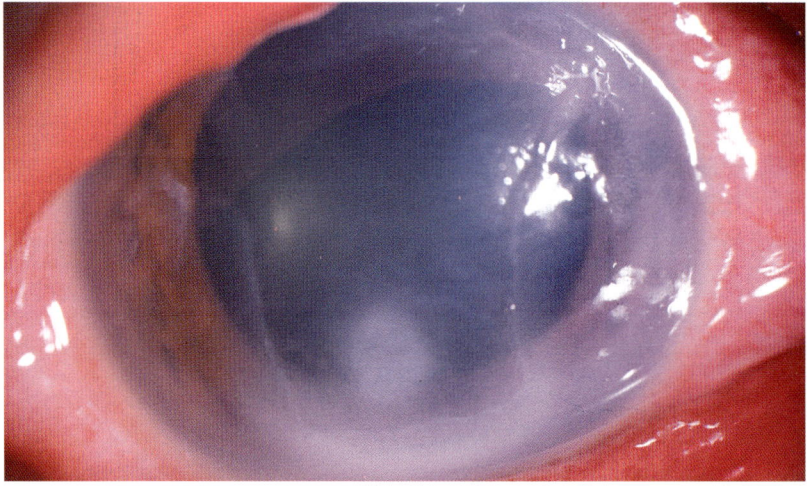

Plate 16 *This patient abused a topical anesthetic agent in order to control his ocular pain. This resulted in a corneal epithelial defect as shown.*

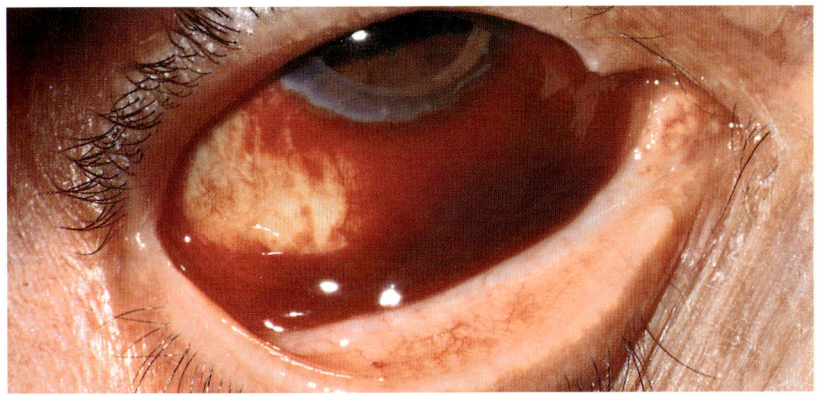

Plate 17 Subconjunctival hemorrhage is seen as blood loculated between the sclera and the conjunctiva.

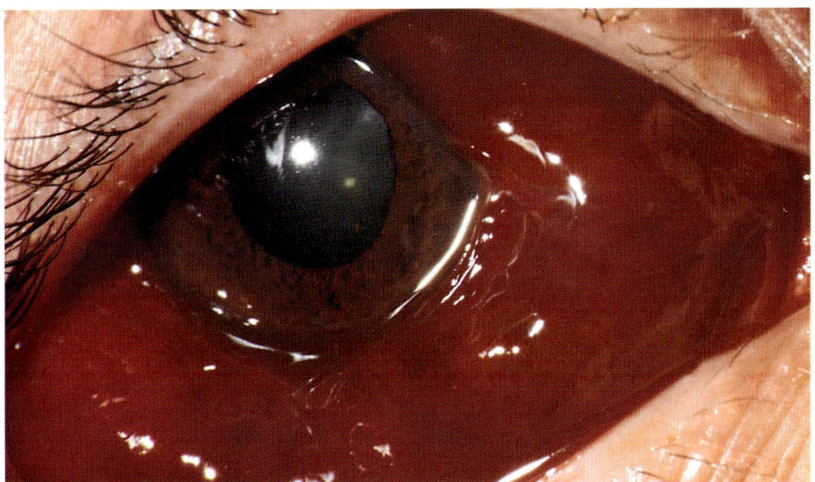

Plate 18 A ruptured globe should be suspected when a subconjunctival hemorrhage is accompanied by chemosis (conjunctival edema).

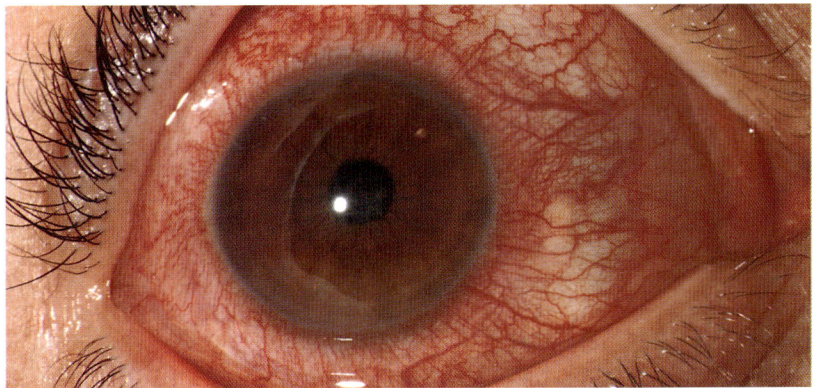

Plate 19 Conjunctival injection with a miotic pupil is suggestive of traumatic iritis.

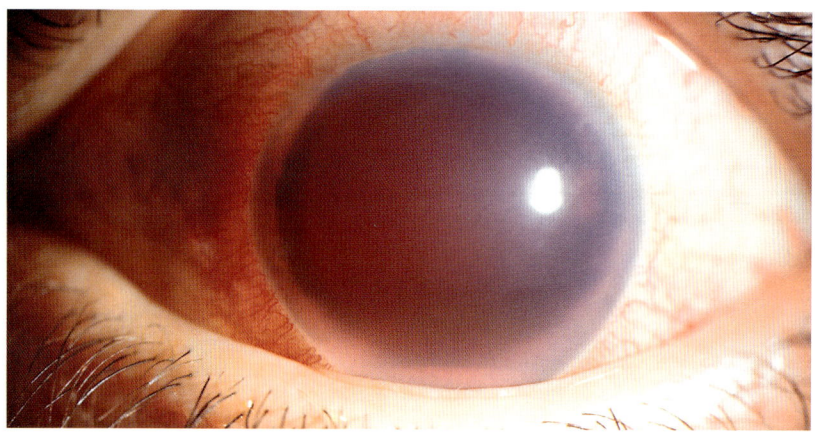

Plate 20 *A large amount of blood can be seen filling the anterior chamber (hyphema).*

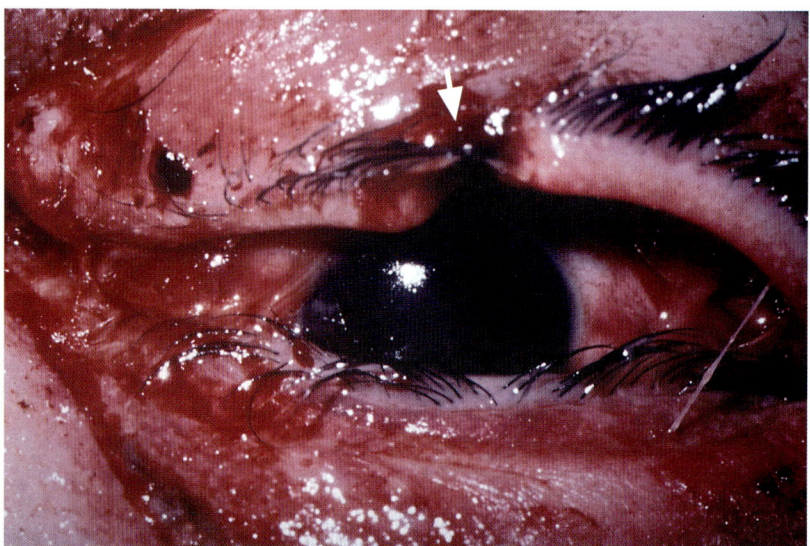

Plate 21 *Laceration of the eyelid which involves the margin (arrow).*

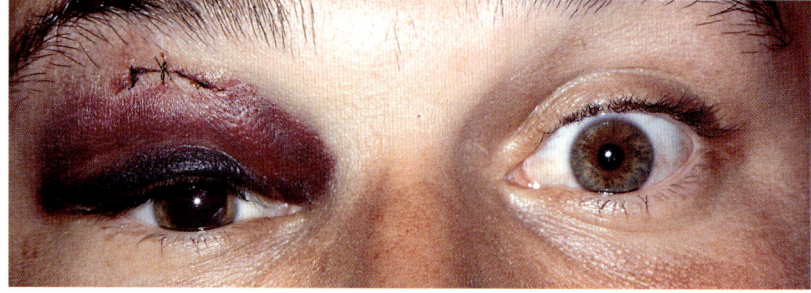

Plate 22 *This patient was elbowed while playing basketball. In addition to the periorbital contusion (edema and ecchymosis), adnexal lacerations were noted. On further testing, a medial wall "blowout" fracture was discovered.*

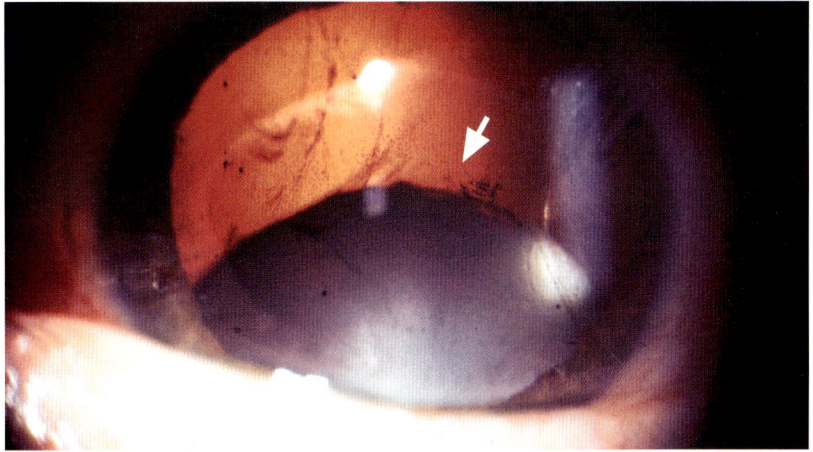

Plate 23 *A subluxated (dislocating lens) (arrow).*

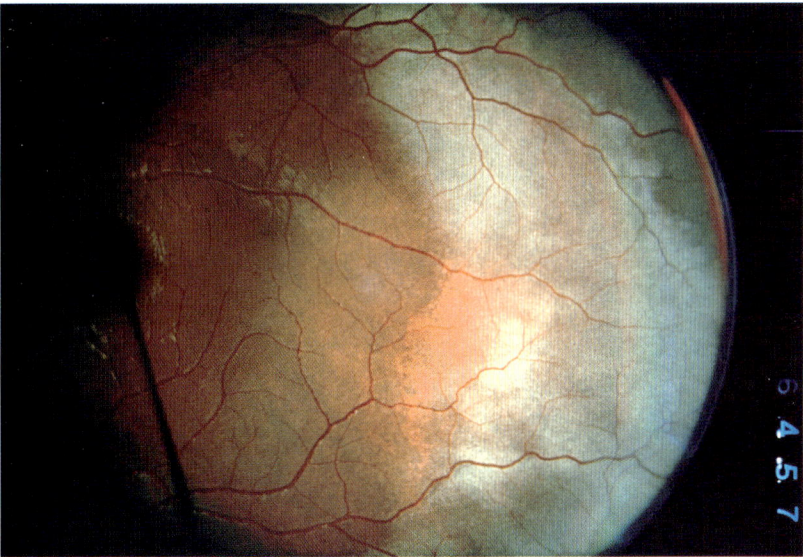

Plate 24 *Peripheral whitening of the retina from a contussive blow to the eye by a baseball. The peripheral retina shows a circumferential area of retinal edema and whitening with some early pigmentatary disturbance at the layer of the retinal pigment epithelial cells.*

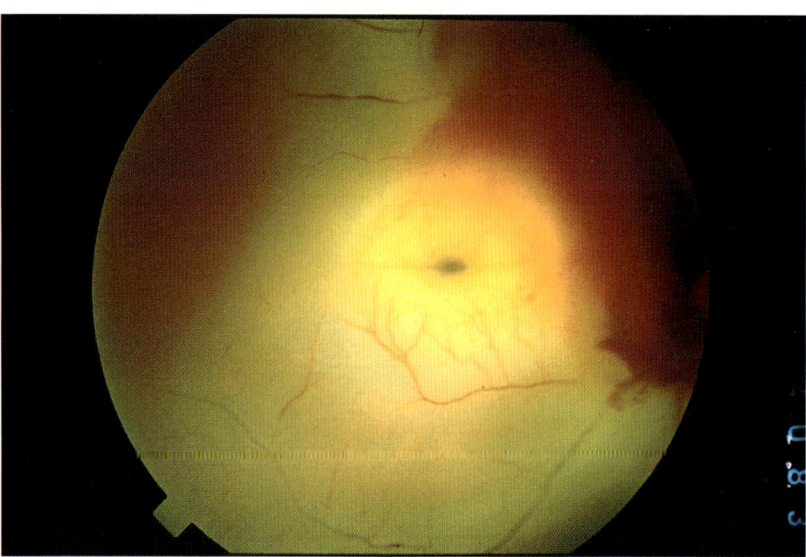

Plate 25 *View of the posterior pole in a patient with severe commotio retinae and hemorrhage. This basketball player suffered an injury to his right eye as a result of another players hand impacting on his eye as he drove toward the basket for a lay-up. His vision at the time of this examination was 20/200. Eventually the commotio and retinal hemorrhage resolved and he regained 20/20-vision in this eye.*

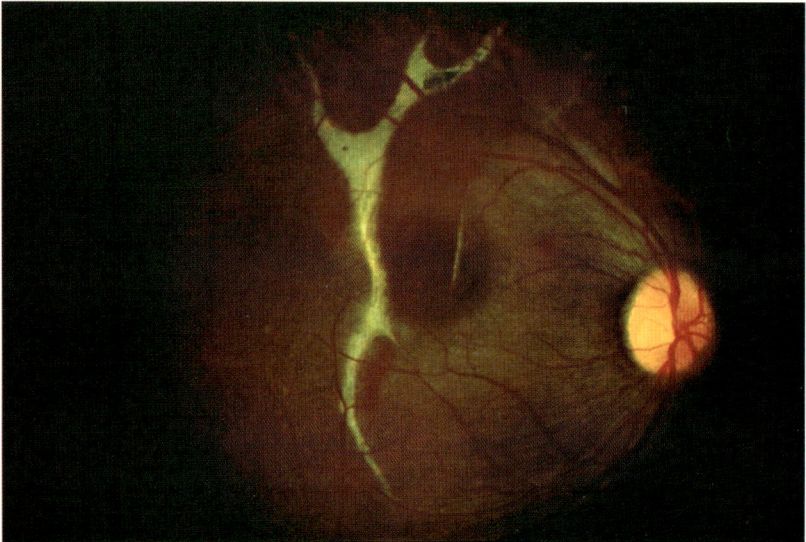

Plate 26 *Longstanding choroidal rupture through the center of the fovea in a 39 year old black male who had suffered a severe blunt trauma to his right eye four years previous to this photograph. His initial injury was due to a golf ball impact to this eye as he watched another golfer tee off. Surprisingly his vision in this eye is 20/25 with a small amount of metamorphopsia.*

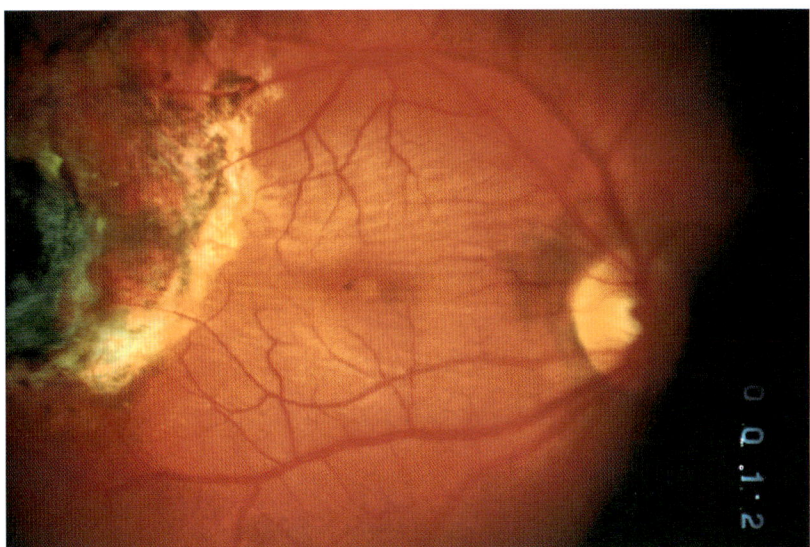

Plate 27 *Fundus of a twenty-two year old hockey player who suffered a high velocity impact to his eye from a hockey puck while playing. There is a large area of chorioretinal scarring and a macular hole. He was not wearing eye protection at the time of the injury.*

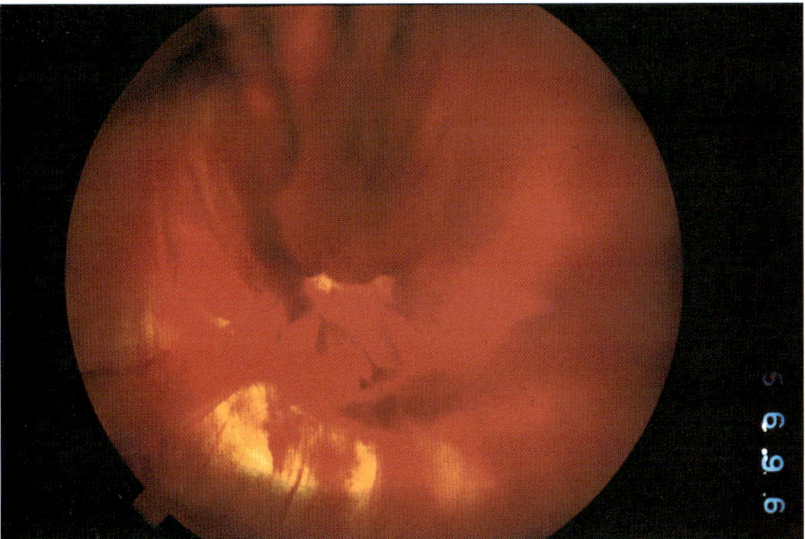

Plate 28 *Vitreous and pre-retinal hemorrhage overlying the retina in a patient who suffered a severe blunt traumatic blow to his eye while playing tennis. Details of the retina and optic nerve are obscured due to this hemorrhage.*

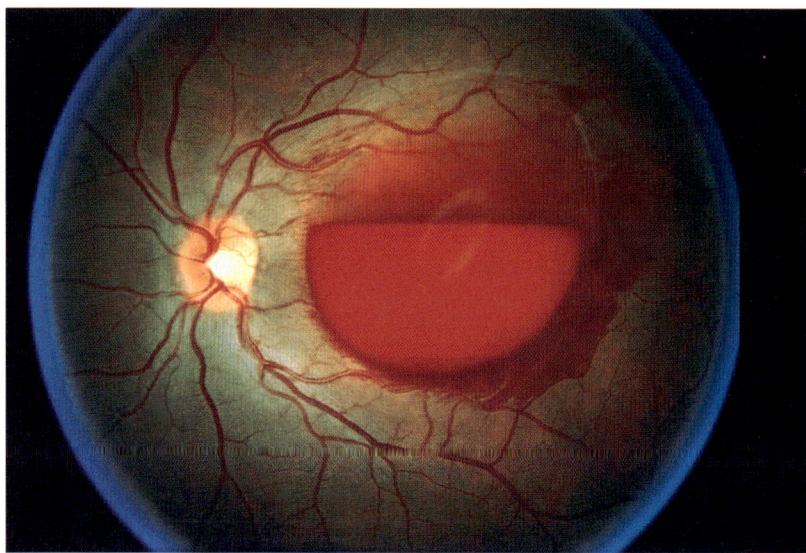

Plate 29 Valsava retinopathy. Note the large area of pre-retinal hemorrhage as well has some deeper hemorrhage in this 23 year old collegiate football player who was lifting weights in the off-season. His vision at the time of this photograph was 20/400. Within 2 months the blood resolved and his vision returned to 20/20.

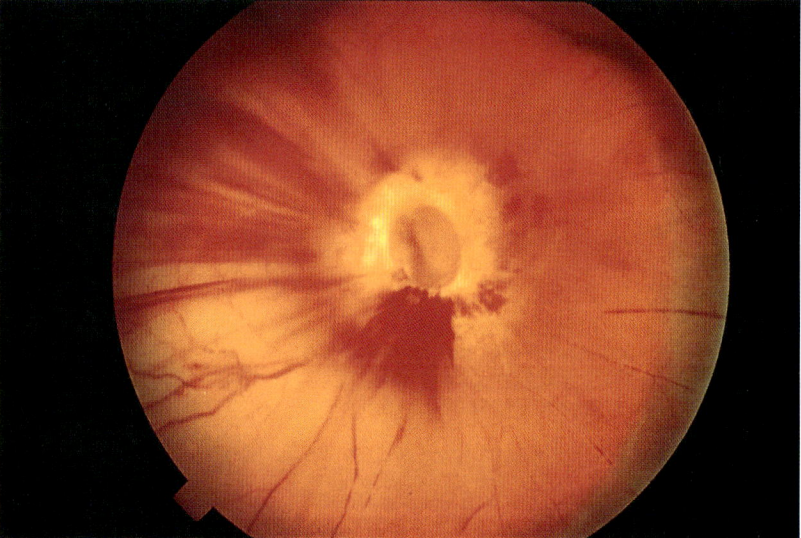

Plate 30 Optic nerve evulsion suffered during an intra-mural college basketball game. This player was struck in the eye by an opponent's elbow while playing. He had on no eye protection at the time of the injury, and his vision was no light perception in this eye.

CHAPTER 8

Golf and Soccer

Wayne I. Larrison

Golf

The game of golf has traditionally been linked to 15th-century Scotland. It is thought to have derived from an ancient Roman game known as paganica after the Roman occupation of Scotland (1,2). Scottish shepherds adapted the game during the 12th century by using bent sticks to strike feather-stuffed leather balls in open fields. The first direct reference to golf came in 1457 when King James II of Scotland issued a proclamation banning "futeball and golfe" as a threat to national security. Apparently, Scottish men were neglecting their practice of archery in favor of "golfe," jeopardizing national defense. The ban was lifted in 1502 after a treaty was signed between England and Scotland. The rules of modern golf were developed in the 1750s at the Royal and Ancient Golf Club in St. Andrews, Scotland. Golfers continued to play with leather balls stuffed with feathers until 1848, when gutta percha, a rubber-like substance, was introduced. Modern rubber golf balls were used near the turn of the century.

During the past 20 years, golf has seen a tremendous surge in popularity (3,4). From 1970 to 1990, participation in the United States jumped from 11.2 million people to over 27.8 million. As in most sports, there is a strong male predominance (78%). More than 1 in 10 Americans now play golf. An estimated 502 million rounds were played in 1990. Despite this surge in popularity, there is a paucity of information regarding golf-related injuries. Virtually all available literature consists of anecdotal case reports of severely traumatized eyes (5–10). From the early report of Millar (5) to the present, the cases have been strikingly similar (i.e., extensive ocular disruption from direct impact of the globe from a high speed golf ball or a companion's club). With the advent of more sophisticated data collection systems associated with the National Eye Injury Surveillance System (NEISS), Consumer Product Safety Commission (CPSC), National Society for the Prevention of Blindness (NSPB), and the United States Eye Injury Registry (USEIR), estimates of the relative frequency of golf injuries are now available.

According to the most recent NSPB fact sheet, there were approximately 969 golf-related ocular injuries in the United States in 1993, accounting for 2.4% of all sports and recreational ocular injuries (11). This places golf ahead of hockey for frequency of injuries. Golf is unique among the sports monitored by the NSPB in that most golf injuries occurred in patients over, rather than under, 25 years of age. Golf ranked first in the actual number of injuries among patients over 64 years old. This reflects the demographic distribution of golfers and the general tendency for continued participation in golf at an age when many other sports have been discontinued. Golfers over age 50 consititute approximately one fourth of the playing population (3) and on average play more frequently than younger players. They account for over 50% of rounds played annually.

The NEISS national estimates represent an extrapolation from a relatively small data sample. The actual 1992 sample count from which the projected 1320 injuries were derived consisted of 21 patients (12). During the period from March 1990 to October 1993, 77 golf-related ocular injuries were recorded. Although detailed descriptions of the types of injuries sustained were not recorded on their standard forms, narrative comments were enclosed, allowing further interpretation of the data. Table 8.1 shows the most common causes of injuries in this group. The most common mode of injury was direct ocular trauma from a struck golf ball, occurring in 29% of cases. When combined with golf club associated injuries, they still represent the minority of cases. A relatively common (22%) yet previously unreported source of injuries were those cases where loose debris (i.e., sand, dirt, or rock) flew up and struck the eye during a golf swing. Three male patients aged 13, 14, and 15 years suffered injuries when cutting into liquid-center golf balls. Case reports from the 1960s and 1970s described numerous cases of ocular surface injuries

Table 8.1 Most common causes of golf-related injuries

MECHANISM OF INJURY	NUMBER (%)
Struck by golf ball	22 (29)
Struck by debris during golf swing	17 (22)
Struck by golf club	11 (14)
Poked by tree branch on golf course	8 (10)
Cut into liquid center of golf ball	3 (4)
Miscellaneous or not identified	16 (21)

resulting from the explosive release of pressurized liquid from golf ball centers (13–15). Granulomatous reactions were identified in the skin and conjunctiva. Lucas et al (15) detailed the histopathologic findings in their series of nine patients. In each of their cases, a birefringent material believed to represent natural baryte crystals was identified in tissue sections. These crystals elicited a localized granulomatous reaction. Some of the earliest liquid-center golf balls contained barium sulfate, soap, and free alkali (16). The alkali component was believed to be the source of the most serious injuries and so was subsequently removed. Information obtained directly from golf ball manufacturers regarding the composition of liquid-center balls was reviewed by Farley (17). Reportedly, the liquid is present at pressures of 2000 to 2500 pounds per square inch and is no longer strongly alkaline. The fluid is generally between pH 7.0 and 8.2. The specific composition of the fluid varies significantly from one manufacturer to another. Some of the various components identified included water, castor oil, corn syrup, sodium sulfate, di-sodium hydrogen phosphate, calsolene oil, polyethylene glycol, glycerine, and lithopone. Fortunately, although it is still possible to obtain liquid-center golf balls, most balls produced today have solid centers and therefore pose no risk of this type of injury.

The USEIR serves as another data collection network that gathers information from individual state registries. Case reports are obtained directly from the local ophthalmologists. Although most states are enrolled in the USEIR, physician participation varies widely. Data obtained from the Eye Injury Registry of Alabama, a state where the level of participation is particularly high, identified six cases of golf-related ocular injuries since 1984. Four patients were struck by the golf ball and two by a club. All six patients suffered intraocular damage. Table 8.2 lists the injuries identified by the treating physi-

Table 8.2 Identified golf-related injuries

PATIENT	MECHANISM OF INJURY	INJURY SUSTAINED
1	Struck by golf club	Hyphema, retinal hemorrhage
2	Struck by golf ball	Hyphema, retinal edema
3	Struck by golf ball	Iridodialysis, cataract, retinal edema, orbital fracture, optic nerve injury
4	Struck by golf club	Hyphema, corneal injury
5	Struck by golf ball	Ruptured globe, corneal injury, retinal detachment, hyphema, cataract, orbital fracture
6	Struck by golf ball	Ruptured globe, hyphema, vitreous hemorrhage

cian. Two of the patients had ruptured globes and a third had severe tissue damage, including optic nerve trauma resulting in less than 5/200 acuity.

A 1981 review of pathology specimens from the Massachusetts Eye and Ear Infirmary obtained over a 20-year period revealed a total of 80 eyes enucleated as a result of sports-related trauma (9). Of these eyes, 11 (14%) were golf-related injuries. Golf balls accounted for 8 of the 11 cases and golf clubs the remaining 3. Only BB guns and darts and arrows accounted for more cases. A subsequent study covering the years from 1980 to 1986 revealed five additional cases of golf-related injuries requiring enucleation, although specific details of the cases are not provided (10).

Millar (5) reported a series of seven patients with golf-related injuries in 1981. Three of the seven patients had ruptured globes, although one of the cases resulted from striking a piece of glass with a golf club. Two other patients had choroidal ruptures after being struck inadvertently by a club. In all, three were struck by the ball and three by the club. Two of the patients with ruptured globes required primary enucleations as a result of extensive tissue disruption. Rousseau (7) identified two golf-related injuries in his general review of ocular injuries in sports. The first case was a ruptured globe with loss of intraocular contents from a golf club injury and the other a sixth nerve palsy secondary to a subdural hemorrhage that resulted from being struck in the head by a golf ball. Gregory (8) and Vinger (18) each reported on two patients with ocular golfing injuries and commented on the severity of golfing injuries without providing specific case details. The Canadian Ophthalmologic Society gathers data from its members on sports-related ocular injuries, including the number of blinding injuries sustained. During the interval from 1976 to 1990, 44 golfing injuries were recorded with 14 (32%) patients suffering blinding injuries (19). This represents the second highest percentage of blinding injuries after war games.

In a retrospective review of perforating or penetrating trauma by Lubniewski et al (6), 4 of 87 cases resulted from golf ball injuries. None of these patients obtained better than light perception vision (6). In a subsequent survey by Berger, Grand, and Lubniewski (unpublished data), several hundred midwestern ophthalmologists were questioned specifically about golfing injuries. Forty golf-related accidents were recorded. Patients ranged in age from 3 to 86 years, with 75% of injuries occurring in males. Four of the patients were hit by the golf club and 34 were struck by a golf ball, including four ricochet injuries. The remaining two patients were accidentally injured by golf balls tossed by a fellow player. In 21 cases, ophthalmologists were able to estimate the distance the injured person was standing from the point at which the ball was struck. Six patients were greater than 100 yards away from the ball's point of origin. None of these patients suffered a ruptured globe. By comparison, 10 of the 15 patients hit at closer range had ruptured globes. The final visual acuities followed a similar pattern with two-thirds of those struck by a golf ball from less than 100 yards away ending up with less than 20/200 vision. Of the four ricochet injuries in this group, three resulted in a final visual acuity of no light perception. In their total series, 33 of 40 patients presented with a hyphema, including all patients struck at close range. Of the 18 patients who had a hyphema without globe rupture, 14 regained 20/40 vision or greater. Of the 15 patients with a concomitant globe rupture, 14 ended up with less than counting fingers vision.

It is clear from the above data that golfing injuries, although relatively infrequent, are often severe. This relates directly to the ability of both golf balls and club heads to fit into the orbital rim (Figs. 8.1 and 8.2). Standard golf balls measure 1.68 inches in diameter. The force of impact when the globe is struck directly exceeds the tensile strength of the scleral collagen, resulting in globe rupture (Plate 4 and Fig. 8.3). Despite the severity of such injuries, the recommendation of safety glasses for all golfers seems neither justified nor cost effective. Simple precautions and common sense would decrease the number of injuries. Checking to ensure that bystanders are well out of the way before beginning a swing and positioning oneself out of

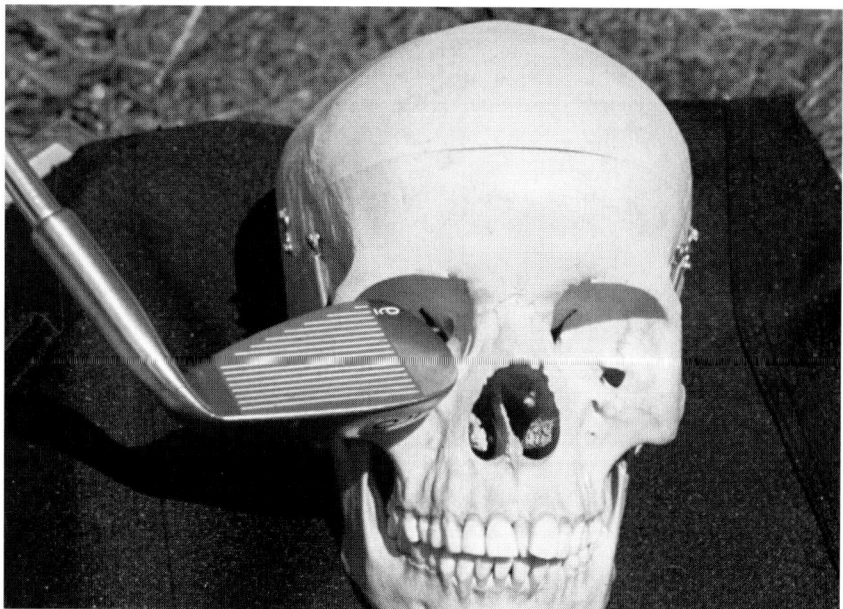

Figure 8.1 *A golf club can easily fit into the orbit as seen here. Irons, which have a narrower profile, may penetrate more readily.*

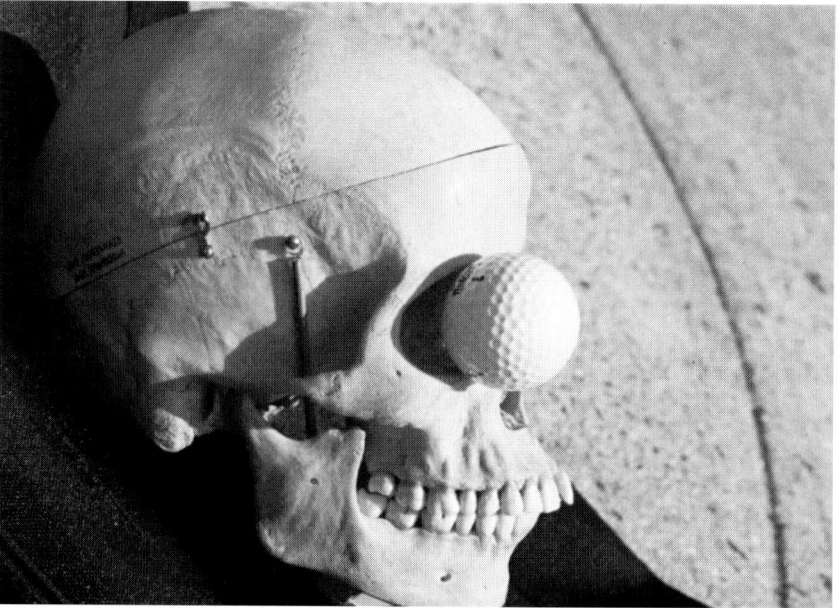

Figure 8.2 *The golf ball is an unusually hard object that travels at high velocity and can result in marked ocular damage.*

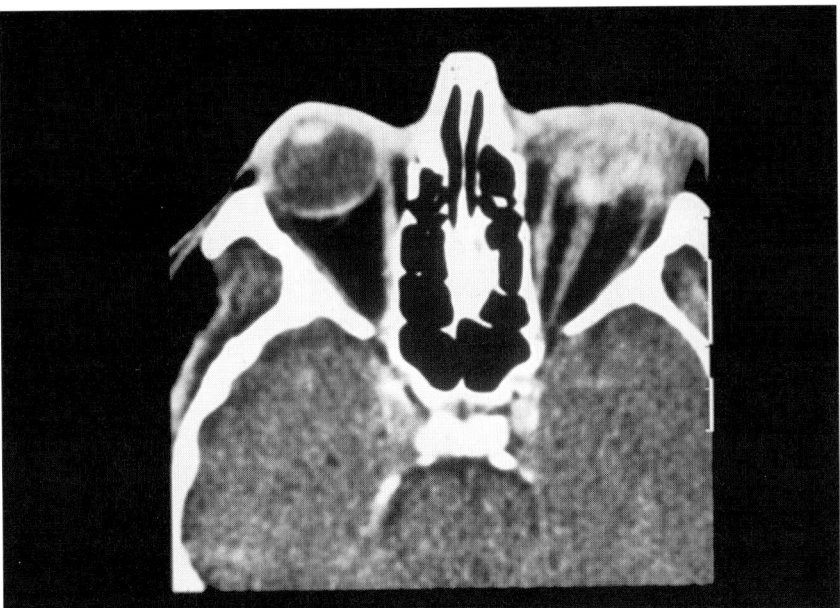

Figure 8.3 *Computerized tomography (CT) shows a disorganized (ruptured) globe in this patient who was hit with a golf ball.*

the line of potential ricocheting balls would help decrease the incidence of blinding injuries.

Soccer

Another sport whose popularity has increased tremendously in the United States since the 1960s is soccer. Outside the United States, soccer is the most popular sport in the world. This is especially true in Europe and Latin America. Although games similar to soccer have existed for hundreds, if not thousands, of years (the Chinese played a similar game as early as 400 B.C.), the first formal rules for soccer were drafted in 1948 at Trinity College in Cambridge, England, where it was and continues to be referred to as "football" (20). The first football association was organized in England in 1863. By the turn of the century, several other European and South American countries had national associations. In 1904, the Federation Internationale de Football Association was organized, paving the way for the first World Cup games in Montevideo, Uruguay, in 1930.

Unlike the demographics of golf injuries, those of soccer injuries more closely parallel those of football and baseball because most soccer players are either children or young adults. According to the NSPB factsheet for 1993, there were an estimated 1319 eye injuries related to soccer (11). This represents 3.2% of all sports injuries. Twenty-eight percent of soccer injuries are estimated to occur in individuals in the 15- to 24-year-old age group. Approximately 55% of injuries occurred in children under 15 years. These incidence figures have remained relatively constant over the past 10 years. In 1982, soccer was the seventh leading cause of eye injuries according to the Consumer Product Safety Commission (CPSC), with an estimated 1665 cases.

Although the opening of the bony orbit in the average adult measures approximately 1.4 × 1.6 inches and the diameter of a standard soccer ball is 8.6 inches (circumference 27 to 28 inches), direct trauma to the globe is readily possible as the orbital opening lies in the plane of the cornea (21). The capability of such a large object to cause direct injury relates to the relative shape (radius of curvature) of the ball and its ability to deform on impact. Even an incompressible round object with a 4.3-inch radius would be capable of direct contact with the globe. The orbital soft tissue and ability of the globe to be retroplaced slightly without significant globe deformation would prevent most nonorbital injuries from incompressible objects. Soccer balls, however, especially if they are somewhat underinflated, can deform on impact and enter the orbital opening, causing more severe globe deformation. This situation is exaggerated even further in children, who have incompletely developed orbital rims with less prominent frontal and maxillary bones. The problem is compounded still further because children play with slightly smaller balls (25-inch circumference). Even in this age group, the orbit still absorbs most of the impact, preventing the types of devastating injuries described with golf balls (e.g., ruptured globes), although serious injuries still occur. In general, the impact force is large enough to deform the intraocular structures without exceeding the tensile strength of the eyewall. As a result, hyphemas, retinal tears and hemorrhages, and commotio retinae are the most frequently encountered injuries. Schneider et al (22) studied the speed of a kicked soccer ball measured at a distance of 10 m and found the impact force may be as high as 200 kp when kicked with full force.

Although occasional injuries occur when players are inadvertently kicked or struck by elbows or hands, most soccer injuries result from the ball striking the orbit or globe. Data collected by the National Electronic Injury Surveillance System (NEISS) between January 1990 and November 1993 recorded 116 soccer injuries (12). The annual projections of the CPSC are derived from this data sample. Narrative comments regarding the mechanism of injury were available in 94 of the cases. Seventy (74%) of the 94 patients were reportedly hit in the eye by a soccer ball and 15 (16%) of the 94 were hit by another player's foot, elbow, or hand. Over 10% of the patients required hospitalization. More detailed injury information was not recorded.

Vinger (23) reported the incidence and mechanism of soccer injuries in patients treated in a private ophthalmology office between January 1981 and December 1983. Twenty-seven soccer injuries were treated. Twenty (74%) of these patients were struck by a soccer ball and 5 (19%) by another player. Although there were no ruptured globes, the spectrum of injuries ranged from minor contusions to retinal detachment. Most injuries occurred in patients between 10 and 19 years of age. Data were also presented from a local public school system estimating the ocular injury rates from selected sports between 1978 and 1979. There were approximately 7000 soccer participants. Seven injuries were recorded, yielding an injury rate of 1 per 1000. This rate is somewhat lower than the estimates from the National Athletic Injury/Illness Reporting System (NAIRS) from 1979 (18). NAIRS collects data on the average annual rate of facial injuries among college athletes. Their 1979 estimates for the preceding 3 years revealed a rate of 2.5%. When only eye-orbit injuries were considered, the rate was 3 per 1000.

Larrison et al (24) reported a prospective evaluation of sports-related ocular injuries from the Massachusetts Eye and Ear Infirmary between 1987 and 1988. Fifteen soccer injuries were identified, accounting for 7.4% of all cases. Five of the 15 patients sustained hyphemas requiring hospitalization. More hyphemas were seen from soccer than any other sport. Eighty percent of the injuries resulted from ball-to-eye contact (25). A 1986 English study by Gregory (8) from the Sussex Eye Hospital of 92 sports-related injuries revealed 19 (21%) soccer injuries. All patients were male and 15 of the injuries resulted from impact by the soccer ball. Seven patients required hospitalization, six of them for hyphemas. Soccer was the leading cause of sports-related admissions to the hospital. Retinal trauma was found in eight patients.

Burke et al (26) reported the results of 23 patients with soccer ball–induced ocular injuries. The patients ranged in age from 6 to 21 years and most (79%) were males. As in the series of Larrison et al (24), hyphema was the most frequently encountered injury. Fifty percent of patients presented with hyphemas. There were no episodes of rebleeding in these cases. Additional anterior segment injuries consisted of angle recession, traumatic iritis, and corneal abrasions. Posterior segment trauma frequently accompanied these anterior segment injuries. Vitreous and/or retinal hemorrhages, retinal edema, and pigmentary retinopathy were recorded in 67% of patients. One patient developed a retinal tear requiring cryotherapy. Of the 12 patients with hyphemas, 6 had posterior segment injuries as well. Retinal injuries were identified in 26% of patients with no evidence of anterior segment trauma.

Orlando (27) identified 13 cases of soccer-related eye injuries in children ages 8 to 15 years during the 3-year period from September 1984 to September 1987. Hyphema was the most common injury, occuring in nine patients. Five patients were found to have angle recession of unspecified degree and seven had retinal injuries, including five patients with commotio retinae and one with choroidal rupture. The latter patient suffered visual loss to the 20/40 level. All other patients recovered visual acuity to the 20/25 level or better. Six of the injuries resulted from balls kicked at close range and three were by the kicking foot of another player. One patient was struck by the head of an opponent attempting to head the ball. Special mention was made of two patients injured by spectacle fragments when their glasses were struck by a kicked ball. Both were defending their goal.

In a review of juvenile retinal detachments by Verdaguer (28), presented before the Pan American Congress of Ophthalmology in 1981, 20 cases of soccer-induced retinal detachments were reported. The patients consisted of Chilean males between the ages of 13 and 30 years. In this Latin American population, where soccer is much more popular than in the United States, soccer ball–related contusive injuries were the most frequent cause (26%) of traumatic retinal detachment. Ten patients suffered superotemporal retinal dialysis with avulsion of the vitreous base. Nine of these 10 patients developed tears along the posterior border of the vitreous base. Seven additional patients had superotemporal retinal holes leading to detachment. Two other patients with high myopia were also described. One patient sustained a giant retinal tear and the other a horseshoe tear-related detachment as well as "many severe traumatic lesions" that precluded return of visual function. As a result, the author specifically warned about the dangers of soccer injuries in highly myopic individuals. The characteristic location of the breaks was attributed to the asymetric elasticity of the sclera and vitreous. The author reviewed the generally accepted model of contusive-type injuries as originally described by Schepens (29). Upon impact of the globe (e.g., by the soccer ball), the anterior-posterior diameter of the globe decreases with simultaneous rapid expansion of the anterior sclera with resultant traction on the vitreous base and retina. Temporally directed contusive forces resulted in temporal dialysis in this model.

Fourteen of the 20 patients were symptomatic within 1 month of injury, and all patients were symptomatic within 3 months. The detachments ranged from localized (seven cases) to complete with proliferative vitreoretinopathy in those with delayed presentation. Vitreous hemorrhages, macular damage, and peripheral atrophy and pigmentary retinal changes were frequently identified. Iris sphincter trauma, corneal abrasions, and iritis were common findings. A traumatic cataract was also reported. Of the 20 cases of retinal detachments, 19 were successfully reattached. Five of these patients were left with less than 20/200 vision.

Conclusion

Both golf and soccer account for a small but significant number of ocular injuries each year. With the continued growth in popularity of both sports, the incidence of injuries is likely to increase. Golf injuries are frequently severe as a result of high impact direct globe trauma from golf balls or club heads. The severity of golf ball injuries is related to the distance from the patient to the point of origin of the ball. Patients struck within 100 yards of where the shot originated, including ricochet injuries, have a much higher risk of ruptured globes and blindness. Golf club injuries also result in devastating trauma. Unlike ball injuries, virtually all club injuries can be prevented by taking simple precautions to ensure that other players and bystanders are out of striking range before beginning to swing. Chemical injuries resulting from mischievous individuals cutting into highly pressurized liquid golf ball centers have become rare as manufacturers have shifted predominantly to solid-center balls.

Soccer injuries, although not as severe as golf injuries, often lead to hyphemas and posterior segment trauma. The mechanism of these contusive injuries is usually contact of the orbit and globe with a kicked ball. Although the orbit often absorbs much of the impact, deformation of the ball and the relative underdevelopment of the orbital rim in younger players allow for direct globe trauma. Serious retinal injuries may be present even in the absence of significant anterior segment pathology, highlighting the importance of a thorough ophthalmologic examination. Intentional heading of the ball, although a cause for concern with regard to neurologic trauma, does not appear to pose a significant ocular risk based on the data available in the literature. The need for protective eyewear in soccer remains far less clear than for other sports, such as hockey or racket sports. Mandatory use of protective eyewear for all soccer players is unlikely to prove beneficial or necessary. The use by children or adolescents with underdeveloped orbital structures may be considered given their increased risk of globe trauma. The use of standard streetwear spectacles or rigid contact lenses without overlying polycarbonate goggles should be prohibited.

References

1. Rochester Golf Week and Sports Ledger, Rochester, New York, January 27, 1989, p. 1.
2. Parascenzo MA. Golf. In: World Book Encyclopedia. vol. 8. 1993:260–267.
3. National Golf Foundation. 1992 Research Summary. Jupiter, FL.
4. Gorman C. On the seventh day he played (golf as sport in the 1990's). Time 1989;133:66–67.
5. Millar GT. Golfing eye injuries. Am J Ophthalmol 1967;64:741.
6. Lubniewski A, Olk RJ, Grand MG. Ocular dangers in the garden. Ophthalmology 1988;95:906–910.
7. Rousseau AP. Ocular trauma in sports. In: Freeman HM, ed. Ocular trauma. New York: Appleton-Century-Crofts, 1979.
8. Gregory PTS. Sussex Eye Hospital sports injuries. Br J Ophthalmol 1986; 70:748–750.
9. Portis JM, Vassallo SA, Albert DM. Ocular sports injuries: a review of cases on file in the Massachusetts Eye and Ear Infirmary pathology laboratory. Int Ophthalmol Clin 1981;21:1–19.
10. Fountain TR, Albert DM. The histopathology of sports-related ocular trauma, 1980–1986. Int Ophthalmol Clin 1988;28:206–210.
11. National Society to Prevent Blindness. 1993 Eye injuries associated with sports and recreational products. Schaumburg, IL: National Center for Sight, 1994.
12. National Electronic Injury Surveillance System Product Summary Report (Soccer and Golf). National Injury Information Clearinghouse, 1990–93.
13. Nelson C. Eye injury from exploding golf balls. Br J Ophthal 1970;54: 670–671.
14. Penner R. The liquid center golf ball: a potential ocular hazard. Arch Ophthal 1966;75:68–71.
15. Lucas DR, Dunham AC, Lee WR, et al. Ocular injuries from liquid golf ball cores. Br J Ophthalmol 1976;60:740–747.

16. Crigler LW. Burn of eyeball due to caustic contents of golf ball. JAMA 1913; 60:1297.
17. Farley KG. Ocular trauma resulting from the explosive rupture of a liquid center golf ball. J Am Optom Assoc 1985;65:310–314.
18. Vinger PF. The incidence of eye injuries in sports. Int Ophthalmol Clin 1981;21:21–46.
19. Pashby TJ. Canadian Ophthalmologic Society survey of eye injuries. Can J Ophthalmol 1990;25:283–284.
20. Polis JE. Soccer. In: World Book Encyclopedia. vol. 18. 1993:544–549.
21. Maus M. Basic anatomy of the orbit. In: Albert DM, Jakobiec FR, eds. Principles and practice of ophthalmology. vol. 3. Philadelphia: WB Saunders, 1994:1871–1880.
22. Schneider PG, Lichte H. Untersuchungen zur Groesse der Krafteinwirkung bein Kopfballspiel des Fussballers. Sportarzut Sportmed 1975;26:10.
23. Vinger PF. The eye and sports medicine. In: Duane TD, Jaeger EA, eds. Clinical ophthalmology. vol. 5. Philadelphia: Lippincott, 1988.
24. Larrison WI, Hersh PS, Kunsweiler T, Shingleton BJ. Sports-related ocular trauma. Ophthalmology 1990;97:1265–1269.
25. Larrison WI. Sports injuries. In: Albert DM, Jakobiec FA, eds. Principles and practice of ophthalmology. vol. 5. Philadelphia: WB Saunders, 1994:3494–3498.
26. Burke MJ, Sanitato JJ, Vinger PF, et al. Soccerball-induced eye injuries. JAMA 1983;249:2682–2685.
27. Orlando RG. Soccer-related eye injuries in children and adolescents. Phys Sportsmed 1988;16:103–106.
28. Verdaguer TJ. Juvenile retinal detachment. Am J Ophthalmol 1982;93:145–156.
29. Schepens CL. Pathogenesis of traumatic rhegmatogenous retinal detachment. In: Freeman HM, ed. Ocular trauma. New York: Appleton-Century-Crofts, 1979:273–284.

CHAPTER 9

Shooting and Water Sports

M. Lisa McHam
Bradford J. Shingleton

Shooting sports and water sports are wide-ranging recreational activities that draw literally millions of participants of all ages every year. Although the ocular injury potential of the shooting sports has been well demonstrated, public awareness of the need for eye protection is lacking. Water sports, including fishing, are becoming increasingly more popular and result in a considerable number of eye injuries every year.

Shooting Sports

Ocular Injuries from Shotgun Sports

It is estimated by the National Rifle Association that 10 to 15 million Americans participate in shotgun sports, including hunting, skeet, trap, and sporting clays. Shotguns are responsible for approximately 5% to 10% of all penetrating eye injuries, and a significant proportion of these occur during shotgun recreational activities. According to the Alabama Eye Injury Registry, 53% of all gunshot-related eye injuries in Alabama since 1982 were accidental and 16% occurred during recreational activities (1). The proportion of shotgun eye injuries due to recreational gun use will vary depending on the setting, with urban centers reporting more violence-related trauma. Clearly, shotgun sports are a major contributor to the total burden of injury.

Although ocular injuries can occur in all shotgun sports, hunting carries the greatest risk. Over a 5-year period in Ireland, there were

20 accidental ocular shotgun injuries requiring hospitalization, at least 75% of which occurred while hunting pheasant (2). Not surprisingly, all injuries occurred in males, as shotgun sports in general have a preponderance of male participants. Interestingly, most hunters involved in accidents considered themselves to be experienced gun handlers. The reason for the increased risk in hunting is most probably attributed to the uncontrolled nature of the sport, with multiple participants, imperfect visibility, and the demand for quick reactions.

In the more structured shotgun sports, including trap, skeet, and sporting clays, clay targets are catapulted by either automated or manually operated mechanical devices. Spectators are commonly present behind the shooter. In trap, shooters stand on a platform and all targets are hurled away from them. In skeet, two clay targets are released, either simultaneously or alternately along fixed intersecting flight paths. There is the risk of wielding the gun in the direction of the spectators, as well as the risk of clay target debris raining down on them. In sporting clays, there is an attempt to simulate hunting, and targets come from all directions in a wooded setting, often with the use of manually operated target throwers. Thus, the injury potential would appear greatest in sporting clays (1).

Despite improved ophthalmic surgical techniques, ocular shotgun injury carries a poor prognosis. A recent review of the literature over the past 20 years revealed 143 cases of shotgun eye injuries, of which 124 were penetrating (1). Among the penetrating injuries, 82% had a visual acuity of 20/200 or worse and only 11% had an acuity of 20/40 or better. The nonpenetrating injuries fared better, with 74% having an acuity of at least 20/40. Overall, the chances of severe permanent visual loss after ocular shotgun injury are high.

The ability of shotguns to produce extensive ocular damage is related to muzzle velocity and the unique characteristics of "shot," or "birdshot," as the ammunition is commonly called. A shotgun cartridge contains numerous small lead pellets within a plastic casing. Ignition of gunpowder upon firing propels the pellets from the gun with a muzzle velocity in the range of 250 m/sec (3), considerably greater than the 103-m/sec velocity needed to perforate the human cornea (4). As they pass down range, the multiple pellets not only fan out, increasing the width of the "spray," but also "string out" to a depth of several feet. As a result, multiple pellets may strike an eye, and bilateral injury is not uncommon (5). One study demonstrated that with head-on aim, the orbital region of a mannequin was hit by at least one pellet 100% of the time at a distance of 40 yards. From the side, the orbit was struck 63% of the time. The pellets will lose some velocity as they proceed down range, but they retain adequate energy for ocular perforation at up to 100 yards (2). Depending on the velocity and trajectory of the pellet, as well as the site of impact, the result may be ocular contusion, ocular rupture without entry of the pellet, single perforation with retained intraocular pellet, or double perforation (6). A single pellet may fragment within the eye, resulting in multiple foreign bodies and even multiple exit wounds (7). Within the orbit, pellets may impinge on the optic nerve and extraocular muscles and cause orbital hemorrhage. A shotgun blast may also cause severe injury to the eyelids, including tissue avulsion.

The most important factor in assessing visual prognosis after ocular shotgun injury is the nature of the direct tissue damage incurred. Direct involvement of the macula or optic nerve, severe ocular disorganization, and no light perception on initial examination are all associated with a poor visual outcome (5). Modern surgical techniques, particularly vitrectomy, have improved the prognosis in injuries that spare the macula and optic nerve by preventing and treating proliferative vitreoretinopathy and secondary retinal detachments. Unfortunately, the initial damage caused by a shotgun blast to the eye is often irreparable.

Because a significant number of ocular shotgun injuries occur during recreational activities, prevention is possible. It has been shown that 3-mm polycarbonate lenses will effectively shield the eyes from a head-on shotgun blast as close as 25 yards (1,8). Three-piece polycarbonate glasses with integral side shields and a headband provide adequate ocular protection from the front and side at 25 yards and beyond (1). The headband is necessary because pellets at the leading edge of the spray can dislodge the glasses, allowing subsequent pellets to strike the eye and orbit. At a distance of 15 yards and closer, safety glasses are generally destroyed and no adequate eye protection is available.

At present, there are no regulations requiring eye protection in hunting, only the recommendation by gun and ammunition manufacturers and hunting organizations to wear eye protection when firing a gun. The organized shotgun sports, including trap, skeet, and sporting clays, require some form of eye protection for participants. There is, however, no specific recommendation regarding the type of protection and no requirement for spectators, who might be at the greatest risk. Because of the often devastating extent of these injuries, prevention is the key to decreasing the morbidity of shotgun-related ocular trauma.

Ocular Injuries from Air Guns

BB and Pellet Guns

BB and pellet guns are popular air-powered firearms that have a high potential for serious ocular injury (9–11). The common BB gun fires a steel sphere, typically 3.0 mm in diameter, with a weight of 0.346 gm (12). The pellet guns are available with a wide variety of ammunition that in general is of greater caliber and weight than the standard BB pellet. Most of these guns can easily attain the muzzle velocity of 103 m/sec necessary to penetrate the human cornea, with a range of 90 to 200 m/sec (3).

The U.S. Consumer Product Safety Commission estimates that air-powered guns are responsible for more than 1000 ocular injuries every year, often of a severe nature (13). Most of these injuries occur in children and adolescents during unsupervised play, with an average age of 15 years (12,14). In a population-based study in Maryland of eye injuries in children under 16 years of age requiring hospitalization, air-powered guns were responsible for 19% of penetrating injuries and 2% of nonpenetrating injuries (15). Although all series show a preponderance of young males, it is likely that the percentage of young females will increase as cultural taboos discouraging gun use by women subside.

Another series of 140 ocular air gun injuries collected between January 1986 and August 1992 through the National Eye Trauma System and the Alabama Eye Injury Registry showed that victims and shooters were predominantly male, 91% and 89%, respectively, with a mean age of 13 years (16). Ninety-five percent of victims knew their assailant; 40% of these assailants were relatives. Eighty-four percent of those with penetrating injuries had visual acuity less than 20/200. Adults were present at the scene of injury in only 11% of cases.

Penetrating ocular BB injury is one of the most devastating forms of sports-related eye trauma. In a retrospective review of all penetrating eye injuries at the Wilmer Institute from 1970 to 1981, an intraocular BB or air gun pellet was associated with the worst visual prognosis, regardless of the size or location of the wound (17). Of a total of 22 eyes with penetrating BB or pellet injury, 19 eyes were ultimately deemed unsalvageable despite extensive surgical intervention and were enucleated to prevent sympathetic ophthalmia. Of the three eyes with penetrating injury that were not enucleated, vision was worse than 5/200. In addition to the 22 eyes with a BB perforation, there were 3 eyes with small corneoscleral lacerations due to shattered glass from the impact of a BB on spectacle lenses, all of which had a final visual acuity of 20/40 or better at 6 months. In patients with penetrating BB injury, the degree of disruption of the intraocular contents, particularly in the posterior segment, tends to be out of proportion to the severity of the entry wound. Histopathology of the 19 enucleated specimens from the Wilmer Institute's study revealed extensive ciliary body damage, vitreous loss and incarceration, and hemorrhagic choroidal and retinal detachments, often with necrosis (14). Double perforation was present in 11 cases and avulsion of the optic nerve head in 3 cases. Anterior segment injuries included corneal edema, hyphema, cataract, and loss of the lens and iris. In another retrospective study demonstrating the severity of these injuries, BB guns accounted for 39% of enucleations due to sports-related trauma at the Massachusetts Eye and Ear Infirmary over a 6-year period (18). Although there are occasional favorable outcomes (19), it is likely that even with advances in ophthalmic surgery, penetrating ocular BB injury will continue to carry a poor prognosis.

A significant number of BB and air gun pellet injuries are nonpenetrating and result in various degrees of blunt ocular trauma. These contusion injuries are often severe but overall have a better visual prognosis than perforating injuries. In one series, the most common findings in order of frequency were hyphema, iridodialysis, vitreous hemorrhage, commotio retinae, choroidal rupture, and cataract (10).

The mechanism by which BB pellets are able to produce such severe ocular injury appears to be related to contusion effects. Using enucleated eyes, Delori et al (20) demonstrated that nonpenetrating BB impact on the cornea resulted in maximal scleral distension in the region of the vitreous base, accompanied by strong shearing forces in the retina. Tillett et al (4) studied perforating ocular BB injury in the rabbit eye by using high-speed photography and found tremendous ocular distortion and displacement. After perforation, there was a primary aqueous and secondary vitreous splash, with oscillation and undulation of the entire globe for up to 100 msec with continued loss of vitreous. In cases of double perforation, the BB passed through the eye within 0.500 msec of impact, but the globe undulation continued for a much longer period of time. Thus,

BB impact transfers considerable energy to the globe, which results in extensive intraocular contusive injury.

Intraorbital BB or air gun pellets can occur either in the presence or in the absence of ocular injury. They often cause morbidity in relation to optic nerve trauma. In fact, most air gun injuries that present with no light perception are due to direct optic nerve injury by the pellet (14). This can occur at the level of the optic nerve head, particularly in double perforating injuries, as the nerve traverses the orbit, or at the orbital apex. The presence of a relative afferent pupillary defect, including a reverse defect, should alert the examiner to the possibility of optic nerve injury. Unfortunately, the localizing value of the pupillary exam is often limited by the severity of the globe injury, which by itself may result in an afferent defect. Intraorbital pellets may also cause contusion, laceration, or avulsion of the extraocular muscles, resulting in motility disturbances or damage to orbital vessels leading to retrobulbar hemorrhage.

If an intraorbital pellet is not in close proximity to the optic nerve or globe, it is generally preferable to leave it in the orbit, as retrieval is often traumatic and difficult. Occasionally, pellets may penetrate the medial orbital wall to lodge in the ethmoid sinus, where they too can be safely left in position. Steel pellets and pellets made of the newer insoluble lead amalgams appear to be well tolerated, without elevating serum lead levels (14,21). However, if a lead-containing pellet is retained in the orbit or sinus, lead levels should be followed closely, especially considering the young age of these patients. Intracranial BB injury is uncommon but life-threatening when it occurs. Rarely, a BB or air gun pellet may traverse the upper eyelid and enter the anterior cranial fossa via the thin bone of the orbital roof, resulting in cerebral injury (22). Sometimes the pellet does not penetrate the bone but causes an orbital roof fracture and a small area of pneumocephalus (Pineda R, personal communication). In these cases, as in most ocular and orbital BB injuries, the external trauma often consists only of a small clean eyelid puncture wound that may mask the severity of the underlying damage. Any patient presenting with air gun–related trauma and an altered mental status should alert the examiner to an occult intracranial injury.

Because of the high incidence of retained pellets, imaging studies are indicated in most cases of ocular and orbital air gun trauma. Conventional radiographs can reveal the presence or absence of a pellet (Fig. 9.1), but more sophisticated techniques are necessary for accurate localization (Fig. 9.2). The study of choice is computed to-

138   Sports Ophthalmology

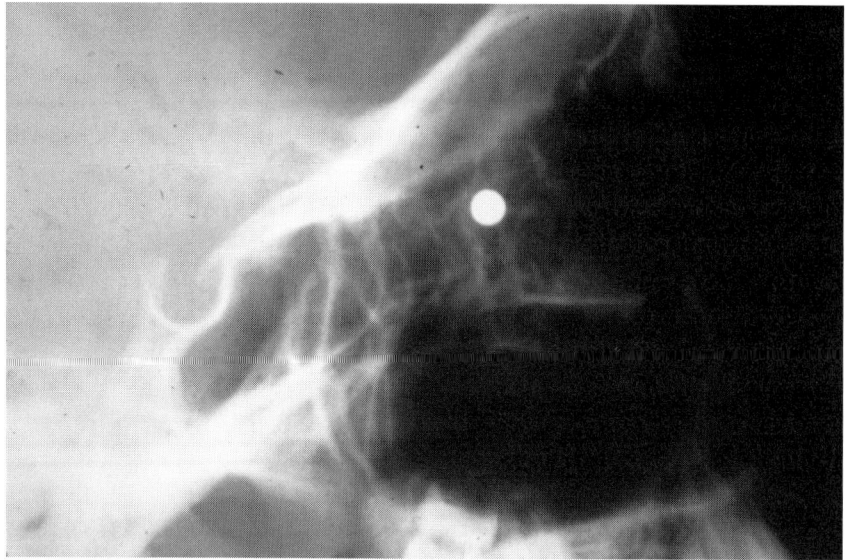

Figure 9.1   *Plain film (x-ray) showing a pellet within the orbit.*

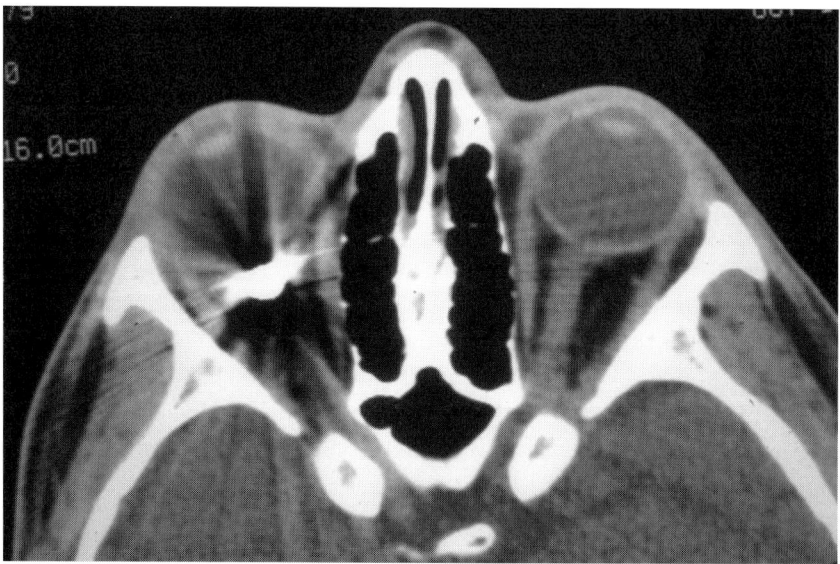

Figure 9.2   *Computerized tomogram shows the exact location of this BB, located in the posterior segment of the right eye at the level of the optic nerve.*

mography, as magnetic resonance imaging is contraindicated in the presence of a metallic foreign body.

It is clear that air guns are responsible for a significant number of devastating eye injuries, mostly among young people. In most cases, the children involved in these injuries reported they were "playing" at the time of the incident, revealing their perception of air guns as toys. In fact, many parents hold the same misperception and freely allow unsupervised use of the guns by their children. Because of the severe nature of ocular air gun injuries, the key to reducing morbidity lies in preventing their occurrence.

Effective prevention must address the problem of air gun misuse. According to the National Rifle Association, BB guns and air-powered pellet guns are good training devices for children in preparation for the safe use of gunpowder-propelled firearms (23). The National Rifle Association advocates education of children in the proper handling of air guns as the best means of prevention. Although the benefit of education is without doubt, it is questionable whether an unsupervised adolescent has the maturity to resist the temptation of "horsing around" with an air gun. Age is no guarantee of responsible behavior, but it would seem prudent to restrict unsupervised use of air-powered as well as gunpowder-propelled firearms to adults and require close supervision of children.

Legislation aimed at regulating the sale and use of air-powered guns has been implemented by only a handful of states (12). Since 1984, only three additional states have adopted laws pertaining to pellet guns, for a total of 14 states. A complete ban on the sale and use of BB guns and air guns is probably untenable considering the strong opposition of the powerful gun lobbies. Even if this were possible, the millions of air guns already in existence would continue to be a source of injury.

Encouraging and possibly requiring eye protection for air gun users may be a practical way to cut down on ocular injuries, although bystanders would continue to be at risk. Currently available polycarbonate protective lenses can reliably withstand the impact of an air gun pellet (Fig. 9.3, A–C). Including protective eyewear with the purchase of a BB or air gun and making it attractive to children who use the guns could significantly increase compliance in wearing eye protection (12).

Alteration of the air-powered gun to reduce its injury potential has been proposed but is probably unrealistic. Decreasing the muzzle velocity sufficiently to prevent ocular injury would severely compro-

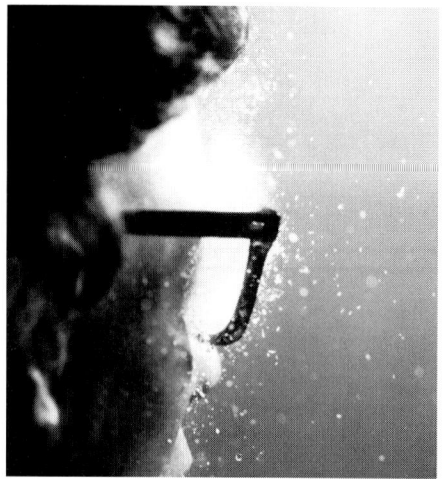

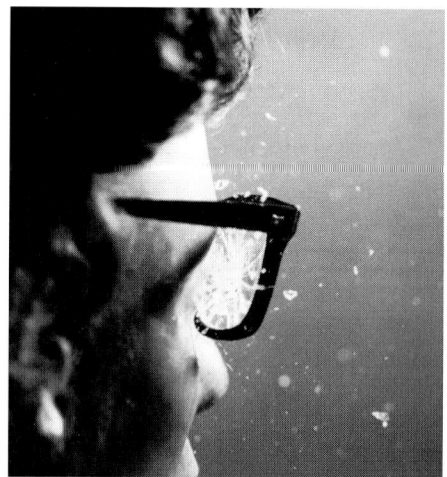

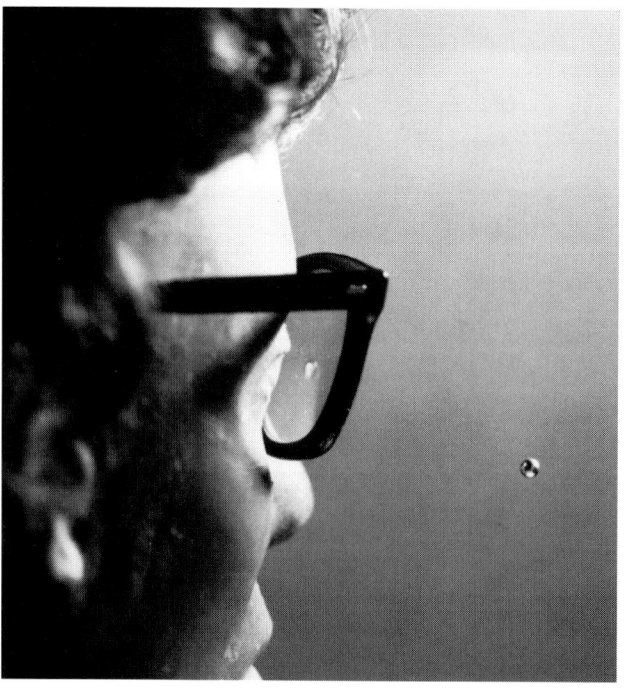

Figure 9.3 Results of the impact of a 0.177-caliber, 0.342-gm steel BB delivered at 500 to 600 feet/sec on 3-mm-thick plano samples mounted on headform.
(A) Tempered glass;
(B) CR-39 (plastic);
(C) polycarbonate.

mise the gun's attractiveness to consumers. Such an impact on sales would be strongly resisted by the industrial lobby.

Educational campaigns informing the public of the dangers of air guns, including the need for protective eyewear and supervision of children, in conjunction with legislation that treats air guns as guns rather than as toys, could have a significant impact on the rate of ocular BB and pellet gun injuries. The impetus for these measures must come from the community, with eyecare professionals, pediatricians, and schools leading the way. An emphasis on prevention is the only realistic hope for making vision loss from ocular BB injuries a thing of the past.

War Games

During the past decade, combat simulation sports have gained popularity throughout many Western countries, including the United States, Canada, the United Kingdom, and Australia, to become a multimillion dollar industry. The sport has a number of different names, such as "war games," "paintball," "survival," and "commando," and involves opposing teams competing in "capture the flag" or similar games. Players use special carbon dioxide–powered guns to shoot paint-filled spheres at opponents, which explode on contact, signifying a wound and eliminating the player from the game. Competitions are generally organized by entrepreneurs who provide a playing field and equipment in exchange for a fee. In general, a consent form is required for individuals younger than 18 years of age.

The carbon dioxide–powered guns used in war games have muzzle velocities in the range of 60 to 90 m/sec (24). Both semiautomatic and fully automatic paintball guns are available. The paintballs consist of spherical gelatin shells filled with glycerin, water, polyethylene glycol, food dye, and titanium oxide. They have a diameter of approximately 1 to 2 cm and are designed to rupture on impact (Fig. 9.4). This diameter is small enough that the full force of the projectile can be transmitted to the eye, resulting in severe blunt injury.

Organizers of war games provide protective eyewear for all participants, but despite this fact, serious eye injuries have plagued the sport. Most of these injuries have occurred when players were not wearing the eye protectors. This occurs during practice with the weapons before the onset of the game and especially during the match, when eyewear becomes fogged or dirty. The typical scenario in reported cases involves fatigued players removing their protective

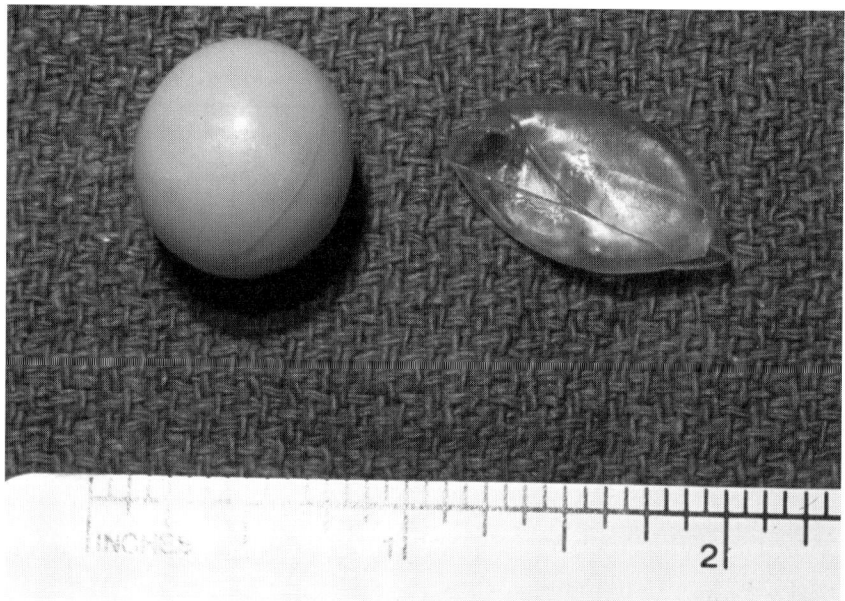

Figure 9.4 *The paintball used in war games, seen here both before and after impact.*

eyewear to clean it or perform some other task, who are then victims of a surprise attack (25). There is one reported case of a paintball fired at close range striking the lateral aspect of protective goggles, displacing them, and causing severe ocular injury (24). Because of their realistic appearance, misuse of paintball guns has also occurred, including one instance of a drive-by shooting of a child in the arm (24).

Over a 3-year period from 1984 to 1987, Canadian ophthalmologists reported 44 ocular injuries to war games participants, none of whom were wearing eye protection (25). Of these, 17 eyes were left legally blind, with a visual acuity of 20/200 or less. Thirteen eyes recovered to less than 20/40, and only 14 regained 20/20 vision. The most common forms of injury were hyphema, retinal damage, and cataract. Two ruptured globes occurred despite the relatively low muzzle velocity of the paintball guns. Any eye involved in a war games–related injury should undergo full ophthalmologic examination (26).

In 1984, 13 cases of eye injury from playing war games were reported (27). All victims were males, with ages ranging from 16 to 41 years old, and their injuries included seven hyphemas, one retinal detachment with a final visual acuity of 20/800, and one ruptured globe with a final visual acuity of no light perception. At the time of injury, none of the 13 patients had on protective eyewear, despite the eyewear being available. They either failed to put them on, lost them during the game, or removed them for cleaning or to leave the game.

Because of the alarming rate of ocular injuries resulting from war games, the Canadian Ophthalmological Society launched an intensive public awareness campaign that succeeded in significantly reducing the number of injuries. They recommend providing new, unscratched polycarbonate eye guards to every player and requiring that eye protection be worn before the distribution of guns and ammunition. Head shots, quick draws, and duels should be forbidden, and alcohol should be banned in the playing area (25). These measures, along with an awareness of the potential for eye injury by participants, could make ocular trauma from war games a rare occurrence.

Water Sports

Water sports encompass a wide variety of activities as diverse as fishing, swimming, sailing, water skiing, water polo, and scuba diving. Ocular trauma can occur while engaging in any water sports activity and should be approached in a similar manner to other sports-related injuries. There are, however, unique features to some water sports–associated ophthalmic problems that require special consideration.

Ocular Problems Related to Sun and Water

Excessive Ultraviolet Radiation

Excessive ultraviolet radiation (UVR) exposure can easily occur while participating in water sports. Reflection from sand, water, and surfaces such as boat decks can significantly increase the amount of UVR incident on the ocular surface, sometimes resulting in phototoxicity to the corneal epithelium. This condition is analogous to "welder's flash" or "snowblindness" and is caused primarily by ultraviolet (UV)B wavelengths, below 315 nm (28). After an initial latent period that varies from 6 to 10 hours, there is the onset of progressively worsening foreign body sensation, pain, and photophobia. Examination reveals conjunctival injection and an irregular corneal epithelium with punctate areas of fluorescein staining (29). Characteristically, the degree of discomfort seems out of proportion to the clinical findings. The usual therapy is supportive and includes cycloplegia, lubrication with an antibiotic ointment, patching, and analgesics. The condition generally resolves within 24 to 48 hours without sequelae. As opposed to acute phototoxicity, long-term exposure to UVR may play a role in pterygium formation, cataractogenesis, and age-related retinal degenerations. Participants in water sports with heavy sun exposure should consider regular use of sunglasses with UV-blocking lenses.

Ocular Irritation and Infection

Swimmers often suffer problems with chemical conjunctivitis due to disinfecting substances such as chlorine used in swimming pools. The wearing of goggles and proper pool maintenance are helpful. Goggles, which do not cover the nose, are useful only for surface swimming, as ocular barotrauma can result from inability to equalize pressure in depths more than several feet. Frequent use of decongestant eye drops should be discouraged because of rebound phenomena.

Another problem associated with swimming pools as well as hot tubs is ocular infection. The most common infection transmitted in this manner is viral conjunctivitis, particularly pharyngoconjunctival fever caused by adenovirus types 3 and 4 (30). In general, persons recovering from viral conjunctivitis should be excluded from swimming pools for 2 weeks after the cessation of symptoms. A serious corneal infection associated with contact lens wear and water sports is *Acanthamoeba* keratitis (Plate 5), which is difficult to treat and frequently results in permanent visual impairment. The organism is a protozoan and is present in fresh water, swimming pools, sea water, and contaminated contact lens solution. It has been cultured in and around hot tubs in association with documented infection (31). In general, water sports and hot tub use should be avoided by any person with a known disruption to the corneal epithelium such as a corneal abrasion or contact lens–related irritation. This disruption may allow entry of microorganisms into the corneal stroma, thus leading to infection.

Contact lenses, both soft and rigid gas permeable, are acceptable for use in swimming as long as the lenses have been well tolerated in daily wear. They do not offer a protective effect from water-associated irritants and infectious agents, as do prescription goggles and masks, and they may increase the risk of acquiring a corneal infection. A more common problem with wearing contact lenses when swimming is losing the lens. In pool water, which is hypotonic, soft contact lens loss may be prevented by splashing pool water into the eyes with the contacts in place before swimming. The lenses then become hypotonic and adhere to the cornea. After leaving a swimming pool, removal of contact lenses should be delayed at least 30 minutes to allow reversal of this effect.

Ocular Injuries in Fishing

Fishing is an extremely popular form of recreation, with over 30 million sport fishing licenses granted annually in the United States alone (32). It is also an important commercial industry providing livelihood to thousands. Not surprisingly, there are a number of mostly minor injuries, usually involving the fingers and hands. Eye injuries are relatively uncommon, but because of the delicate nature of the ocular structures, they are often serious when they do occur.

Fishing-related eye injuries occur in all age groups, including elderly persons and children (15). Overall, however, these injuries are associated with an older average age than most other forms of sports-related ocular trauma. In one study, fishing-related eye injuries had the highest mean age (32 years) of all sports-related injuries (18). This likely relates to the appeal of the sport to a broad range of the population.

Most eye injuries in fishing are due to trauma from the implements of the sport. Of the 10 fishing-related ocular injuries reported in a trauma series at the Massachusetts Eye and Ear Infirmary, six resulted from flying hooks, two from fishing line, and one from a fish pick (18). In one case, the mechanism was unknown. Although penetrating injuries are usually the most serious, blunt trauma, particularly from fishing weights, can be visually significant. We have seen complete dislocation of the lens into the vitreous cavity in an elderly woman struck by another fisherman's weight while casting. Lid lacerations are also common, especially as a result of fish hooks (Plate 6). In these cases, ocular penetration is less likely, presumably because the lid effectively protects the globe (32).

Penetrating ocular fish hook injuries are more common in the anterior segment than the posterior segment (32). Typically, the hook pierces the cornea and may involve the iris and lens. Removing a fish hook is problematic because of the barb located at the tip of the hook. If the hook has penetrated beyond the barb, special care must be taken in removing it, because backing out a barb through the cornea may cause considerable tissue disruption. In anterior segment injuries, a useful technique involves advancement of the barb through a second surgical wound followed by removal of the barb with metal cutters. The remainder of the hook can then be atraumatically backed out of the entry site (32–34). If performed away from the visual axis of the cornea, the second wound can usually be accomplished without a negative impact on the visual prognosis. This is substantiated in a series from the Wilmer Institute in which four cases managed with this technique all had final visual acuities of 20/30 or better (32). When a fish hook penetrates the posterior segment, the "advance and cut" technique is less useful because of the problems involved in making a second wound in the retina. In some cases, it is possible to advance the tip of the hook through the pars plana (35), but generally, the "needle-cover" technique is the method of choice for removing hooks from the vitreous and retina (36). This consists of surgically enlarging the entry wound and passing a large-bore needle along the shank of the hook until engaging the barb (Fig. 9.5). The hook and needle are then removed together, the barb being covered in the lumen of the needle. This technique may also be useful in some cases of anterior segment fish hook penetration.

Ocular trauma in a marine environment carries a significant risk of infection. Penetrating injuries such as fish hook wounds may be complicated by endophthalmitis secondary to unusual pathogens such as *Vibrio* parahaemolyticus (37). In one reported case, an anterior segment fish hook perforation with a 48-hour delay in wound closure developed *Enterobacter cloacae* panendophthalmitis. Corneal injuries from nylon fishing line may be at risk for fungal keratitis (38). There is one reported case of pseudomembranous conjunctivitis

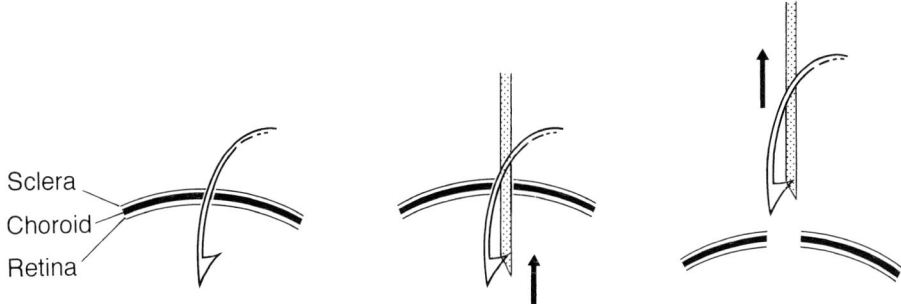

Figure 9.5 *Fish hook penetrating the eye and entering the vitreous. Removal is facilitated by passing a needle through the retina to engage the barb of the hook before withdrawing them out of the eye.*

in a debilitated patient due to *Vibrio alginolyticus* presumably acquired from handling seashell fragments (32). Prophylactic broad spectrum antibiotics along with close observation should be used in any patient with a penetrating ocular injury acquired in an aquatic setting. Overall, casting appears to be the highest risk activity for trauma in fishing. Precautions should be taken, such as adequate spacing of fisherman while casting. When this is not possible, warning bystanders and fellow fishermen in preparation for casting could likely avoid a large number of mishaps. Wearing eye protection would also prevent injuries and could serve an additional purpose as photoprotection.

Ocular Jellyfish Stings

Most reported cases of ocular jellyfish stings have occurred among fishermen and swimmers in the Chesapeake Bay. The responsible organism, *Chrysaora quinquecirrha*, or sea nettle, has tentacles coated with nematocysts that discharge a venomous thread on contact (Fig. 9.6). If a nematocyst contacts the eye, the poisonous thread can penetrate the corneal epithelium. In one study, 90 of 110 Chesapeake Bay watermen gave a history of an ocular sea nettle sting at some point during their career, usually while hauling crab traps into their boats (39). Symptoms consist of the acute onset of intense burning pain, photophobia, and tearing. Examination may reveal conjunctival and limbal injection, chemosis, punctate epithelial keratitis, corneal stromal edema, and mild anterior chamber flare (40). Occasionally, jellyfish nematocysts may be seen adhering to the cornea, often in cases of underlying anterior stromal edema. Because manipulation can result in further discharge of venom, it is generally best to allow the nematocysts to slough spontaneously (40). Symptoms and findings usually resolve within 48 hours. Watermen often carry topical proparacaine on their boats in the event of an ocular jellyfish sting. Obviously, this may be a dangerous practice since the anesthetic may mask other serious pathology.

Rarely, a severe iritis with elevated intraocular pressure may develop that responds to topical corticosteroids, cycloplegia, and temporizing pressure-lowering agents (39). In these cases, mydriasis and loss of accommodation are common. Iris transillumination defects, peripheral anterior synechiae, and chronic unilateral glaucoma have also been observed. The mechanism for this severe reaction may be hypersensitivity or a direct action of the jellyfish venom. Interestingly, three of the five documented cases with severe inflammation had a

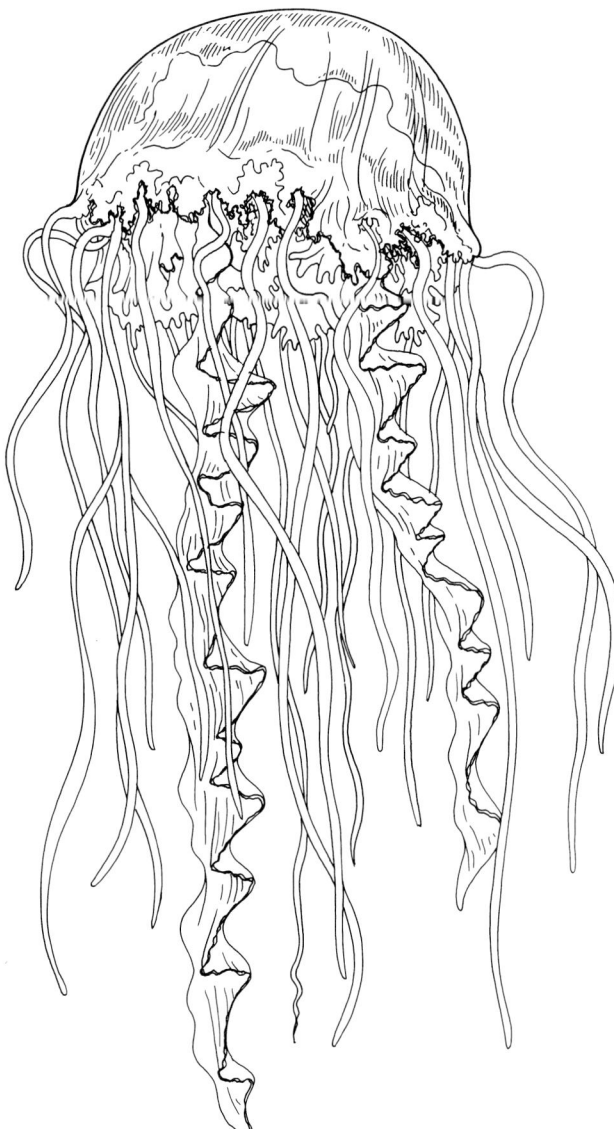

Figure 9.6 *This sea nettle* (Chrysaora quinquecirrha) *has tentacles that can discharge a venomous thread.*

history of allergy to seafood or iodinated contrast dye, although none of them demonstrated any systemic reaction to the jellyfish sting.

It is likely that wearing eye protection would lessen the frequency of ocular jellyfish stings in the Chesapeake Bay watermen by preventing contact of the nematocysts with the ocular surface. Swimmers should always exercise caution when in waters known to have a significant jellyfish population.

Ophthalmic Considerations in Scuba Diving

Scuba diving is a growing recreational activity that has become increasingly more accessible to the general population. With it come significant hazards, especially to the inexperienced diver. Ocular trauma can occur in a variety of circumstances, although the use of facemasks in diving substantially decreases this risk. The most important ophthalmic considerations in diving are adequate underwater vision and problems related to decompression.

Optical Correction

Without optical aids, an emmetropic human is approximately 42 diopters hyperopic when underwater (30). This is because the usual air-cornea interface is replaced by a water-cornea interface, with subsequent focusing of light rays behind the retina. By wearing a facemask or goggles, the air-cornea interface is restored and acuity improved. Refraction of light at the water-glass-air interface of the mask results in a magnification effect of about 25%, which can interfere with distance estimation. For divers with refractive errors, it is possible to have a correction ground into the face plate, but most prefer to wear soft contact lenses under nonprescription masks. Soft contact lenses appear to be well tolerated in diving. Divers should be aware that contact lens loss into a facemask is possible and may place them at risk during a dive because of impaired visual acuity. Hard contact lenses are contraindicated in deep dives because of problems during decompression (41,42). It should be noted that misuse of commercial mask defogging agents can cause a delayed toxic reaction of the corneal epithelium (43). This punctate epithelial keratopathy has occurred after copious application of defogging agents without proper buffing or drying of the mask before diving. The onset of severe ocular burning and photophobia typically occurs a few hours after exposure, usually after completion of the dive. Treatment involves patching, with resolution of symptoms within 24 hours. No permanent sequelae have been reported.

Ocular Squeeze

Ocular squeeze is a phenomenon that occurs because of air compression within a goggle or mask at depths greater than about 3 m (30). With a facemask, it is possible to neutralize the compression effect by blowing air into the mask through the nose. With goggles this is not possible, unless they are specially modified, as are those of Ama divers of Korea and Japan (44). Ocular squeeze results in subconjunctival hemorrhage (Plate 7), which can be quite excessive and uncomfortable but rarely causes serious ocular pathology.

Decompression Effects

During the ascent phase of a deep dive, the partial pressure of dissolved nitrogen in body fluids can exceed the ambient pressure, resulting in bubble formation in many different tissues. This bubble formation in vessels, joints, and the spinal white matter and resultant ischemia gives rise to the clinical syndrome known as the "bends," or decompression sickness. There is also evidence that hyperbaric conditions may lead to a hyperviscosity syndrome and may contribute to vascular occlusions independent of decompression effects. In any event, extensive infarctions can occur, leading to severe central nervous system damage and death.

There are occasional reports of transient visual loss and fundus hemorrhages in divers, consistent with ocular ischemia due to bubble formation and hyperviscosity. In a study comparing retinal fluorescein angiograms of 84 professional divers with those of age-matched controls, the divers had a statistically significant decrease in macular capillary density relative to controls (45). Divers also had pigment epithelial changes and microaneurysms in the posterior pole that were not present in the nondivers. With one exception, all divers with a history of decompression sickness had pigment epithelial lesions, but those without such a history still had a high incidence of abnormalities. These findings are typical consequences of retinal and choroidal ischemia. Thus, scuba divers, particularly those who undertake frequent deep dives with long decompression cycles, may be experiencing multiple microvascular occlusions in the retinal and choroidal circulation. The practical significance of this in terms of risk of vision-threatening complications is unknown.

Bubble formation during decompression is also a problem for hard contact lens wearers (41,42). Nitrogen comes out of solution in the precorneal tear film during decompression and accumulates beneath hard lenses, which are relatively impermeable to nitrogen. This interferes with normal tear exchange, resulting in focal areas of epithelial edema. Divers experience soreness, decreased acuity, and halos around lights, symptoms that persist for as long as 2 hours after the completion of the dive. Placing a small fenestration in the center of a hard contact lens prevents bubbles from building up and alleviates the problem. Soft contact lenses have better gas exchange and are generally well tolerated even during deep dives.

Diving After Ocular Surgery

There are several special considerations for individuals who wish to dive after ocular surgery (46). Exposure to waterborne pathogens may increase the risk of devastating infection in the postoperative period after intraocular surgery, such as cataract extraction, penetrating keratoplasty, and vitrectomy. This increased risk presumably normalizes with healing of the incisions. In glaucoma-filtering surgery, however, a permanent ocular fistula is created and thus the increased risk of intraocular infection with swimming and diving may be longstanding.

Pressure effects can also be important after ocular surgery, especially when an intraocular air or gas bubble is present. This could theoretically lead to severe intraocular barotrauma as the bubble contracts and expands. Thus, diving is contraindicated in any patient with intraocular air or gas until the bubble has been completely resorbed. The ocular squeeze effect, which occurs with goggles or masks in which pressure has not been equalized, can result in subconjunctival hemorrhage and therefore threaten the function of glaucoma-filtering operations. There is no evidence that diving has a deleterious effect on glaucoma patients without a history of surgery. Although the absolute pressure within the globe increases with underwater depth, there is no change in the pressure differential as long as ocular squeeze is prevented by nasal exhalation into a facemask. Similarly, the theoretical risk of radial keratotomy wound rupture because of barotrauma is low as long as ocular squeeze is avoided and the pressure differential across the cornea is not significantly altered.

Conclusion

This chapter addresses the ophthalmic considerations of shooting sports, war games, fishing, and scuba diving. The common theme has been the preventable nature of most injuries. All of these activities require a certain amount of skill for proficiency, but the acquisition of skill in no way obviates the need for caution in using often dangerous implements. The simple use of eye protection could prevent most serious ocular injuries in these sports and should be encouraged.

References

1. Varr WF, Cook RA. Shotgun eye injuries: ocular risk and eye protection efficacy. Ophthalmology 1992;6:867–872.
2. Roden D, Cleary P, Eustace P. A five year survey of ocular shotgun injuries in Ireland. Br J Ophthalmol 1987;71.449–453.
3. Drummond J, Kielar RA. Perforating ocular shotgun injuries: relationship of ocular findings to pellet ballistics. South Med J 1976;69:1066–1068.
4. Tillet CW, Rose HW, Herget C. High-speed photographic study of perforating ocular injury by the BB. Am J Ophthalmol 1962;54:675–688.
5. Morris RE, Witherspoon CE, Feist RM, et al. Bilateral ocular shotgun injury. Am J Ophthalmol 1987;103:695–700.
6. Hill JC, Peart DA. The visual outcome of ocular birdshot injuries. S Afr Med J 1986;70:807–809.
7. Ford JG, Barr CC. Penetrating pellet fragmentation: a complication of ocular shotgun injury. Arch Ophthalmol 1990;108:48–50.
8. John G, Feist RM, White MF, et al. Field evaluation of polycarbonate versus conventional safety glasses. South Med J 1988;81:1534–1536.
9. Kreshon MJ. Eye injuries due to BB guns. Am J Ophthalmol 1964;58:858–861.
10. Bowen DI, Magauran DM. Ocular injuries caused by airgun pellets: an analysis of 105 cases. Br Med J 1973;1:333–337.
11. Batch AJG. The air rifle: a dangerous weapon. Br Med J 1981;282:1834.
12. Sternberg P, De Juan E, Green WR, et al. Ocular BB injuries. Ophthalmology 1984;91:1269–1277.
13. Strahlman E, Sommer A. The epidemiology of sports-related ocular trauma. Int Ophthalmol Clin 1988;28:199–202.
14. Sharif KW, McGhee CNJ, Tomlinson RC. Ocular trauma caused by airgun pellets: a ten year survey. Eye 1990;4:855–860.
15. Strahlman E, Elman M, Daub E, Baker S. Causes of pediatric eye injuries. Arch Ophthalmol 1990;108:603–606.
16. Schein OD, Enger C, Tielsch JM. The context and consequences of ocular injuries from air guns. Am J Ophthalmol 1994;117:501–506.
17. DeJuan E, Sternberg P, Michels RG. Penetrating ocular injuries: types of injuries and visual results. Ophthalmology 1983;90:1318–1322.
18. Fountain TR, Albert DM. The histopathology of sports-related ocular trauma. Int Ophthalmol Clin 1988;28:206–210.
19. Conlon MR, Canny CLB. Favourable outcome in a patient with penetrating intraocular BB pellet injury. Can J Ophthalmol 1992;27:251–253.
20. Delori F, Pomerantzeff O, Cox MS. Deformation of the globe under high-speed impact: its relation to contusion injuries. Invest Ophthalmol 1969;8:290–301.
21. Jacobs NA, Morgan LM. On the management of retained airgun pellets: a survey of 11 orbital cases. Br J Ophthalmol 1988;72:97–100.

22. Guthkeich AN. Apparently trivial wounds of the eyelids with intracranial damage. Br Med J 1960;2:842–844.
23. Sheets W, Vinger P. Ocular injuries from airguns. Int Ophthalmol Clin 1988;28:225–227.
24. Wrenn KD, White SJ. Injury potential in "paintball" combat simulation games: a report of two cases. Am J Emerg Med 1991;9:402–403.
25. Easterbrook M, Pashby TJ. Ocular injuries and war games. Int Ophthalmol Clin 1988;28:222–224.
26. Mamalis N, Monson C, Farnsworth ST, White GL. Blunt ocular trauma secondary to "war games." Ann Ophthalmol 1990;22:416–418.
27. Tardif D, Little J, Mercier M, et al. Ocular trauma in war games. Phys Sportsmed 1986;14:90–93.
28. Sliney DH. Ocular injury due to light toxicity. Int Ophthalmol Clin 1988;28:246–250.
29. Gentile DA, Auerbach PS. The sun and water sports. Clin Sports Med 1987;6:674–684.
30. Seiff SR. Ophthalmic complications of water sports. Clin Sports Med 1987;6:684–685.
31. Samples JR, et al. *Acanthamoeba* keratitis possibly acquired from a hot tub. Arch Ophthalmol 1984;102:707.
32. Aiello LP, Iwamoto M, Guyer DR. Penetrating ocular fish-hook injuries. Ophthalmology 1992;99:862–866.
33. Aiello LP, Iwamoto M, Taylor HR. Perforating ocular fishhook injury. Arch Ophthalmol 1992;110:1316–1317.
34. Bartholomew RS, MacDonald M. Fish hook injuries of the eye. Br J Ophthalmol 1980;64:531–533.
35. Mandelcorn MS, Crichton A. Fish hook removal from vitreous and retina. Arch Ophthalmol 1989;107:493.
36. Grand MG, Lobes LA. Technique for removing a fishhook from the posterior segment of the eye. Arch Ophthalmol 1980;98:152–153.
37. Lessner AM, Webb RM, Rabin B. *Vibrio alginolyticus* conjunctivitis. Arch Ophthalmol 1985;103:229–230.
38. Clinch TE, Robinson MJ, Barron BA, et al. Fungal keratitis from nylon line lawn trimmers. Am J Ophthalmol 1992;114:437–440.
39. Rapoza PA, West SK, Newland HS, Taylor HR. Ocular jelly fish stings in Chesapeake Bay watermen. Am J Ophthalmol 1986;102:536–537.
40. Glasser DB, Noell MJ, Burnett JW, et al. Ocular jellyfish stings. Ophthalmology 1992;99:1414–1418.
41. Simon DR, Bradely ME. Corneal edema in divers wearing hard contact lenses. Am J Ophthalmol 1978;85:462–464.
42. Simon DR, Bradely ME. Adverse effects of contact lens wear during decompression. JAMA 1980;244:1213–1214.
43. Wright WL. Scuba diver's delayed toxic epithelial keratopathy from commercial mask defogging agents. Am J Ophthalmol 1982;93:470–472.
44. Hong S, Rahn H. The diving women of Korea and Japan. Sci Am 1967;216:34–43.
45. Polkinghorne PJ, Cross MR, Sehmi K, et al. Ocular fundus lesions in divers. Lancet 1988:1381–1383.
46. Butler FK. Diving and hyperbaric ophthalmology. Surv Ophthalmol 1995;39:347–366.

CHAPTER 10

Anatomy

Brian S. Biesman
Albert Hornblass

The Bony Orbit

The orbits are paired bony cavities located on either side of the midline sagittal plane. They contain the globes and their surrounding soft tissue, supporting structures including fat, extraocular muscles, neurovascular tissues, and most of the lacrimal system. The orbit provides structure, support, and protection for the soft tissues contained within, thus enabling the eye to function properly.

Each orbit is formed by seven bones: frontal, zygoma, sphenoid, maxilla, lacrimal, ethmoid, and palatine (Fig. 10.1). These bones form a pear-shaped structure that is nearly rectangular at its opening and becomes rounded and narrow at its apex. The medial walls are nearly parallel, whereas the lateral walls make an angle of approximately 90 degrees with each other. The total volume of the adult orbit is approximately 30 mL, of which the globe itself occupies nearly 25%, or about 6.5 to 7.0 mL. This has an important clinical correlation because the standard orbital implants used after enucleation (removal of the eye) have a volume of only about 2.5 to 3.0 mL, thus creating a volume deficit in the orbit. It is for this reason that many patients who have undergone enucleation have a deep superior sulcus, a challenging problem to correct (1).

The orbital rim or margin is the strong anterior border of the bony orbit. It is nearly quadrilateral in shape, interrupted only by the lacrimal fossa. The entrance to the adult orbit is slightly greater in horizontal (40 mm) than in vertical dimensions (35 mm). The superior

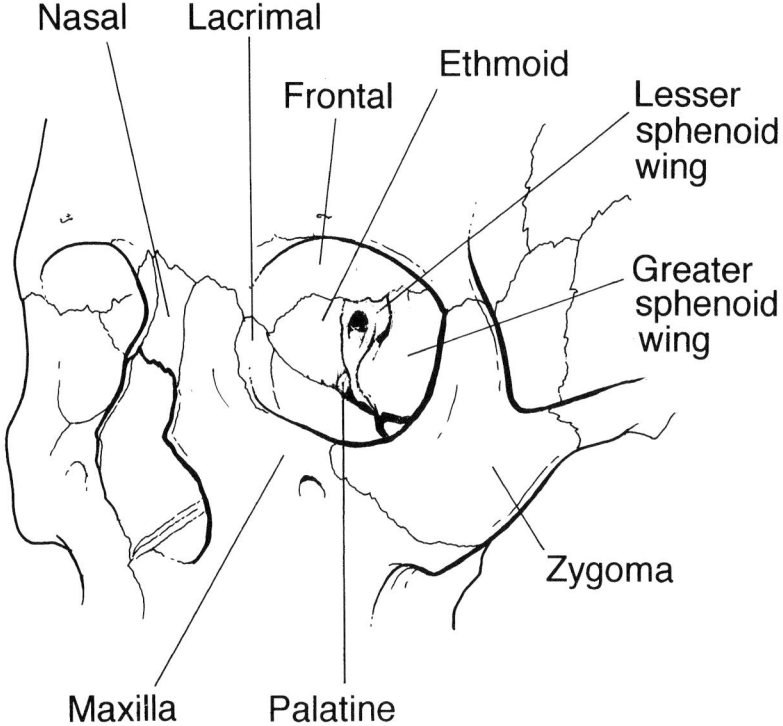

Figure 10.1 *Bones of the orbit.*

rim is formed by the frontal bone and is interrupted by the supraorbital notch (which may be an enclosed foramen in 25% of cases). Medially, the superior orbital rim becomes continuous with the posterior lacrimal crest, comprising a portion of the medial orbital rim. The remainder of the medial rim is formed by the anterior lacrimal crest, an extension of the frontal process of the maxilla. The medial rim of the orbit is thus discontinuous, with a space present between the anterior and posterior lacrimal crests. This space is the lacrimal fossa and is an important surgical landmark because it houses the lacrimal sac. The frontal process of the maxilla and the maxillary process of the zygoma form the inferior orbital rim. The infraorbital foramen is located approximately 7 to 10 mm inferior to the zygomaticomaxillary suture. The infraorbital nerve, artery, and vein exit from this foramen. The lateral orbital margin is formed by the frontal process of the maxilla and the maxillary process of the frontal bone, the frontomaxillary suture marking the joining of these bones. This suture line, along with the zygomaticomaxillary suture, is the fracture site in a so-called tripod fracture. The tripod fracture is a common injury after significant blunt trauma to the lateral orbital rim and is manifest by flattening of the malar eminence, inferior displacement of the lateral canthal angle, step-offs when palpating the contour of the rim, and trismus (Fig. 10.2) (2).

Three walls of the orbit are roughly triangular in shape, whereas the medial wall is rectangular; each contains special modifications to accommodate vital structures. The roof of the orbit is formed by the orbital plate of the frontal bone and the lesser wing of the sphenoid (Fig. 10.3). Special modifications of the roof include a fossa for the lacrimal gland, located behind the zygomatic process of the frontal

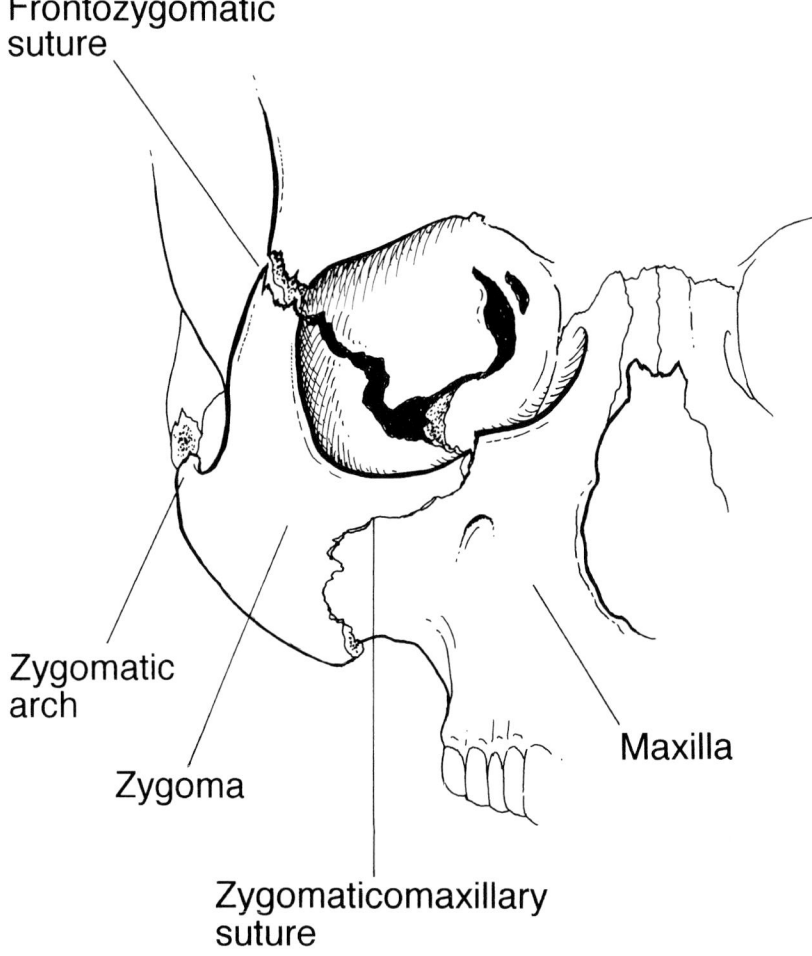

Figure 10.2 *Anatomy of a tripod fracture. Note the fractures at the zygomaticomaxillary suture, frontozygomatic suture, and the zygomatic arch.*

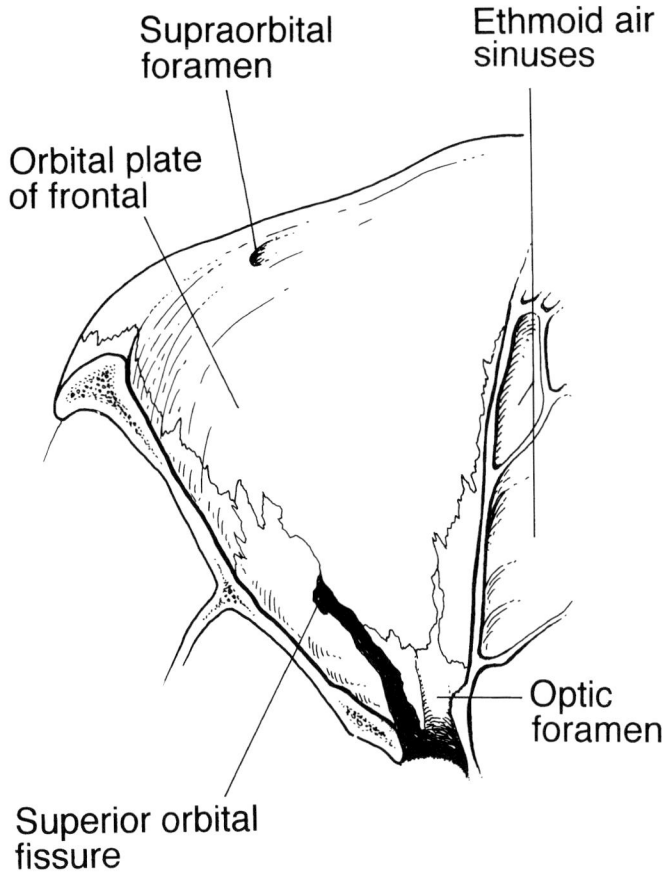

Figure 10.3 *Roof of the orbit.*

bone, and a small depression in the anteromedial aspect near the rim, called the fovea, for the trochlea of the superior oblique muscle. The optic foramen is a modification of the lesser wing of the sphenoid that transmits the optic nerve, the central retinal vessels, and sympathetic nerve fibers.

The medial orbital wall is the thinnest, measuring approximately 0.2 to 0.5 mm in thickness (Fig. 10.4). It is formed by the lacrimal, ethmoid, maxillary, and sphenoid bones. It separates the ethmoid sinuses from the orbit and is often fractured after blunt orbital trauma. Fortunately, these fractures are usually asymptomatic (3). Special structures of the medial wall include the anterior and posterior ethmoidal foramina. These transmit the anterior and posterior ethmoidal arteries and nerves. The average distance from the optic

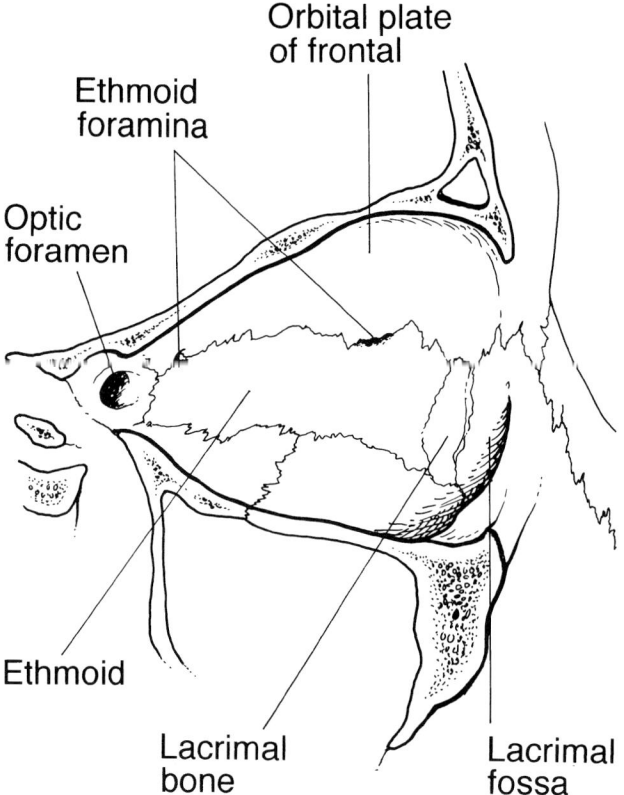

Figure 10.4 *Medial wall of the orbit.*

foramen to the posterior ethmoidal foramen is 6 mm, and the average distance between the ethmoidal foramina is 12 mm.

The orbital floor is formed by the maxillary, zygomatic, and palatine bones and lies immediately superior to the maxillary sinus (Fig. 10.5). The floor is also rather thin, averaging approximately 1 mm in thickness in its thinnest part. Therefore, it is quite susceptible to fracture after direct and indirect trauma. Floor fractures are more often symptomatic than medial wall fractures and may present with diplopia, enophthalmos, and/or numbness in the distribution of the infraorbital nerve that passes, in conjunction with the infraorbital vessels, through the infraorbital groove, canal, and foramen (4). Posterolaterally, the floor is bounded by the inferior orbital fissure that terminates approximately 20 mm posterior to the orbital rim and transmits the inferior ophthalmic vein, the infraorbital and zygomatic nerves, and the nerve to the pterygopalatine ganglion.

The lateral orbital wall is by far the sturdiest. The anterior third

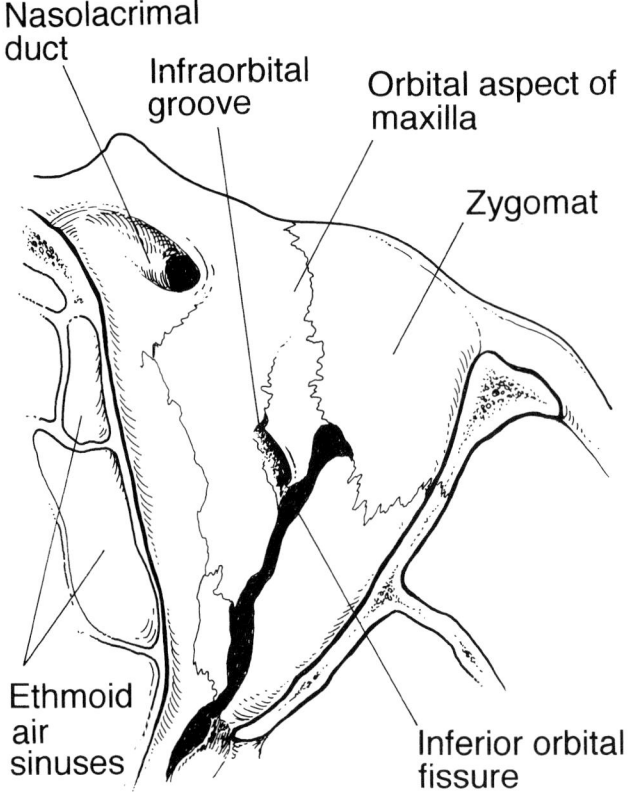

Figure 10.5 *The floor of the orbit.*

is formed by the zygoma and the posterior two-thirds by the greater wing of the sphenoid (Fig. 10.6). Posteriorly, the lateral wall is separated from the roof by the superior orbital fissure, an opening between the greater and lesser wings of the sphenoid bone. The superior orbital fissure transmits the lacrimal, frontal, trochlear, and abducens nerves; the superior and inferior divisions of the third cranial nerve; and the superior ophthalmic vein. The superior orbital fissure is divided by the annulus of Zinn, a fibrous ring continuous with the periorbita that serves as the origin of the horizontal and vertical recti muscles. The lateral orbital tubercle (of Whitnall) is a small elevation on the orbital aspect of the zygoma, approximately 10 mm below the frontozygomatic suture. This marks the site of attachment of the check ligament of the lateral rectus muscle, the suspensory ligament of the eyeball (Lockwood's ligament), and the lateral horn of the levator muscle (5).

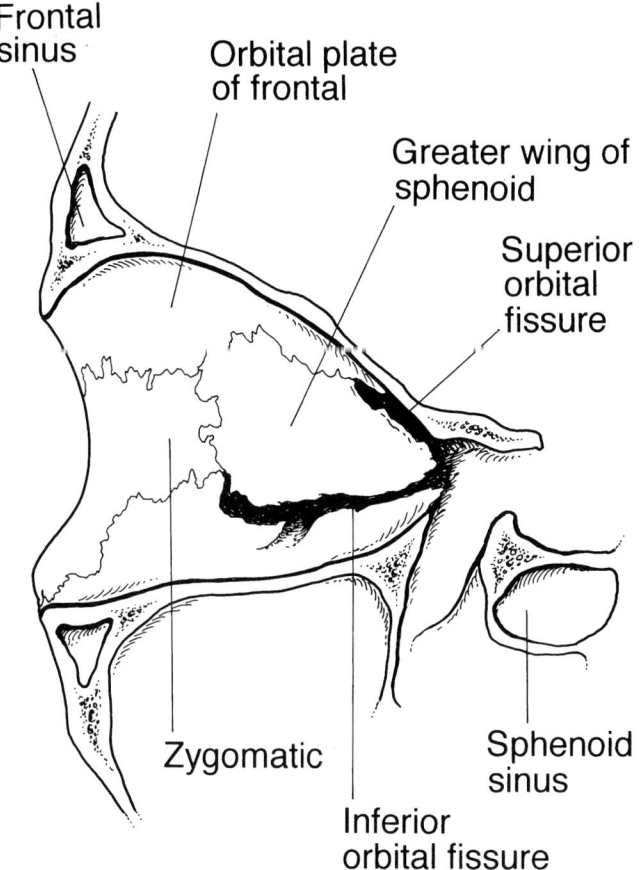

Figure 10.6 *Lateral wall of the right orbit.*

The Orbital Contents

Periorbita

> The periosteum lining the orbital bones is known as the periorbita. It is loosely adherent over most of the orbit but adheres tightly over bony sutures, around the orbital fissures and foramina, at the lacrimal fossa and posterior lacrimal crest, and at the orbital rim, where it forms a thickened band known as the arcus marginalis. The arcus marginalis blends with the periosteum of the facial bones and serves as the origin of the orbital septum. The periorbita becomes continuous with the dura mater at the superior orbital fissure, optic foramen, and the anterior ethmoidal foramen.

The Globe

The globe itself is located somewhat superiorly and laterally in the orbit. It is an oblong structure formed by the fusion of two spheres. The anterior clear sphere (the cornea) comprises approximately 15% of the globe and has a radius of curvature of 8 mm, whereas the remaining 85% is made up of a posterior opaque sphere (the sclera) with a radius of curvature of 12 mm. The position of the globe within the bony orbit protects it from trauma caused by large blunt objects (e.g., basketball, softball) but does not protect it from smaller objects that fit within the orbital margins (e.g., golf ball, squash ball) or compressible objects (e.g., racquetball, underinflated soccer ball). The ocular injuries with the most serious sequelae usually result from trauma directed in a superonasal direction, striking the globe inferolaterally. The sclera is thinnest beneath the insertions of the extraocular muscles (Fig. 10.7). It is here and at the limbus that scleral ruptures resulting from athletic injuries are most likely to occur (6).

Orbital Fascia

An intricate and complicated fascial system supports the globe and other orbital structures, maximizing their function and maintaining their appropriate anatomic relationships. Koorneef (7–9) provided the current understanding of the orbital connective tissue system by performing meticulous thick-section analysis of decalcified orbits. He described three orbital fascial systems: Tenon's capsule, which surrounds the globe and extraocular muscles anteriorly; tissue connecting Tenon's capsule to the periorbita anteriorly; and a system derived from the fascial sheaths of the extraocular muscles.

Tenon's capsule is composed of dense connective tissue surrounding the eye and extraocular muscles anteriorly. It inserts approximately 2 mm from the limbus and extends posteriorly to the optic nerve, where it blends with the periorbita. The entrance of the recti muscles into Tenon's capsule divides it into anterior and posterior portions. The anterior portion, approximately one-third of the capsule, fuses with the intermuscular septae arising from the fascial sheaths associated with the extraocular muscles. Tenon's capsule separates the globe and muscles from the intra- and extraconal orbital fat pads, and its traumatic or surgical violation may result in a prolapse of orbital fat anteriorly. The surface of Tenon's capsule that faces the globe is smooth, thus enhancing ocular motility.

The anterior connective tissue system helps to support the globe within the orbit with connections between the globe and periorbita.

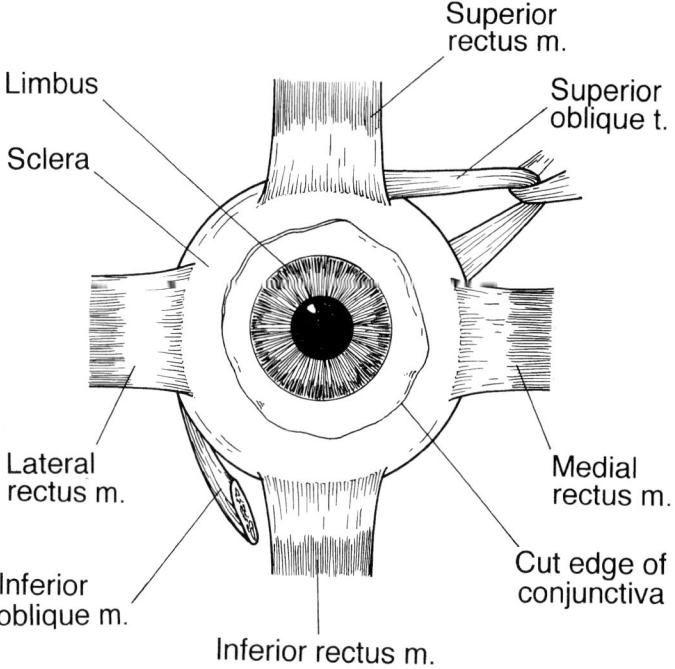
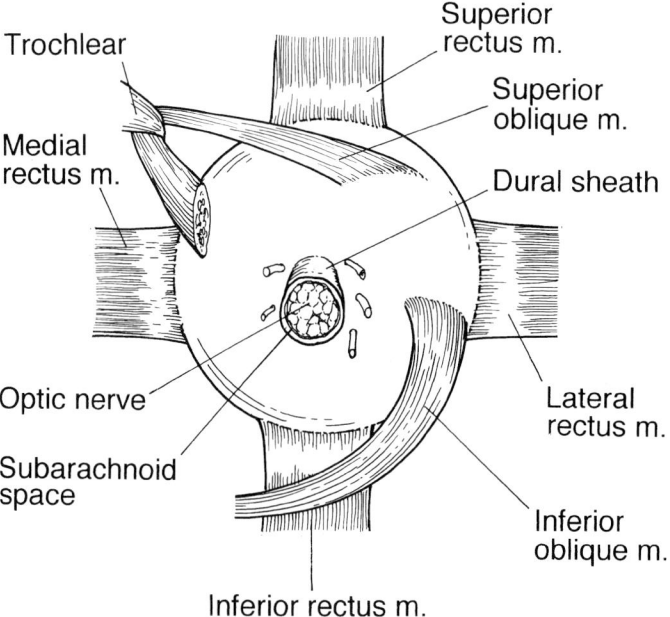

Figure 10.7 *Extraocular muscles of the eye. Key: m = muscle, t = tendon.*

This system also contributes to the suspensory ligament of the globe (Lockwood's ligament). Thus, support and stability are contributed by the anterior connective tissues.

The extraocular muscle connective tissue system is derived from the fascial sheaths of the extraocular muscles. Anteriorly, these fascial sheaths fuse together to form the intermuscular septum. In addition, the sheaths of each of the recti muscles have unique modifications contributing to the support and function of the globe. Extensions from the medial and lateral rectus muscle sheaths form the medial and lateral check ligaments, respectively. The connective tissue surrounding the superior rectus gives rise to a supporting network for the superior ophthalmic vein, and that surrounding the inferior rectus gives rise to the capsulopalpebral fascia, an important retractor of the lower eyelid (7–9).

Orbital Vessels

The blood supply to the orbit is derived primarily from the ophthalmic artery (Fig. 10.8), a branch of the internal carotid, with relatively minor contributions from maxillary and facial arteries of the

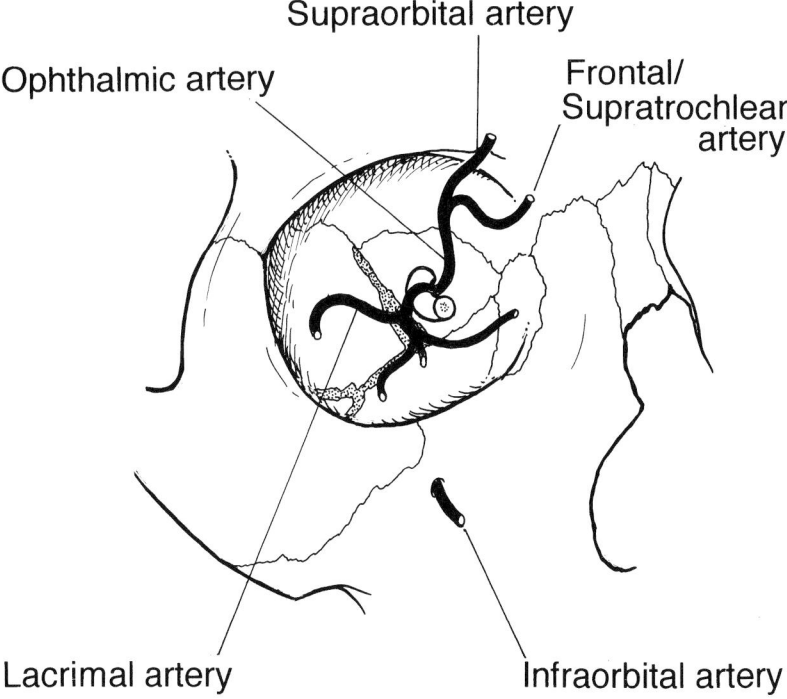

Figure 10.8 *Major branches of the ophthalmic artery within the orbit.*

external carotid system. The ophthalmic artery, the first branch of the internal carotid, initially lies beneath the optic nerve. It travels forward and medially, assuming a position on top of the nerve as it gives off its first principal branch, the central retinal artery, which enters the nerve some 10 mm behind the globe. As the ophthalmic artery travels in close proximity to the optic nerve, it gives off small branches contributing to its blood supply.

The medial and lateral long posterior ciliary arteries are the next branches of the ophthalmic artery. They travel anteriorly, branching into numerous small vessels that perforate the sclera at the posterior aspect of the globe. Two of these multiple small vessels travel anteriorly in the 3 and 9 o'clock meridians as the long posterior ciliary arteries, providing blood supply to the iris, ciliary body, and a portion of the choroid.

The ophthalmic artery continues forward within the orbit, giving rise to its intraorbital branches, the muscular, lacrimal, and supraorbital arteries (Fig. 10.8). Two muscular arteries supply each rectus muscle with the exception of the lateral rectus, which receives only one branch. The lacrimal artery passes anteriorly along the lateral orbital wall, accompanied by the lacrimal nerve, lying superior to the lateral rectus muscle. It divides into the recurrent meningeal artery as well as into several smaller branches before supplying the lacrimal gland. It then passes through the orbital septum, terminating as the lateral palpebral arteries. The supraorbital artery and nerve proceed forward in the superomedial aspect of the orbit, near the superior rectus muscle, exiting through the supraorbital foramen and supplying the muscles of the forehead, glabella, and brows.

The ophthalmic artery continues anteriorly in the medial orbit, dividing into the anterior and posterior ethmoidal and supratrochlear arteries. It then divides into the medial palpebral arteries, paired vessels that subsequently anastomose with the lateral palpebral arteries, thus forming the palpebral arcades, a critical source of blood supply to the eyelids.

The terminal branches of the ophthalmic artery are the supratrochlear and dorsal nasal arteries. The supratrochlear artery supplies the brow superior to the trochlea, whereas the dorsal nasal artery forms a communication between the internal and external carotid circulations, anastomosing with the angular artery in the medial canthal region (see Fig. 10.9) (10–13).

The infraorbital artery, the terminal branch of the internal maxillary artery, is also an important orbital vessel. It enters through the

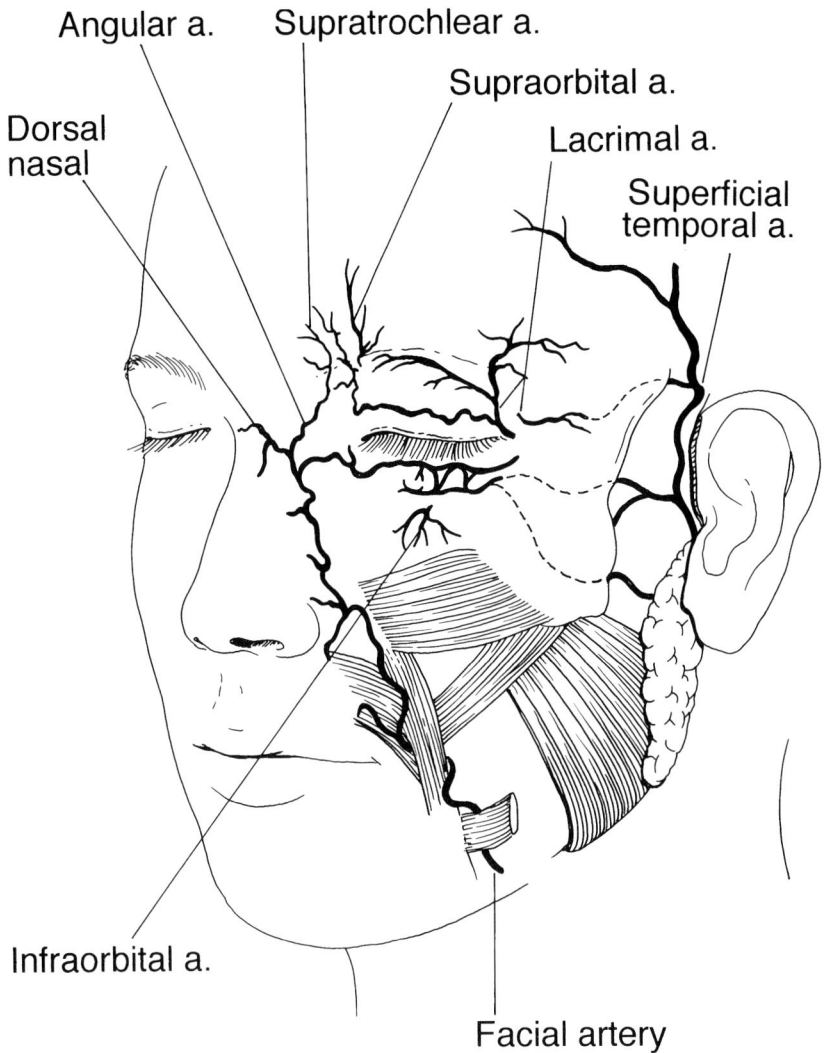

Figure 10.9 *Superficial arteries of the ocular region. Key: a = artery.*

inferior orbital fissure, passes along the orbital floor within the infraorbital groove, and exits through the infraorbital foramen along with the infraorbital nerve. It may be damaged after fracture of the orbital floor. The infraorbital artery contributes to the blood supply of the lacrimal gland, inferior rectus and oblique muscles, and the lacrimal sac before anastomosing with terminal branches of the facial artery.

As opposed to most other anatomic regions, the orbital venous system is independent of the arterial supply (Fig. 10.10). The principal source of venous drainage is the superior opthalmic vein, a large vessel formed in the superior medial orbit by the angular and supraorbital veins. The superior ophthalmic vein passes posteriorly in close association with the superior rectus muscle before piercing the muscle cone and exiting the orbit through the superior orbital fissure and emptying into the cavernous sinus.

The inferior ophthalmic vein is formed from a venous plexus on the orbital floor. It passes posteriorly in the orbit and joins the superior ophthalmic vein before its entering the cavernous sinus. A smaller branch enters the pterygoid plexus. The central retinal vein is parallel to the central retinal artery and provides venous drainage for the globe (14).

The classic teaching is that lymphatics are not found within the orbit. Recently, however, lymphatic channels have been identified within the lacrimal gland. This may explain the occurrence of lymphoid tumors, including malignant lymphoma, that are well-recog-

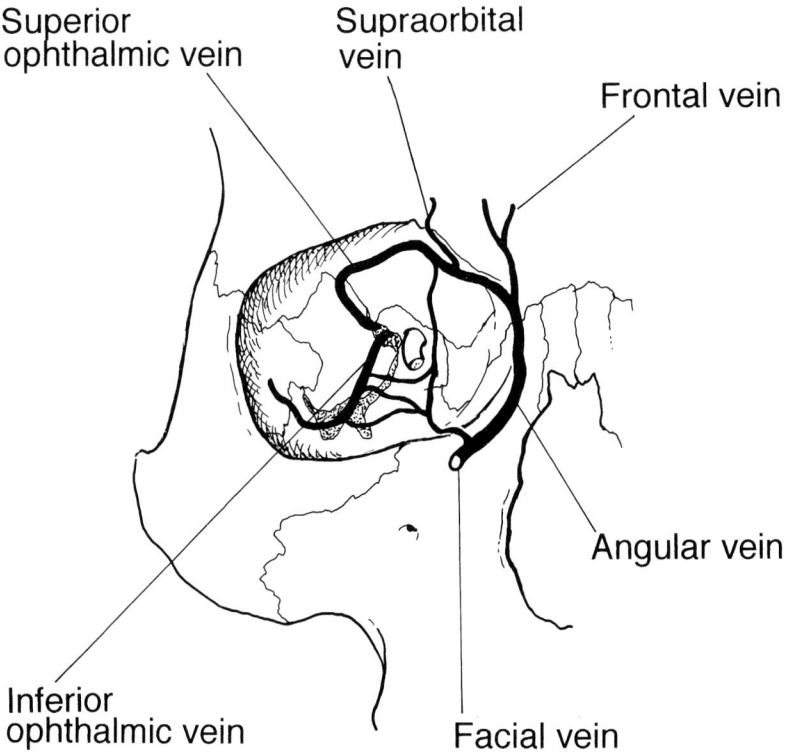

Figure 10.10 *Venous drainage of the orbit. Note that the orbital venous drainage is not parallel to the arterial supply.*

nized primary orbital processes. The lymphatic drainage of the eyelids is to the preauricular and submandibular lymph nodes (Fig. 10.11) (15).

Orbital Nerves

The orbit contains a complex variety of motor, sensory, and autonomic nerves (Fig. 10.12). In addition to the optic nerve (cranial nerve II), which is actually an extension of the brain, cranial nerves III, IV, and VI terminate within the orbit, and portions of cranial nerve V innervate vital orbital structures.

The optic nerve originates in the optic chasm and enters the orbit via the optic foramen, an opening in the lesser wing of the sphenoid. It is within this foramen that the nerve is believed to be susceptible

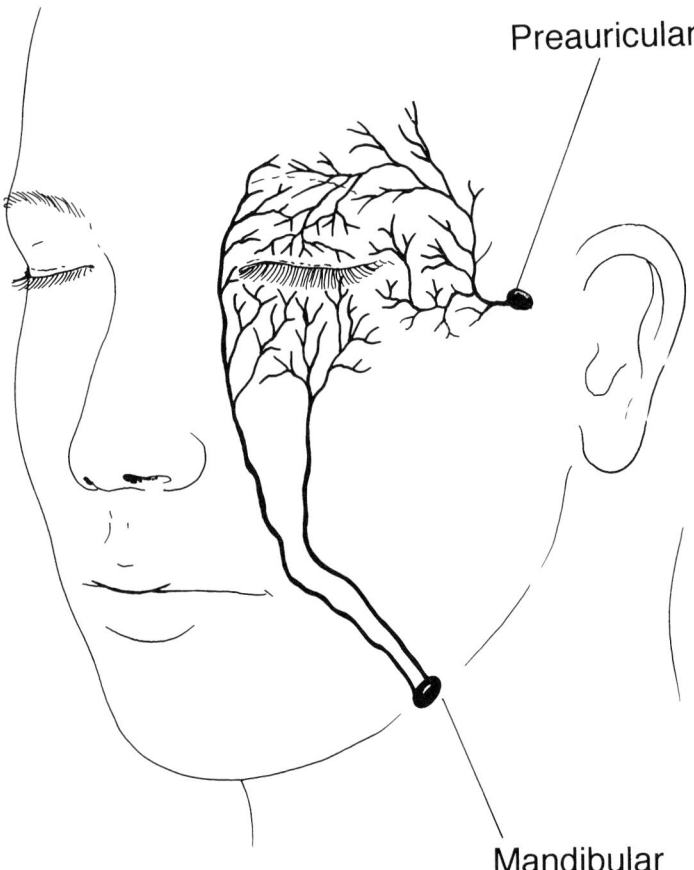

Figure 10.11 *Lymphatic drainage of the eyelids.*

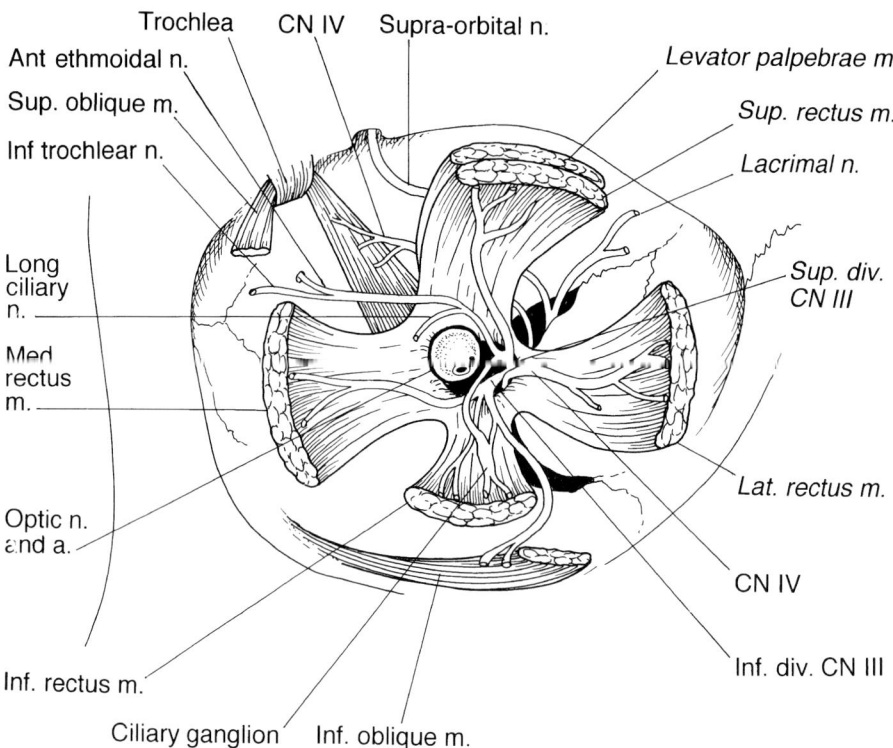

Figure 10.12 *The left orbital apex. Cranial nerves II, III, IV, VI, and VII, as well as the autonomic nerves, enter the orbit at the apex. Key: m = muscle, n = nerve, a = artery.*

to ischemic necrosis after severe blunt orbital trauma (16). The intraorbital portion of the nerve is approximately 30 mm in length and somewhat S-shaped. This configuration allows for full rotation of the globe without compromise of the nerve. The optic nerve enters the globe medial to the visual axis. The diameter of the intraocular portion of the nerve is 1.5 mm, whereas that of the orbital portion is approximately 4 mm because of the myelination of these retrobulbar axons. Within the orbit, the optic nerve is covered by dura mater, the arachnoid membrane, and pia mater. The blood supply to the optic nerve is derived from the internal carotid, ophthalmic, and posterior ciliary arteries.

The third cranial (oculomotor) nerve arises in the midbrain, passes between the posterior cerebral and superior cerebellar arteries, travels alongside the posterior communicating artery, where it is vulnerable to compression from an aneurysm, passes through the cavernous sinus, and enters the orbit through the superior orbital fissure. Soon after entering the orbit, it divides into superior and inferior branches. Both divisions pass through the annulus of Zinn, within which they are separated by the nasociliary nerve. The superior branch provides motor innervation to the superior rectus and levator palpebrae superioris muscles, whereas the inferior branch innervates the inferior and medial recti and the inferior oblique muscles. The oculomotor nerve also carries parasympathetic fibers that travel with the branch to the inferior oblique muscle and that synapse in the ciliary ganglion. Postganglionic parasympathetic fibers enter the globe and contribute to pupillary function.

The ciliary ganglion lies on the lateral aspect of the optic nerve approximately 10 mm anterior to the orbital apex. As mentioned above, parasympathetic fibers constricting the pupil synapse within the ganglion. Sympathetic fibers that dilate the pupil pass through the ciliary ganglion without synapsing. Sensory fibers from the nasociliary nerve also pass through the ciliary ganglion before continuing as the short ciliary nerves.

The fourth cranial (trochlear) nerve arises from the dorsal brain stem and then courses anteriorly, passing through the cavernous sinus en route to the orbit. It enters the orbit via the superior orbital fissure and carries motor innervation to the superior oblique muscle. The trochlear nerve has the longest intracranial course of all the cranial nerves and is relatively easily damaged after blunt head trauma.

The fifth cranial (trigeminal) nerve has both sensory and motor fibers. It arises from several subnuclei within the brain stem and spinal cord and has three major branches: ophthalmic, maxillary, and mandibular. The first two of these branches supply orbital and ocular structures. The ophthalmic branch travels within the cavernous sinus, where it divides into the lacrimal, frontal, and nasociliary nerves (Fig. 10.13). The lacrimal nerve enters the orbit through the superior orbital fissure, above the annulus of Zinn, and courses along the lateral orbital wall, where it is joined by fibers from the zygomatic nerve carrying parasympathetic innervation to the lacrimal gland. The lacrimal nerve then exits the orbit and provides sensory innervation to the skin of the lateral upper eyelid. The frontal nerve, the largest of the three branches of the ophthalmic nerve, also enters the orbit through the superior orbital fissure, above the annulus of Zinn. This nerve travels along the orbital roof between the levator and the periorbita. It divides into its two terminal branches, the supraorbital and supratrochlear nerves that exit the orbit, providing innervation to

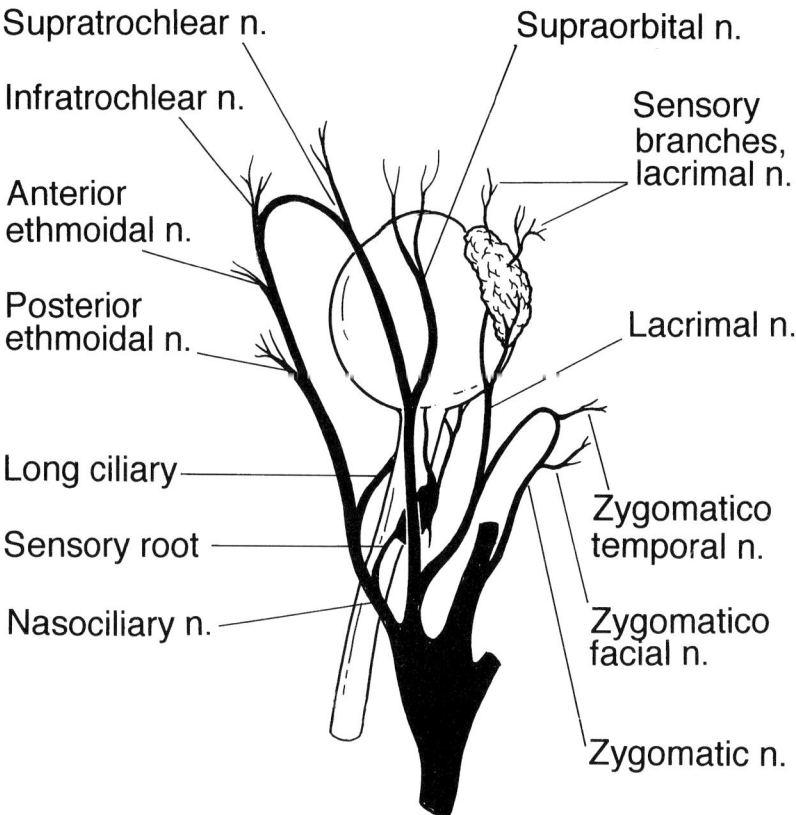

Figure 10.13 *The distribution of the ophthalmic division of the fifth cranial nerve within the orbit. Key: n = nerve.*

the remainder of the upper eyelid and brow. The third branch of the ophthalmic nerve is the nasociliary nerve. It also enters the orbit through the superior orbital fissure; however, in contrast to the lacrimal and frontal nerves, it passes through the annulus of Zinn. It then turns toward the medial orbital wall and divides into the ciliary ganglion (see above). As the nasociliary nerve travels along the medial orbital wall, it gives rise to the long ciliary nerves, which provide sensation to the globe and carry sympathetic fibers to the dilator muscle of the iris. The nasociliary nerve continues anteriorly in the medial orbit, where it produces the anterior and posterior ethmoidal and infratrochlear nerves. These nerves supply the ethmoidal and nasal mucosa. The infratrochlear nerve, the terminal branch of the nasociliary nerve, exits the orbit to supply sensory innervation to the lacrimal sac, conjunctiva, and skin of the medial canthal region.

The sixth cranial (abducens) nerve arises in the ventral pons, courses anteriorly through the cavernous sinus, and enters the orbit through the superior orbital fissure. It passes through the annulus of Zinn before delivering motor nerve supply to the lateral rectus muscle. The long course of the abducens nerve makes it vulnerable to injury from a variety of conditions, including tumors, infections, inflammation, and microvascular infarctions.

The maxillary nerve, the second branch of cranial nerve V, travels briefly within the cavernous sinus before exiting through the foramen rotundum to enter the pterygopalatine fossa. It is here that the zygomaticotemporal nerve branches off, carrying parasympathetic fibers that will join the lacrimal nerve before entering the lacrimal gland. The terminal branch of the maxillary nerve is the infraorbital nerve that runs anteriorly in the infraorbital groove before exiting the maxilla several millimeters below the inferior orbital rim. In its location on the orbital floor, the infraorbital nerve is susceptible to injury when orbital floor fractures occur, as is common after blunt trauma. Symptoms of infraorbital nerve damage include numbness of the lower eyelid, side of the nose, upper lip, and upper teeth on the involved side. In some cases, these may be the only symptoms of an orbital fracture. The third division of the trigeminal nerve does not innervate orbital or adnexal structures and is not discussed here.

Although not a nerve of the orbit, the seventh cranial (facial) nerve innervates the muscles of the brow, eyelids, and face and thus bears discussion here. The facial nerve arises from nuclei within the brain stem and carries motor, sensory, and parasympathetic fibers to the face and brow. It travels within the temporal bone, where it is susceptible to injury from inflammation, trauma, and tumors before exiting the skull at the stylomastoid foramen. Parasympathetic secretory innervation is carried to the submandibular, sublingual, and lacrimal (via the maxillary nerve) glands. The motor fibers of the facial nerve divide into upper and lower trunks that then distribute to the muscles of the brow, orbicularis oculi muscles of the eyelids, and the muscles of facial expression. The facial nerve lies in close proximity to the parotid gland.

The autonomic nerve supply to the orbit, consisting of sympathetic and parasympathetic fibers, has already been discussed in the sections above. To briefly review, ocular parasympathetic fibers originate in the third nerve nucleus, travel with the inferior division of the oculomotor nerve within the orbit, and enter the globe with the short posterior ciliary nerves. These fibers control pupillary constriction, and damage anywhere along their course will result in a dilated pupil. Parasympathetic fibers also travel to the orbit with the facial nerve for secretomotor innervation of the lacrimal gland. Sympathetic fibers supplying the orbit innervate the iris dilator muscle and Müller's muscle, a retractor of the upper and lower lids. These fibers originate in the hypothalamus and travel to the orbit after synapsing in the cervical spinal cord and the superior cervical ganglion. They enter the skull via their close association with the internal carotid artery and are carried to their final destination by smaller blood vessels. Interruption of ocular sympathetic fibers results in blepharoptosis (drooping of the eyelid) from lack of innervation of Müller's muscle, miosis (small pupil) from loss of innervation to the iris dilator, and sometimes anhydrosis (loss of sweating) if the fibers traveling with branches of the external carotid artery that supply sweat glands are involved. This constellation of symptoms is known as Horner's syndrome and may be seen in a number of clinical situations (17).

Muscles of the Orbit

The extraocular muscles, levator palpebrae superioris, and Müller's muscle are all found within the orbit. There are six extraocular muscles, four rectus muscles and two obliques (see Fig. 10.7), that work together in a complicated but well-coordinated fashion in allowing the eyes to look simultaneously at a given object, move together in all directions, and move in opposite directions (convergence or divergence) when necessary.

The medial and lateral recti are the horizontal rectus muscles. They arise from the annulus of Zinn and insert 5.5 and 6.9 mm from the limbus, respectively. Their primary action produces rotation of the globes in the horizontal plane. The medial rectus is innervated by the inferior division of the oculomotor nerve, and its blood supply is from muscular branches of the ophthalmic artery. The lateral rectus is innervated by the abducens nerve and is the only rectus muscle to receive its blood supply from a single muscular artery. The vertical rectus muscles consisting of the superior and inferior recti act primarily to provide ocular rotation in the vertical plane. They also arise from the annulus of Zinn and pass forward to insert 7.7 and 6.5 mm posterior to the limbus, respectively. The levator palpebrae superioris, the primary elevator of the upper eyelid, travels in close association with the superior rectus, as does the superior ophthalmic vein. The superior rectus muscle receives innervation from the superior division of the oculomotor nerve, whereas the inferior rectus is innervated by the inferior division of cranial nerve III.

The oblique muscles are slightly more complex. Their primary action is torsion of the globe, the superior oblique allowing intorsion and the inferior oblique extorsion. The superior oblique muscle arises from the greater wing of the sphenoid and passes anteriorly in the superomedial orbit, where it becomes tendinous. The tendon passes through the trochlea, a cartilaginous structure located inside the superior orbital rim that acts as a pulley and changes the direction of force applied to the globe from vertical to horizontal. After passing through the trochlea, the tendon inserts on the sclera in the superolateral quadrant of the globe. The superior oblique is innervated by the trochlear nerve, and its blood supply is from branches of the ophthalmic artery. The inferior oblique originates from the periosteum of the maxilla, passes beneath the inferior rectus muscle, and inserts in the inferolateral quadrant of the globe. It is innervated by the inferior division of cranial nerve III and receives its blood supply from the ophthalmic and infraorbital arteries (18).

The levator palpebrae superioris originates from the lesser wing of the sphenoid and passes anteriorly above the superior rectus muscle until it becomes tendinous, approximately 10 mm posterior to the orbital septum (Figs. 10.14 and 10.15). The tendon then passes anteriorly and inferiorly to insert on the anterior, superior third of the tarsus, and on the skin, thus forming the eyelid crease. Before its insertion on the tarsus, the levator tendon fuses with the orbital septum. The levator receives support from the insertion of its medial and lateral extensions (known as horns), which insert on the posterior lacrimal crest and lateral orbital tubercle, respectively. The lateral horn of the levator muscle divides the lacrimal gland into its orbital and palpebral lobes. Whitnall's ligament is a special modification of the levator muscle. This fibrous structure acts as a check suspensory ligament, preventing excessive posterior movement of the levator and providing mechanical support for the levator. The orientation of the muscle fibers changes in the region of Whitnall's ligament from anterior-posterior to superior-inferior. The ligament is an important landmark in eyelid surgery and in repairing severely traumatized lids (19). The lower eyelid analogue of Whitnall's ligament is Lockwood's suspensory ligament. Lockwood's ligament is a fibrous structure formed by fascial contributions from Tenon's capsule, the intermuscular septum, and capsulopalpebral fascia. It inserts laterally at the lateral retinaculum, a structure consisting of the lat-

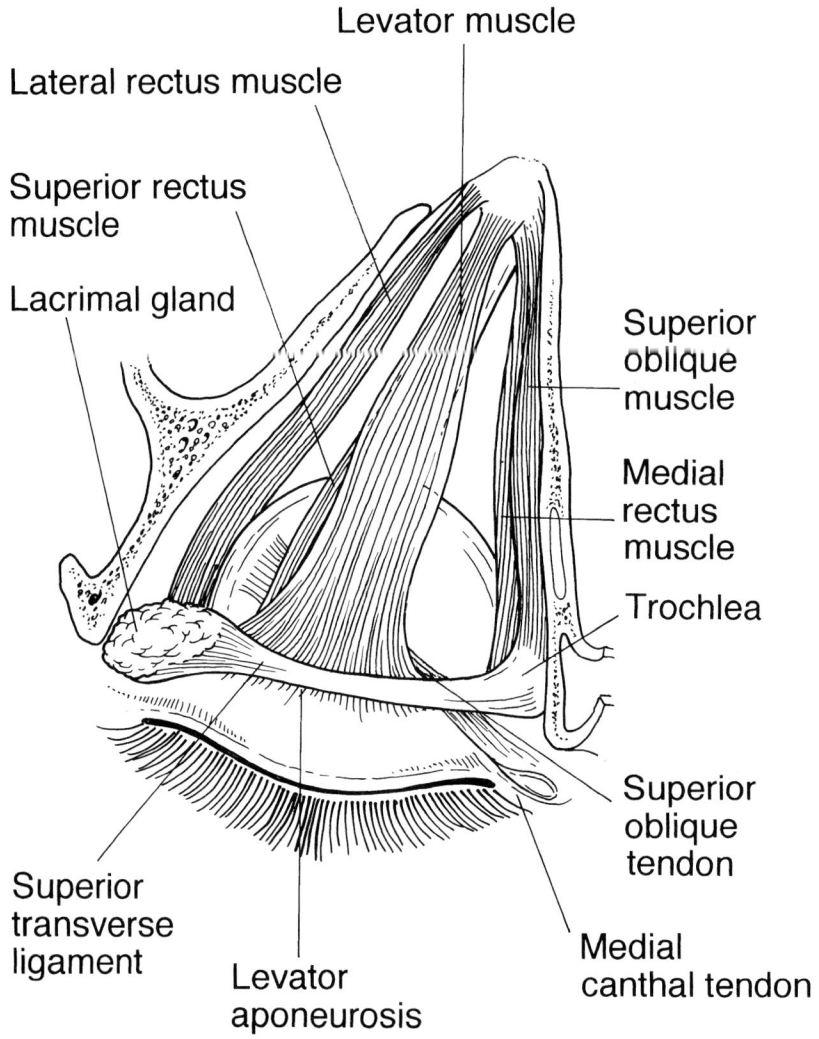

Figure 10.14 *Right orbit as viewed from above.*

eral canthal tendon, lateral horn of the levator aponeurosis, Lockwood's ligament, and the check ligament of the lateral rectus muscle (20).

Müller's superior tarsal muscle and its lower lid counterpart, the inferior tarsal muscle, are the only orbital muscles that are formed from smooth as opposed to striated muscle. Müller's muscle arises from the posterior aspect of the levator aponeurosis near Whitnall's ligament and therefore is located between the conjunctiva and levator aponeurosis. It inserts onto the superior tarsal border and acts as a

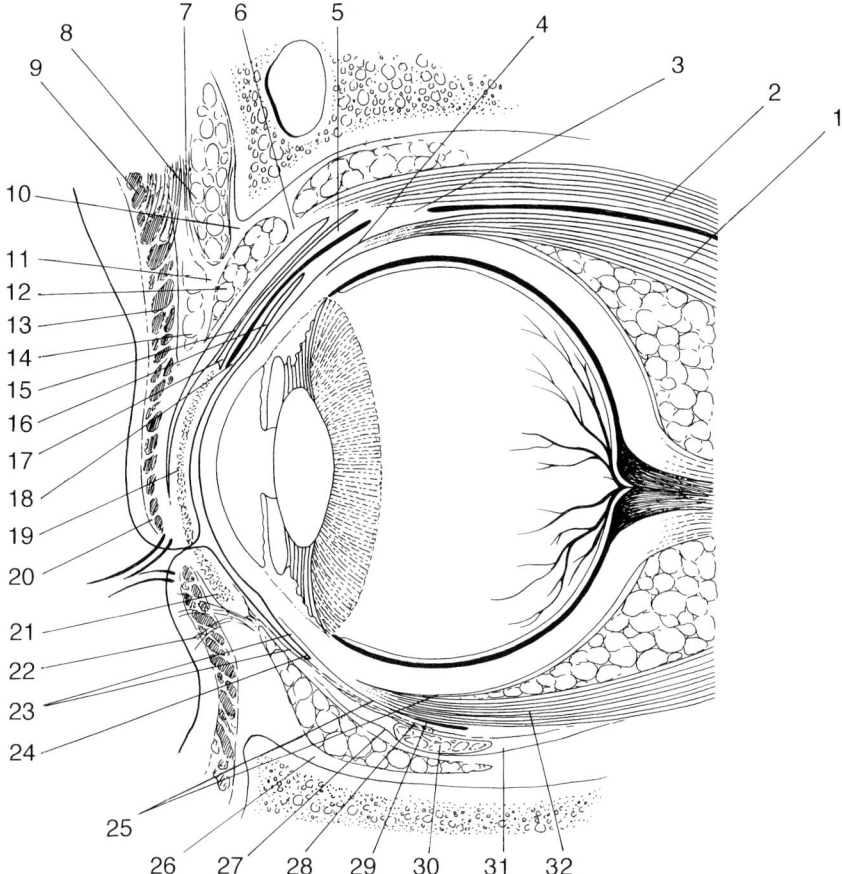

Figure 10.15 *Parasagittal section showing anterior orbital structures. 1, Superior rectus muscle; 2, levator palpebrae superioris muscle; 3, conjoining of superior rectus muscle with levator muscle sheath; 4, Tenon's capsule; 5, suspensory ligament of superior fornix; 6, Whitnall's ligament; 7, frontal muscle; 8, brow fat pad; 9, orbital orbicularis; 10, arcus marginalis; 11, orbital septum; 12, aponeurotic fat pad; 13, preseptal orbicularis; 14, postorbicularis fascia; 15, levator aponeurosis; 16, superior conjunctival fornix; 17, Müller's muscle; 18, conjunctiva; 19, superior tarsus; 20, pretarsal orbicularis; 21, inferior tarsus; 22, musculocutaneous retractor insertion; 23, conjunctiva; 24, inferior conjunctival fornix; 25, Tenon's capsule; 26, inferior septum; 27, Lockwood's ligament; 28, inferior tarsal muscle; 29, suspensory ligament of inferior fornix; 30, inferior oblique muscle; 31, capsulopalpebral fascia; 32, inferior rectus muscle.*

protractor of the lid. The inferior tarsal muscle is often less well defined. Both Müller's muscle and the inferior tarsal muscle are sympathetically innervated (21).

Orbital fat occupies any space not occupied by other orbital structures. In the posterior orbit, the fat can be separated into the intraconal and extraconal fat. The intraconal fat lies within the muscle cone and is separated into lobules by fibrous septae and Tenon's capsule. The extraconal fat is located between the muscles and periorbita and is limited by the septum anteriorly. There are two fat pads in the anterior orbit superiorly and three fat pads inferiorly. The medial and middle fat pads in the lower lids are separated by the inferior oblique muscle.

Eyelid Soft Tissues

The eyelids are important structures that help to protect the globe from injury. Along with the conjunctiva, the eyelids play a critical role in maintaining the integrity of the ocular surface. They blend in smoothly with the eyebrows above and the cheeks below.

The eyelids are separated by the tarsal plate into orbital and tarsal portions. The upper eyelid crease is formed by the insertion of the anterior portion of the levator aponeurosis into the eyelid skin (Fig. 10.16, A and B). In the occidental eyelid, the upper lid crease is usually located 8 to 11 mm above the eyelid margin and is somewhat higher in women than in men. In contrast, the upper lid crease is much lower in the Asian eyelid because of the low fusion of the orbital septum with the levator aponeurosis. In many Asian patients, the upper lid fold will overhang the crease, obscuring it. In the lower eyelid, the crease is less well defined and is formed by the attachment of the orbicularis oculi muscle to the skin. The upper and lower eyelids become fused at the medial and lateral canthi, and traumatic or involutional disruption of these areas can lead to significant eyelid dysfunction or malposition. The opening between the eyelids is known as the palpebral fissure and averages 10 to 12 mm in adults, whereas the horizontal distance between the medial and lateral canthi in normal adults is approximately 30 mm (22). The upper and lower eyelids are lined by a double or triple row of eyelashes, short hairs that normally curve away from the eye. After trauma or other eyelid injury, the lashes may become misdirected such that they turn toward the globe, potentially causing serious disruption of the ocular surface.

The eyelid margin marks the transition from the nonkeratinized epithelium of the conjunctiva to the keratinized epithelium of the

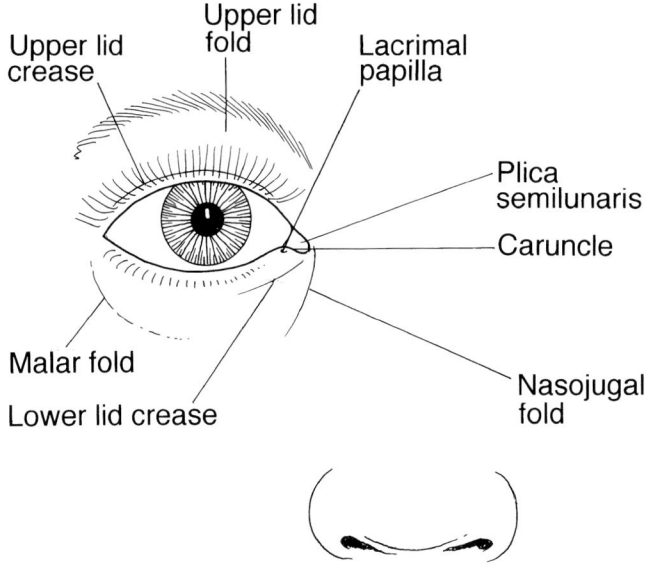

Figure 10.16 *(A) External view of the eyelids with important anatomic landmarks. (B) Sagittal view of upper eyelid, demonstrating the relationship of Müller's muscle and the levator aponeurosis to the tarsus. The formation of the eyelid crease is created by the insertion of the anterior leaf of the levator aponeurosis into the eyelid skin.*

eyelid skin. Convention divides the eyelid margin into anterior and posterior lamellae, the anterior lamella consisting of skin and orbicularis muscle and the posterior lamella consisting of tarsus and conjunctiva. The division between these lamellae is known as the grey line. Within the tarsus lie the meibomian glands, which are sebaceous glands that contribute to the tear film. Other sebaceous glands, known as Zeis' glands, are found at the base of the eyelash follicles.

The skin of the eyelids is one of the thinnest in the body, with very little subcutaneous tissue present. Beneath the eyelid skin is the orbicularis oculi muscle (Fig. 10.17). This muscle is divided into pre-

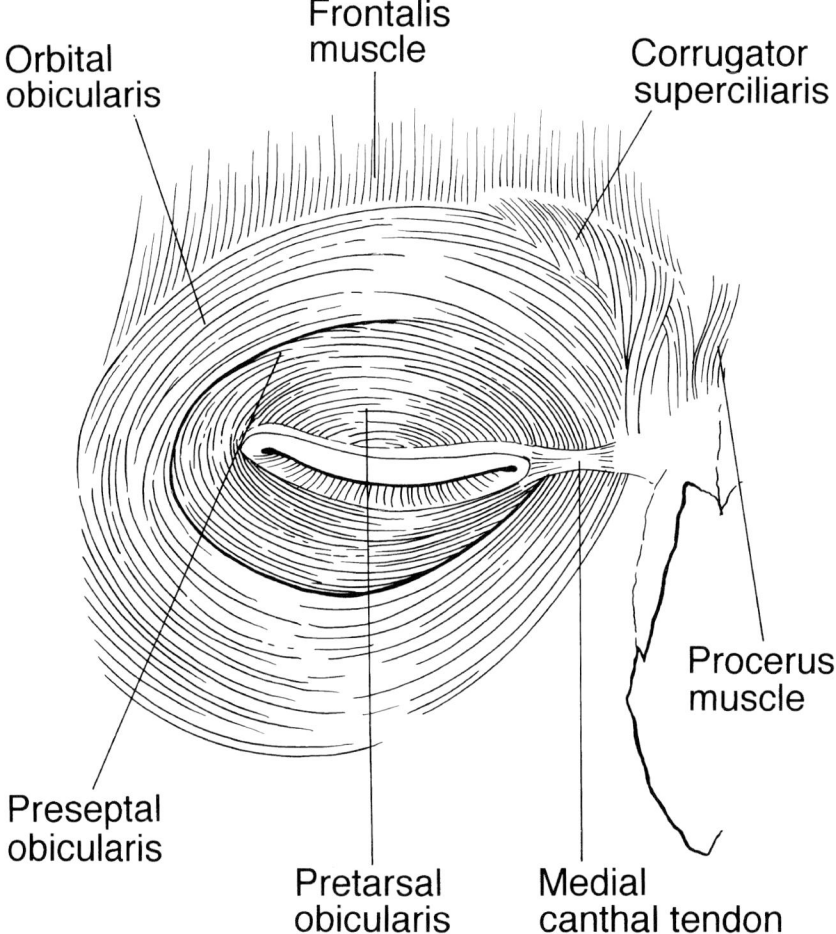

Figure 10.17 *The orbicularis oculi muscle. Note the three divisions of the muscle and the relationship of the orbicularis fibers to the muscles of the eyebrow and forehead.*

tarsal, preseptal, and orbital components. The orbital portion blends with the frontalis, procerus, and corrugator supercilii muscles of the eyebrow superiorly and the temporalis and cheek muscles laterally. Medially, the orbital orbicularis fibers arise from the orbital rim. The preseptal orbicularis overlies the orbital septum and sends deep fibers to insert on the lacrimal sac (Jones' muscle), whereas the pretarsal orbicularis is just anterior to the tarsal plate, a firm structure formed by compressed collagen fibers that acts as the "skeleton" of the eyelids. At its medial aspect, the pretarsal orbicularis splits into superficial and deep heads, the superficial head forming the anterior limb of the medial canthal tendon and inserting on the anterior lacrimal crest, and the deep head (Horner's muscle) inserting on the posterior lacrimal crest and contributing to the posterior limb of the medial canthal tendon. Laterally, the pretarsal orbicularis fibers from the upper and lower eyelids join to form the lateral canthal tendon. This structure may be less well defined than the medial canthal tendon and inserts onto the lateral orbital tubercle. Disruption of either the medial canthal or lateral canthal tendon will result in marked eyelid malposition and/or canthal deformities. Contraction of the orbicularis muscle results in eyelid closure (23).

Deep to the orbicularis lies the orbital septum (Fig. 10.18). The septum is a tough fibrous structure arising from the arcus marginalis at the orbital margin and extending toward the tarsal plates, separating the orbital contents from the eyelids (24). In the upper eyelid, the orbital septum fuses with the levator aponeurosis before their combined insertion onto the anterior surface of the tarsus. In the occidental lid, this fusion occurs several millimeters above the superior tarsal border, whereas in the Asian lid it occurs anterior to the tarsal plate. In the lower eyelid, the orbital septum fuses with the lower lid analogue of the levator aponeurosis, the capsulopalpebral fascia (see "Orbital Fascia," p. 160), before inserting on the tarsal plate (25). The tarsal plates are firm structures composed of condensed collagen that give structure and support to the eyelids. The vertical height of the upper lid tarsus is approximately 10 mm, as compared with 4 mm in the lower lid (25).

The eyelids are lined by conjunctiva, a fine, moist mucous membrane that reflects upon itself superiorly and inferiorly, thus forming the superior and inferior fornices. The conjunctiva provides a surface conducive to normal ocular function. The conjunctiva is lined with a stratified squamous nonkeratinizing epithelium interspersed with unicellular mucus-producing goblet cells.

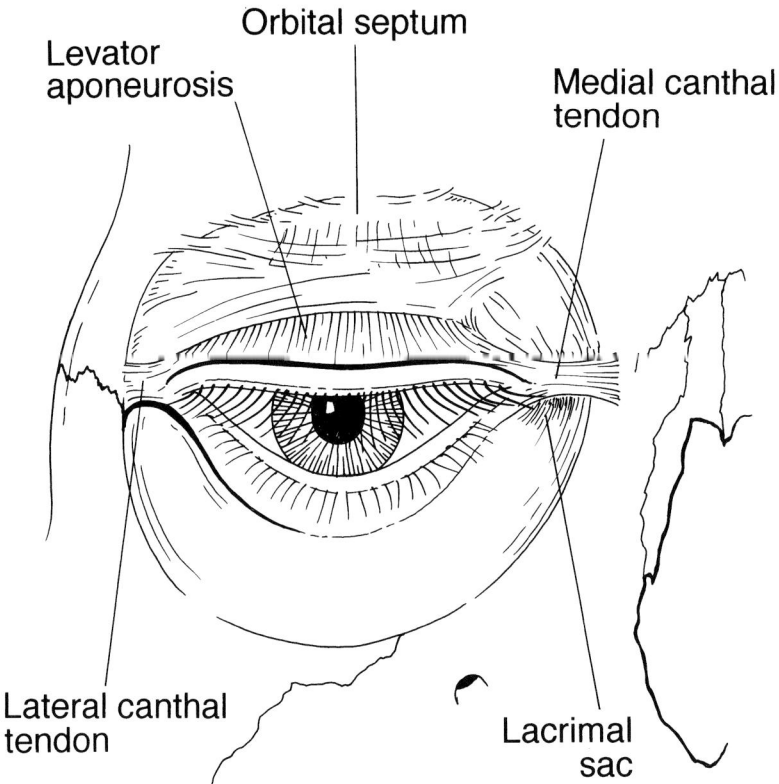

Figure 10.18 *The orbital septum is visible after the orbicularis oculi muscle has been removed. The septum fuses with the levator aponeurosis in the upper eyelid and the capsulopalpebral fascia in the lower eyelid.*

The Lacrimal System

The lacrimal system can be divided for the purpose of description into secretory and excretory components. Together, these components produce a tear film that adequately moisturizes and maintains the external ocular surface.

The lacrimal secretory system is composed primarily of the accessory and main lacrimal glands. The accessory lacrimal glands, Krause's and Wolfring's glands, are found within the conjunctiva, Krause's glands located in the fornices and Wolfring's glands near the tarsal border. A greater number of accessory lacrimal glands are found in the superior than in the inferior fornix. The accessory lacrimal glands are believed to be responsible for baseline tear production.

The main lacrimal gland lies within the lacrimal fossa in the su-

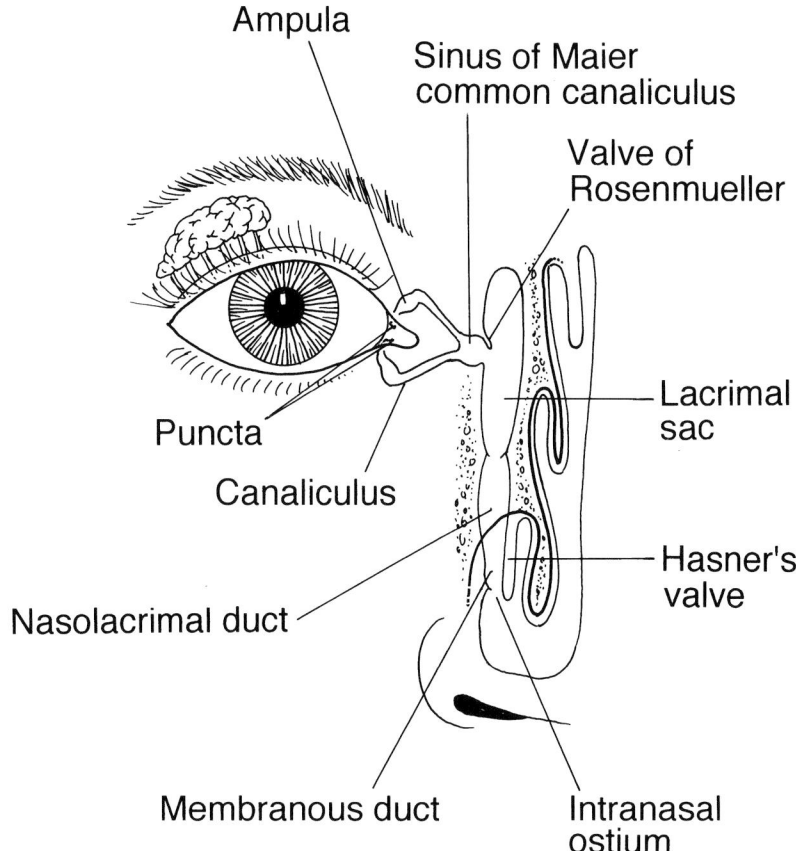

Figure 10.19 *Anatomy of the lacrimal drainage system.*

perolateral orbit (Fig. 10.19). It is divided into a larger superior (orbital) lobe and a smaller inferior (palpebral) lobe by the lateral horn of the levator aponeurosis. At the microscopic level, the lacrimal gland is found to consist of numerous lobules that drain into an anastomosing system of lacrimal ducts. The ducts serve to drain secretions from the gland into the superior fornix, with all ducts passing through the palpebral lobe. Thus, damage to the palpebral lobe will disrupt the flow of secretions from the entire gland. Approximately twelve ducts empty into the superior fornix. As discussed earlier, the lacrimal gland's sensory innervation is provided by the lacrimal nerve, whereas parasympathetic secretomotor fibers reach the gland via the zygomatic nerve. It is believed that tear production by the main lacrimal gland is stimulated centrally (i.e., emotionally) and reflexively in response to stimulation of the fifth cranial nerve.

The lacrimal excretory system functions to drain tears from the eye in a regulated fashion such that the ocular surface is kept moist while at the same time spillover onto the eyelids and cheek is prevented. Along the upper and lower eyelid margins, approximately 5 mm from the medial canthal angle, are elevated nipple-like structures known as the lacrimal papillae. Each papilla represents the opening into the lacrimal canaliculus, an epithelial-lined structure that serves as a conduit for tears from the external surface of the eye to the lacrimal sac. The lacrimal canaliculi have a vertical component measuring 2 mm and a horizontal component measuring 8 mm (see Fig. 10.19). Near the lacrimal sac, the upper and lower canaliculi usually fuse, forming the common canaliculus, which then enters the lacrimal sac. The lacrimal sac is a tubular structure lined with respiratory epithelium and is found in the lacrimal fossa between the anterior and posterior lacrimal crests. Superiorly, it extends a few millimeters above the medial canthal tendon, and inferiorly it is continuous with the nasolacrimal duct. As they blink, the eyelids interact with the lacrimal excretory system in a complicated fashion to drain tears into the lacrimal sac. From the sac, tears then drain inferiorly into the nasopharynx, where they are swallowed. Injury to the medial aspect of the eyelids may result in disruption of the lacrimal excretory system. If such injuries are not recognized and properly repaired, permanent destruction of the lacrimal drainage system may result (26,27).

References

1. Kronish JW, Gonnering RS, Dortzback RK, et al. The pathophysiology of the anophthalmic socket. Part II. Analysis of orbital fat. Ophthal Plast Reconstr Surg 1990;6:88.
2. Bosniak SL, Tizes BR. Trimalar fractures: diagnosis and treatment. Adv Ophthal Plast Reconstr Surg 1987;6:403–414.
3. Dodick JM, Galin MA, Littleton JT, Sod LM. Concomitant medial wall fracture and blowout fracture of the orbit. Arch Ophthalmol 1971;85: 273–276.
4. Smith B, Regan WF. Blowout fracture of the orbit. Am J Ophthalmol 1957; 44:733–739.
5. Doxanas MT, Anderson RL. Clinical orbital anatomy. Baltimore: Williams and Wilkins, 1984:28–29.
6. Warwick R, ed. Eugene Wolff's anatomy of the eye and orbit. Philadelphia: WB Saunders, 1976:130–135.
7. Koorneef L. New insights in the human orbital connective tissue: results of a new anatomic approach. Arch Ophthalmol 1977;95:1269–1273.

8. Koorneef L. Orbital septa: anatomy and function. Ophthalmology 1979; 86:876–885.
9. Koorneef L. Orbital connective tissue. In: Duane TD, Jaeger EA, eds. Biomedical foundations of ophthalmology. vol. 1. Philadelphia: Harper and Row, 1988:1–23.
10. Hayreh SS, Dass R. The ophthalmic artery. I. Origin and intracranial and intracanalicular course. Br J Ophthalmol 1962;46:65–98.
11. Hayreh SS. The ophthalmic artery. III. Branches. Br J Ophthalmol 1962;46: 217–247.
12. Hayreh SS. Arteries of the orbit in the human being. Br J Surg 1963;50: 938–953.
13. Hayreh SS, Dass R. The ophthalmic artery. II. Intraorbital course. Br J Ophthalmol 1962;46:165–185.
14. Brisman J. Orbital phlebography. III. Topography of orbital veins. Acta Radiol 1974;15:577–594.
15. Sherman DD, Gonnering RS, Wallow IHL, et al. Identification of orbital lymphatics: enzyme histochemical light microscopic and electron microscopic studies. Ophthal Plast Reconstr Surg 1993;9:153–169.
16. Anderson RL, Panje WR, Gross CE. Optic nerve blindness following blunt forehead trauma. Ophthalmol 1982;89:445–455.
17. Thompson HS, Mensher JH. Horner's syndrome. Am J Ophthalmol 1974; 78:739.
18. Scott AB. Ocular motility. In: Duane TD, Jaeger EA, eds. Biomedical foundations of ophthalmology. vol. 2. Philadelphia: Harper and Row, 1988:1–60.
19. Anderson RL, Beard C. The levator aponeurosis attachments and their clinical significance. Arch Ophthalmol 1977;95:1437–1441.
20. Hawes MJ, Dortzbach RK. The microscopic anatomy of the lower eyelid retractors. Arch Ophthalmol 1982;100:1313–1318.
21. Beard C. Müller's superior tarsal muscle: anatomy, physiology, and clinical significance. Ann Plast Surg 1985;14:324–333.
22. Callahan M, Beard C, eds. Beard's ptosis. 4th ed. Birmingham: Aesculapius, 1990:22–37.
23. Doxanas MT, Anderson RL. Clinical orbital anatomy. Baltimore: Williams and Wilkins, 1984.
24. Putterman AM, Urist MJ. Surgical anatomy of the orbital septum. Ann Ophthalmol 1974;6:290–294.
25. Wesley RE, McCord CD, Jones NA. Height of the tarsus of the lower eyelid. Am J Ophthalmol 1980;90:102–105.
26. Jones LT. The lacrimal secretory system and its treatment. Am J Ophthalmol 1966;62:47–60.
27. Iwamoto T, Jakobiec FA. Lacrimal glands. In: Duane TD, Jaeger EA, eds. Biomedical foundations of ophthalmology. vol. 1. Philadelphia: Harper and Row, 1988:1–21.

CHAPTER 11

Anterior Segment Injuries

Roopinder K. Grewal
Deepinder K. Dhaliwal
Peter S. Hersh
Bruce M. Zagelbaum

Sports-related trauma is a significant cause of ocular morbidity. Of the more than 2.4 million eye injuries that occur in the United States annually, 100,000 are sports related (1). Each year, hospital emergency departments treat over 40,000 eye injuries that are sports and recreation related (2). Eye injuries are often disabling and create enormous costs to both the victim and society (3). In a 1-year prospective study of sports-related ocular trauma conducted at the Massachusetts Eye and Ear Infirmary, 202 patients were evaluated; 13.8% required hospitalization, and 5.6% required intraocular surgery (4). Overall, 12.8% of these patients sustained permanent ocular sequelae, including 3.5%, who suffered visual loss.

Clinical Evaluation

Many minor sports-related eye injuries can be treated by health care professionals (i.e., trainers, team physicians, team ophthalmologists) with the appropriate medical equipment and supplies (5). Initial evaluation of the eye trauma patient must be performed in a timely manner because rapid diagnosis and treatment are essential to optimize visual outcome. Although most sports-related ocular injuries are minor in nature, a high index of suspicion for occult and more serious damage is critical for properly dealing with the injured athlete.

A thorough eye examination should always be performed on both eyes when any ocular injury occurs. Moreover, it is important to prevent further damage by avoiding manipulation of the globe and inappropriate examination techniques. For example, if a ruptured globe is suspected given the history and initial examination findings, precautions must be taken to reduce the possibility of extrusion of intraocular contents. A rigid eye shield should be taped over the eye to eliminate external pressure on the globe and prevent further inadvertent injury. The patient should be given appropriate medications to prevent nausea, vomiting, coughing, and straining, which may increase pressure on the eye. No ocular medications should be instilled until the diagnosis of ruptured globe has been excluded, and the patient should be immediately transferred to a medical center for further evaluation and treatment by an ophthalmologist.

The Anterior Segment

History

After all life-threatening and neurologic conditions that require immediate medical management are addressed, a history of the events surrounding the injury should be elicited. Inquiries should be made regarding the sports environment, mechanism, and time of injury. The use of contact lenses, spectacles, or protective eyewear should be determined, and if used, these items should be examined for any damage. Past ocular history, including previous visual acuity and any preexisting ocular conditions such as amblyopia, previous trauma, or ophthalmic surgery, is important. The patient's general medical history should also be obtained, including medications and allergies. In most instances, the initial examination of an athlete with an eye injury will take place at the sporting event. For this reason, an emergency first-aid kit for ocular examination should always be available (Table 11.1). The primary objective of the physical examination is to determine the extent of injury, enabling planning for treatment and referral as needed.

Examination

External Examination

Face and Eyelids: The physical examination of a patient with eye trauma should begin with the external examination. The eyelids and periorbital area should be inspected for abrasions, lacerations, puncture wounds, erythema, hemorrhage, subcutaneous emphysema, or any particulate matter. Any bleeding from skin wounds should be controlled with tamponade, taking care not to place pressure on the

Table 11.1 Eye injuries: first-aid kit for evaluation and treatment

Emergency telephone numbers
  Local hospital emergency room/team ophthalmologist
Near-reading card
Occluder
Penlight with cobalt blue filter
Wire lid speculum, adult and pediatric
Schiotz tonometer or tonopen (if possible)
Topical anesthetic (i.e., 0.5% proparacaine solution)
Dilating agents (i.e., 2.5% neosynephrine ophthalmic solution and 1% tropicamide ophthalmic solution)
Fluorescein strips
Cotton-tipped applicators (sterile)
Eye pads/eye shield (plastic or metal)
Tape
Sterile ocular irrigant (squeeze bottle)
Topical antibiotics (i.e., tobramycin ophthalmic solution)
Contact lens case and solutions
Sterile gauze sponges
Sterile hemostat and straight scissor

globe if a rupture is suspected. The skin may be gently cleansed with a sterile gauze sponge and sterile saline solution to facilitate examination of the injured tissue and to detect small wounds. If an eyelid laceration is present, its location and borders should be described. Lacerations through the lid margin and involvement of the lacrimal drainage system should be noted because they will require special surgical repair.

Fractures of the orbital bones or sinuses may be indicated by subcutaneous emphysema or abnormal positioning of the globe relative to other facial structures. The orbital and facial bones may be palpated for a "step-off," or area of discontinuity. The patient's upper cheek on the affected side should be checked for any skin anesthesia that may indicate orbital fracture with involvement of a branch of the trigeminal nerve.

Ocular Surface and Adnexa: Overall initial external examination of the globe should include inspection of the eye and ocular adnexa (Figs. 11.1 and 11.2). The examiner should carefully look for any foreign bodies, including the presence of contact lenses if worn. Large foreign bodies remaining in the orbit or globe should not be removed until a full examination is performed by an ophthalmologist. Sub-

Anterior Segment Injuries 187

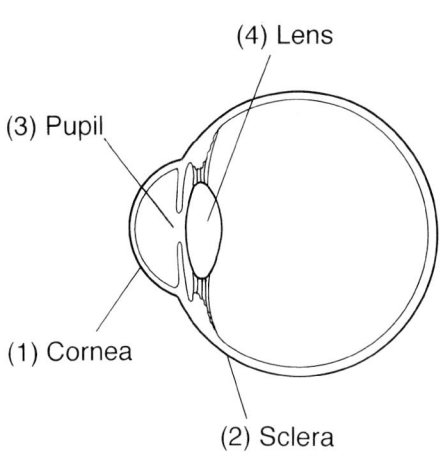

Figure 11.1 Side view of the globe showing the (1) cornea, (2) sclera, (3) pupil, and (4) lens.

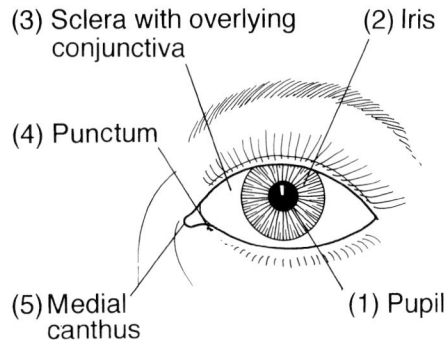

Figure 11.2 External view of the left eye showing (1) the pupil, (2) iris, (3) sclera with overlying conjunctiva, (4) punctum, and (5) medial canthus.

conjunctival edema, hemorrhage, conjunctival/corneal lacerations, and the presence of an obvious hyphema should be noted. If intraocular contents are noted outside the globe or an obvious rupture is noted, further damage to the globe should be prevented by placement of an eye shield over the eye (Fig. 11.3A). If an eye shield is not available, one may be fashioned by cutting the base off a paper cup (Fig. 11.3B). Further examination should be performed by an ophthalmologist.

Visual Acuity

Visual acuity should be assessed after the initial overall evaluation. The examiner should test both eyes independently, checking one eye while the other is covered, even if the injury involves only one eye. In an emergency setting, a near card (Fig. 11.4) may be used to obtain an estimate of baseline visual acuity. The patient should be questioned regarding the use of reading glasses, and, if applicable, they should be worn when testing near visual acuity. Each eye is covered separately and the patient is asked to read the smallest line visible at his or her optimal reading distance. If a near card is unavailable, a newspaper or magazine can be used. If a patient is unable to read any letters, the examiner should ask the patient to count the number of fingers held up at different distances. A determination of hand movement or light perception vision using a penlight or flashlight should be made if the patient is unable to count fingers. If unable to

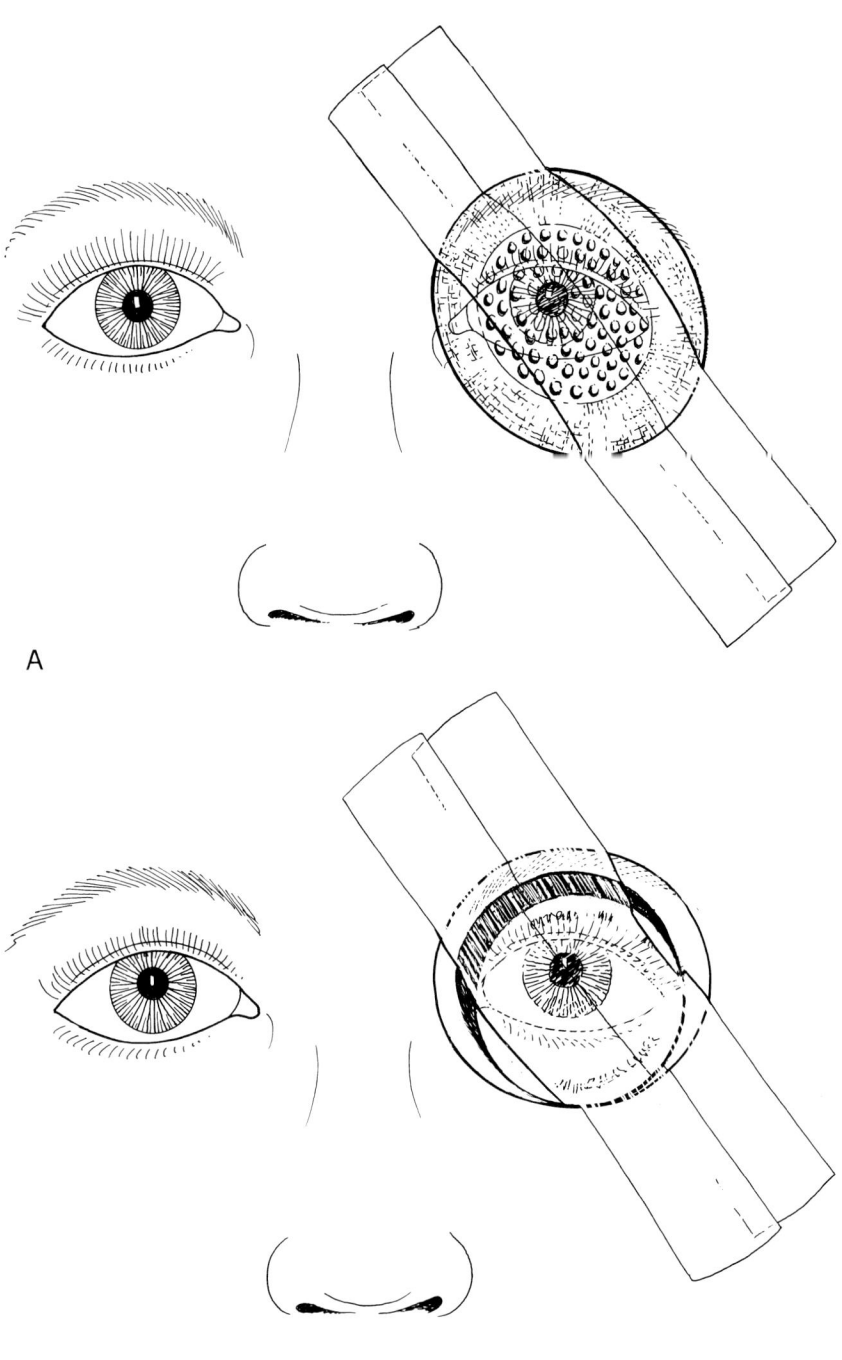

Figure 11.3 If there is any suspicion of a ruptured globe, a protective shield should be placed over the eye immediately. (A) A rigid shield is placed over the affected eye with tape running in an oblique fashion. (B) If a shield is not available, the bottom of a cup (i.e., styrofoam) may be used to protect the eye.

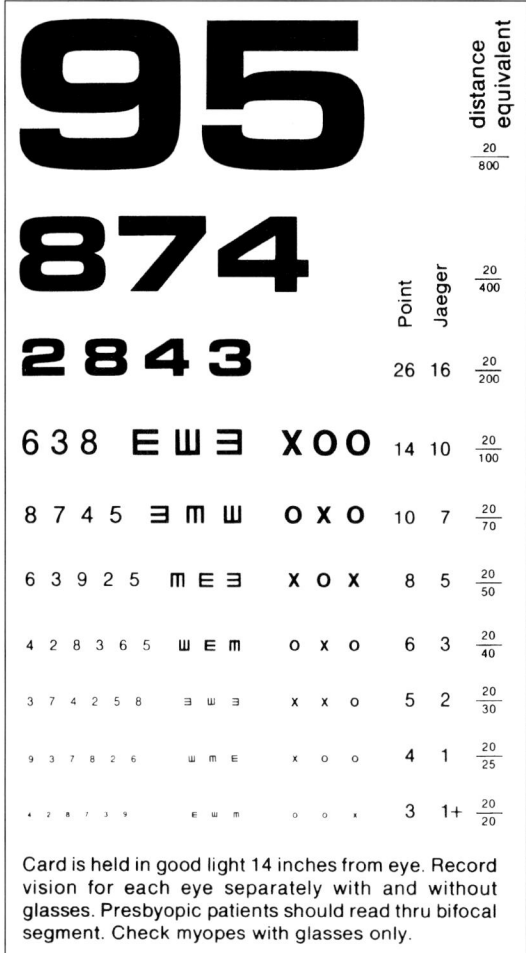

Figure 11.4 *When checking visual acuity, a near card may be used. Be sure to test each eye individually.*

detect bright light, the patient's visual acuity is referred to as no light perception. There should be careful documentation of the manner in which visual acuity is tested, including the use of corrective lenses (i.e., glasses) and whether distance or near vision was tested. One of the primary goals of the eye examination is to explain the cause of the visual decrease noted.

Pupils

Most pupillary irregularities are associated with a pathologic process. Using a penlight, the examiner should inspect both pupils for size, shape, and reaction to light. Blunt injury characteristically may create either a small constricted pupil (miosis) (Fig. 11.5A) or a large dilated pupil (mydriasis) (Fig. 11.5B). A dilated pupil in a head-injured patient may indicate increased intracranial pressure with associated neurologic abnormalities. Mydriasis may also be caused by iris pupillary sphincter tears or pharmacologic agents.

Direct and consensual pupillary responses to light are important aspects of the pupillary examination. The direct response is determined by observing the reaction of the pupil to a bright light shone directly in one eye and then the other while the patient is fixating on a distant target (Fig. 11.6). Fixating on a near target will invoke the accommodative response, causing the pupils to constrict. The swinging light pupil test will determine the presence of a relative afferent pupillary defect (RAPD) (6). A light is held over one eye for 3 seconds and then quickly moved to the opposite eye for the same length of time. The light is swung back and forth in this manner while carefully observing the pupillary response. Classically, the affected pupil will dilate when light is shone upon it, indicating a defect in the afferent optic nerve function. The presence of an RAPD is a significant finding in any trauma patient; it may signify optic nerve trauma and requires further investigation.

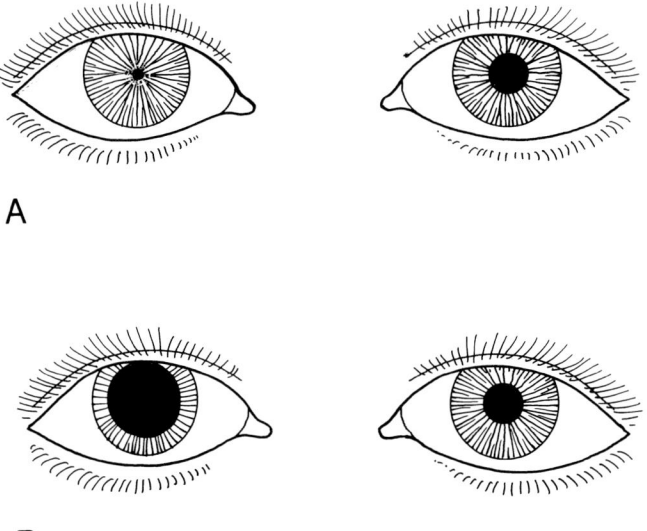

Figure 11.5 *In the examination, check the pupils for any irregularity. (A) A constricted (miotic) right pupil; (B) a dilated (mydriatic) right pupil.*

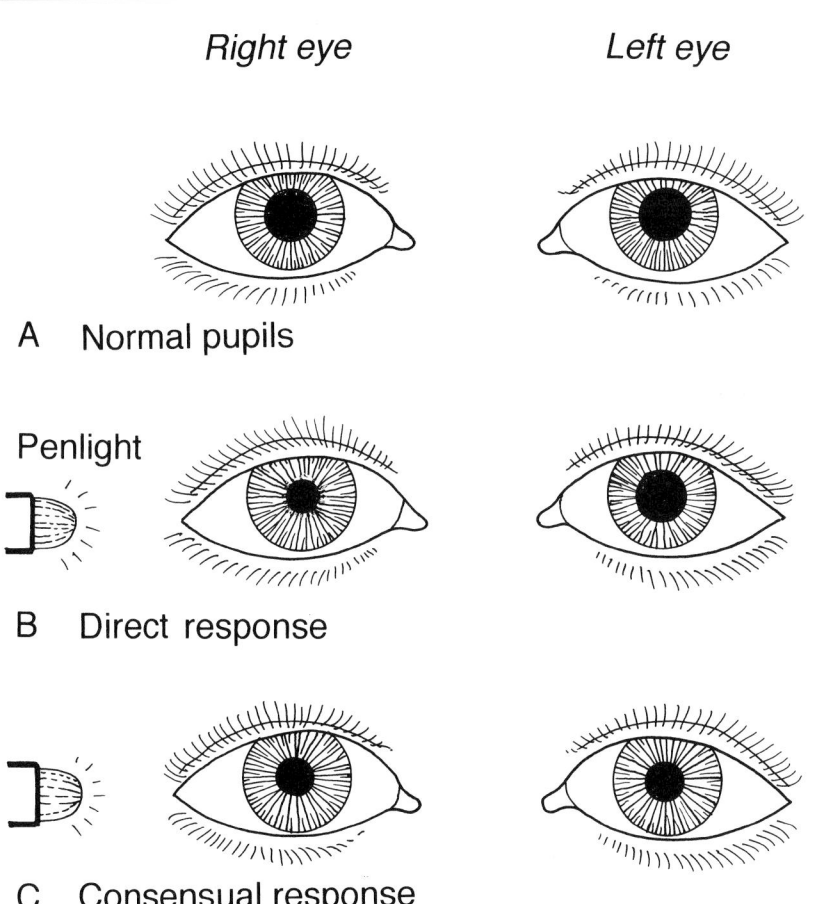

Figure 11.6 *Shining a penlight in one eye should cause direct pupillary constriction in one eye as well as a consensual response (constriction) in the other eye.*

Extraocular Movements

Abnormalities in extraocular motility may indicate the presence of orbital wall and/or floor fractures, nerve injury, injury to the muscle itself, or restriction from intraorbital edema. Motility is assessed by asking the patient to look up, down, right, and left with careful observation of any signs of restriction or paresis of movement (Plate 8). Motility should not be tested if a ruptured globe is suspected, because contraction of the extraocular muscles may cause sufficient elevation of intraocular pressure with extrusion of intraocular contents.

Anterior Segment Examination

Examination of the anterior segment should be performed in a methodical fashion. The examiner should not jump directly to the most obvious site of injury. In the field, a penlight examination is acceptable.

After the external evaluation, the conjunctiva should be inspected, beginning with the eyelid margins and proceeding to the palpebral conjunctiva, fornices, and bulbar conjunctiva. The presence of foreign bodies, lacerations, hemorrhage, edema, and injection is noted. The presence of any darkly pigmented material under the conjunctiva should be viewed with suspicion because this may represent the eye's intraocular contents protruding through a scleral perforation.

The cornea is then examined with a penlight for clarity and the presence of abrasions, foreign bodies, or lacerations. If the patient is in pain, a drop of topical anesthetic (i.e., 0.5% proparacaine) may be instilled. After initial examination of the cornea, a fluorescein strip may be dampened with a drop of sterile saline and touched to the inner surface of the lower eyelid (Fig. 11.7). Care should be taken to avoid touching the cornea directly with the fluorescein strip because this may cause a corneal abrasion. The patient is then asked to blink several times to distribute the fluorescein dye over the surface of the eye. Fluorescein stain is taken up by the de-epithelialized cornea, thus indicating the presence of a corneal abrasion. The use of a penlight will help identify an area with absent corneal epithelium (corneal abrasion) that will appear bright green. If accessible, a cobalt blue filter should be placed over the penlight to facilitate visualization of areas of fluorescein staining. Fluorescein may also be used to identify conjunctival abrasions (Plate 9).

If a corneal foreign body or laceration is identified, the patient should be carefully examined at a slit-lamp by an ophthalmologist to determine the depth of corneal penetration. Corneal edema secondary to injury will appear as a clouding (haze) of the cornea (Plate 10).

Examination of the anterior chamber is best performed with a slit-lamp. In the field, however, a penlight can be used to assess the anterior chamber depth by shining the light obliquely from the temporal side and judging the distance between the cornea and the iris (Fig. 11.8). The presence of a hyphema (blood in the anterior chamber, which is usually seen to layer inferiorly) should be identified (Plate 11). Slit-lamp examination allows the examiner to identify the presence of traumatic iritis by noting a cell-and-flare reaction in the anterior chamber. Such a reaction is a consequence of breakdown of the blood-aqueous barrier with liberation of inflammatory cells and molecules into the anterior chamber.

Next, the iris is inspected for any irregularities in the shape and size of the pupils. Peaking of the pupil may represent an occult scleral rupture with prolapse of intraocular contents (Plate 12). An irregular pupillary border may be secondary to pupillary sphincter tears, which may also affect the ability of the pupil to react to light. Iris sphincter tears are best evaluated under high magnification using a slit-lamp.

Intraocular Pressure

Determination of intraocular pressure is particularly important in the presence of a hyphema or retrobulbar hemorrhage. Intraocular pressure should never be measured in the presence of a ruptured globe because this may cause further injury to the globe or extrusion of

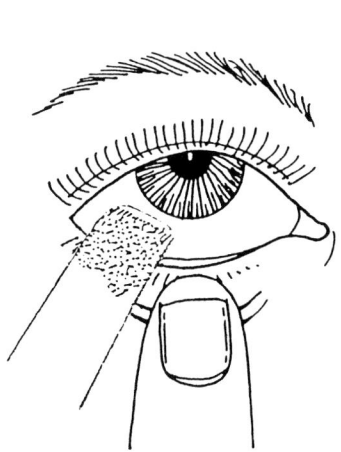

Figure 11.7 *The correct method of applying fluorescein stain is to touch the moistened fluorescein strip to the lower conjunctiva while the patient looks up.*

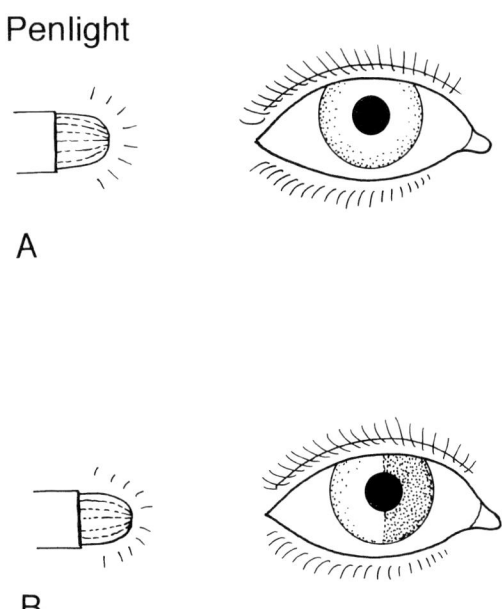

Figure 11.8 *Estimating the depth of the anterior chamber is assessed by shining a penlight from the temporal side. (A) A deep anterior chamber shows the iris completely illuminated, whereas (B) a shallow anterior chamber shows a shadow on the far side.*

intraocular contents. Intraocular pressure can be measured using a Schiotz tonometer or tonopen, if available, after instilling a drop of anesthetic. A more accurate method would be applanation tonometry using a slit-lamp.

Diagnosis and Management

Corneal Abrasions

Corneal abrasions are defects in the corneal epithelium. Symptoms include pain, photophobia, foreign-body sensation, and tearing. Diagnosis is made by the use of fluorescein sodium dye that is taken up by de-epithelialized tissue. The presence of bright green fluorescence identifies the area of absent corneal epithelium (Plate 13). If a corneal stromal infiltrate (whitening) is associated with an epithelial defect (Plate 14), the patient should be immediately referred to an ophthalmologist to rule out an infectious corneal ulcer. Other signs associated with a corneal abrasion include conjunctival injection (redness), anterior chamber inflammation (iritis), and eyelid edema. Vertical linear abrasions on the cornea should alert the examiner to look for a foreign body under the eyelid. The eyelids should be everted to rule out the presence of a foreign body that may be lodged in the fornices or embedded under the lids (Fig. 11.9 and Plate 15). The patient should also be carefully questioned regarding the use of contact lenses, which can predispose the patient with a corneal abrasion to develop a corneal ulcer.

Treatment of a corneal abrasion consists of using a broad-spectrum topical antibiotic (i.e., tobramycin ophthalmic ointment), a cy-

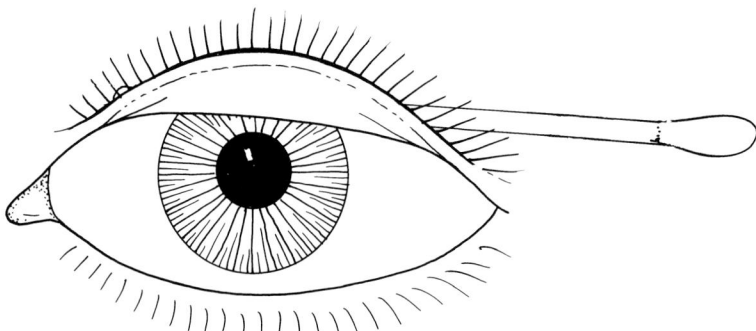

Figure 11.9 *If a foreign body is suspected, inspection of the inside of the upper eyelid should be performed by everting the eyelid with the back end of a cotton-tipped applicator.*

cloplegic agent (i.e., 1% cyclopentolate hydrochloride), and the application of a pressure patch if the patient is not a contact lens wearer (Table 11.2). If the abrasion occurs in a contact lens wearer, a patch should not be applied to avoid developing infectious keratitis (i.e., *Pseudomonas* corneal ulcer). In these cases, an antibiotic with good gram-negative coverage (i.e., tobramycin) should be used four times daily until the abrasion heals. Contact lenses should not be used while an abrasion exists unless an ophthalmologist chooses to use a therapeutic "bandage lens" to promote healing.

A pressure patch is applied by first placing a folded sterile eye pad over the closed eyelids followed by a second unfolded eye pad (Fig. 11.10, A–C). The patch is securely taped from the forehead to the cheek so that the patient is unable to open the lids under the patch. The patch should be removed the following day and the abrasion reassessed. Again, any patient with a history of contact lens wear should never be patched. Corneal abrasions heal relatively quickly, usually within a few days depending on the size of the epithelial defect. The patient should be followed daily until the corneal abrasion has healed. Repeat pressure patching may be considered if the abrasion is still present. After discontinuing the patch, topical antibiotics four times daily may be continued for a few days. Artificial tear lubricants may be given as needed.

A corneal abrasion may be extremely painful. Typically, a combination of patching (in the non–contact lens wearer), cycloplegia, and over-the-counter analgesics (i.e., acetaminophen) is sufficient for adequate pain control. Under no circumstances should a topical anesthetic be prescribed for pain control because this may result in disastrous sequelae. Topical ocular anesthetic abuse is a serious disorder that can result in persistent epithelial defects, permanent corneal damage, and visual loss (Plate 16) (7).

Table 11.2 Management of corneal abrasions

Broad-spectrum topical antibiotic (e.g., 10% sulfacetamide, gentamicin, tobramycin, or ophthalmic solution or ointment)
Cycloplegia (i.e., 1% cyclopentolate hydrochloride)
Pressure patch only if patient does not wear contact lenses
In contact lens wearer, treat the abrasion without patching using an antibiotic with good gram-negative coverage (i.e., tobramycin) four times daily
Oral analgesic (i.e., acetaminophen) as needed for pain
Follow-up daily until the abrasion has healed
Refer to ophthalmologist at any time

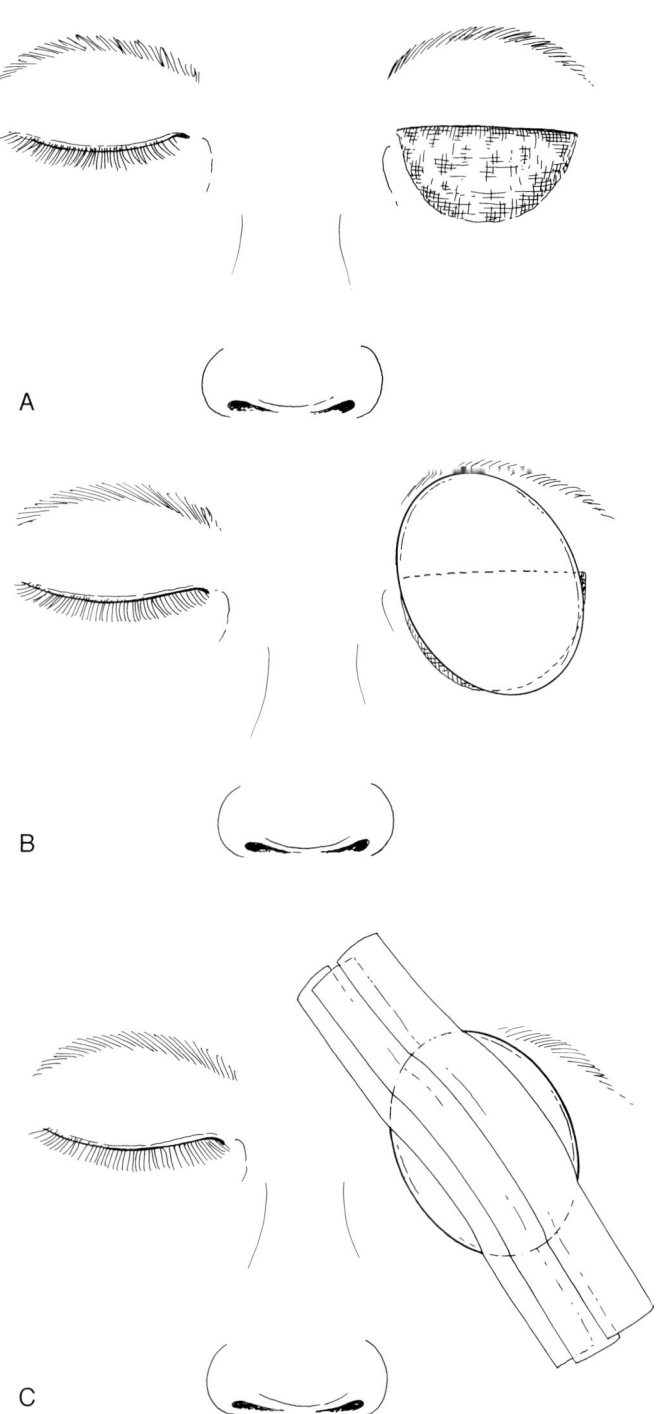

Figure 11.10 *Correct method to apply a pressure patch. (A) With the patient's eyes closed, the first patch is folded in half and placed over the affected eye. (B) The second patch is then placed directly over the first patch and held in place. (C) Tape is applied with pressure over both patches as shown.*

Conjunctival Lacerations

Conjunctival lacerations may be associated with subconjunctival hemorrhage, chemosis (edema), or prolapse of underlying tissue. All conjunctival lacerations should be carefully explored after topical anesthetic is instilled, to determine the extent of damage and to evaluate underlying scleral integrity. A dilated fundus examination should also be performed with particular attention to the corresponding area of external injury. Small conjunctival lacerations (<1 cm) require only conservative treatment with topical antibiotic ointment. Larger conjunctival lacerations may be sutured with absorbable or nylon sutures, ensuring good wound apposition (8).

Subconjunctival Hemorrhage

Damage to a conjunctival vessel may result in a localized or diffuse collection of blood beneath the conjunctiva (Plate 17). The patient may be asymptomatic or complain of some minor irritation. Signs include redness of the eye that obscures the conjunctival and episcleral vessels. No treatment is required, and the patient should be reassured that the subconjunctival hemorrhage will gradually resolve, usually in 10 to 14 days. It is important to exclude a rupture of the globe beneath the area of subconjunctival hemorrhage, particularly in the presence of marked chemosis (conjunctival edema) (Plate 18).

Traumatic Iritis

Traumatic iritis (iridocyclitis) is an inflammation of the iris and ciliary body that may result from blunt trauma to the anterior segment. Symptoms include photophobia, pain, and tearing. Common findings on examination include perilimbal hyperemia, pupillary miosis (Plate 19), a lower intraocular pressure compared with the other eye, and the diagnostic finding of cells and flare in the anterior chamber seen on slit-lamp examination.

Treatment of traumatic iritis consists of using a cycloplegic agent (i.e., 1% cyclopentolate hydrochloride) (Table 11.3). Topical steroid drops (i.e., 1% prednisolone acetate) may also be added, depending

Table 11.3 Management of iritis

Cycloplegia (i.e., 1% cyclopentolate hydrochloride)
Topical steroids in moderate to severe cases (i.e., 1% prednisolone acetate)
Follow-up as per ophthalmologist

on severity of inflammation. Follow-up examinations with an ophthalmologist are essential. Disruption of the angle structures (angle recession) and retinal tears and/or detachment should be excluded in follow-up examinations by gonioscopy and dilated fundus examination with scleral depression.

Hyphema

Hyphema is the term for blood in the anterior chamber of the eye (Plates 11 and 20). It is usually the result of blunt trauma, whereby a compressive force to the ocular surface results in a disruption of the arterial system and bleeding into the anterior chamber (Fig. 11.11). A microhyphema is defined as a suspension of red blood cells in the aqueous humor without the gross accumulation of blood. Schein et al (9) noted that sports injuries may account for up to 60% of all traumatic hyphemas. Twenty-five percent to 35% of patients with hyphema also have damage to other structures of the eye (10).

Decreased vision and pain are common symptoms. A hyphema can be diagnosed in the field by careful penlight examination, with the examiner looking for the accumulation of blood in the anterior chamber. Microhyphema must be diagnosed by slit-lamp examination. The extent of the hyphema is described in terms of the percentage of the anterior chamber that is filled with blood. After a ruptured globe has been excluded, it is important to determine the vision, measure the intraocular pressure, and perform a dilated fundus examination.

Hyphema patients should avoid strenuous exercise, and their activity should be restricted (Table 11.4). The head of the bed should be elevated 30 degrees to allow the blood to settle. A rigid eye shield is placed over the eye at all times, cycloplegia is administered (i.e., 1% atropine t.i.d.), and aspirin-containing compounds are avoided. Oral steroids or antifibrinolytic agents such as aminocaproic acid may be used in selected cases to avoid rebleeding (11). If the intraocular pressure is elevated, pressure-lowering agents should be prescribed (the agent prescribed depends on the degree of intraocular pressure elevation and the patient's sickle cell status). Patients may require hospitalization if daily follow-up is not ensured.

All hyphema patients should be questioned about bleeding diathesis, the use of aspirin or other anticoagulants, and sickle cell status. Carbonic anhydrase inhibitors (used for treatment of elevated intraocular pressure) are relatively contraindicated in patients with a history of sickle cell trait or disease because the use of these drugs may

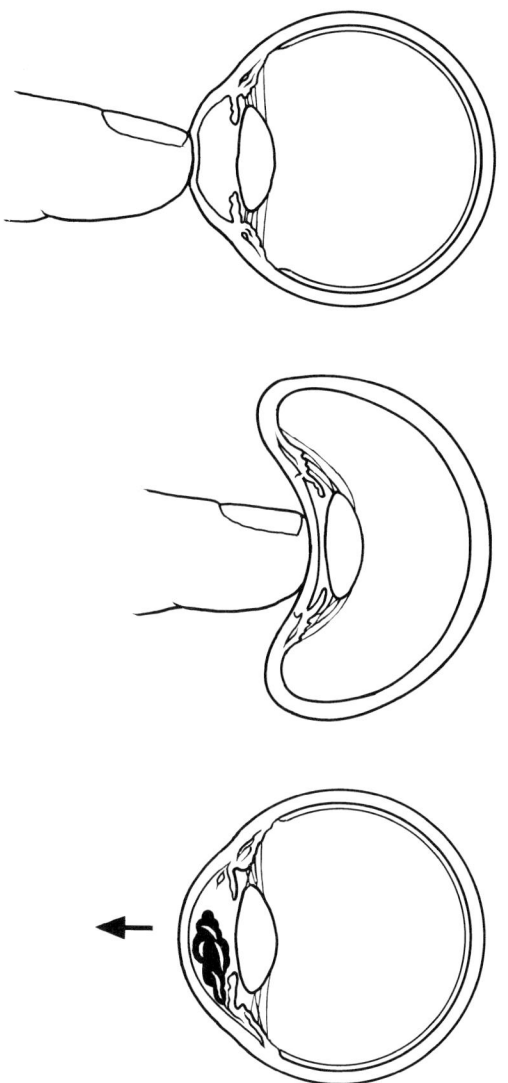

Figure 11.11 *Blunt trauma (i.e., finger poke) to the eye may result in disruption of the arteries and bleeding into the anterior chamber.*

precipitate sickling of the red blood cells and preclude clearing of the hyphema.

With hyphemas, there is a risk of rebleeding that most frequently occurs 2 to 5 days after the injury (12). In cases of persistently elevated intraocular pressure, corneal blood staining, or delayed clearing of the clot, the patient may require surgical evacuation of the hyphema (8). All hyphema patients should be closely followed by an

Table 11.4 Management of hyphema

Rigid eye shield should be worn at all times
Limit activities
Head of bed elevated to 30 degrees to allow settling of blood
Cycloplegia (i.e., 1% atropine t.i.d)
Avoid aspirin-containing compounds
Oral corticosteroids or antifibrinolytic agents such as aminocaproic acid in selected cases
If intraocular pressure is elevated, appropriate agents are prescribed
Determine patient's sickle cell status; if positive for sickle cell, avoid carbonic anhydrase inhibitors and osmotic agents
Follow-up daily with ophthalmologist

ophthalmologist. The athlete may return to his or her sport after the hyphema is cleared, the eye is quiet, and all associated injuries are identified and treated, but he or she should wait at least 2 weeks after the initial injury (see Table 11.4).

Eyelid Lacerations

All patients with eyelid lacerations should be considered for tetanus prophylaxis. When evaluating an eyelid laceration, the skin may be gently irrigated with sterile saline solution. The exact location and extent of injury should be determined. It is important to document involvement of the eyelid margin (Plate 21). Care should be taken to avoid manipulating the tissues until a ruptured globe can be ruled out. What seem to be small superficial lid lacerations may very well extend deep into the orbital structures, resulting in significant damage (Plate 22). A thorough ocular examination should be performed before repair of any lid laceration (Table 11.5).

A sterile gauze pad moistened with sterile saline solution should be placed over the laceration to prevent excessive drying of the tissues before repair. If corneal exposure is noted secondary to the lid laceration and a ruptured globe is excluded, sterile ophthalmic antibiotic ointment may be placed in the eye under the moistened gauze pad. An ophthalmologist should perform the surgical repair of eyelid lacerations in which the 1) lid margin is involved, 2) medial aspect of the eyelid is involved, to rule out canalicular damage, 3) upper eyelid is involved, as damage to underlying structures such as the levator palpebrae superioris muscle or its aponeurosis may be present, or 4) upper or lower lids, when the injury involves excessive tissue loss or full-lid thickness.

Table 11.5 Management of eyelid lacerations

Determine involvement of lid margin/exclude a ruptured globe
Place a sterile gauze pad moistened with sterile saline over the laceration to prevent drying of the tissue before repair
If corneal exposure is noted, place sterile ophthalmic antibiotic ointment in the eye under the gauze pad
Consider tetanus prophylaxis
Refer the following eyelid lacerations to the ophthalmologist
    Margin involved
    Medial aspect of the lid involved (possible canalicular tear)
    Upper eyelid involved
    Excessive tissue loss or full-thickness laceration
Clean the affected area with povidone-iodine
Apply a local anesthetic (i.e., 2% lidocaine with epinephrine)
Close (suture) deeper layers with absorbable sutures
Close (suture) skin with 6-0 or 7-0 nylon or silk
Consider oral antibiotics and topical antibiotic ointment
Remove skin sutures in 5 to 7 days; remove lid margin sutures in 10 to 14 days

After cleaning with povidone-iodine, local anesthetic (2% lidocaine with epinephrine) should be administered. If deeper layers require closure, this should be done first with absorbable suture (Fig. 11.12). The overlying skin should be well approximated and closed with 6-0 or 7-0 nylon or silk (Fig. 11.13). The use of an oral antibiotic should be considered. After the laceration is repaired, topical

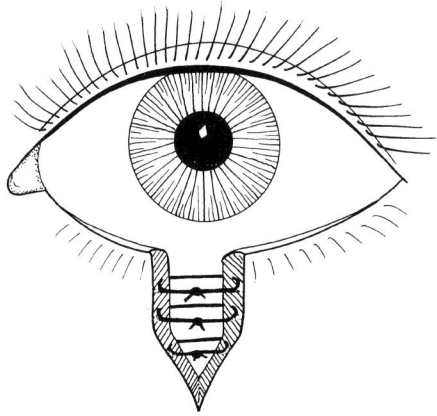
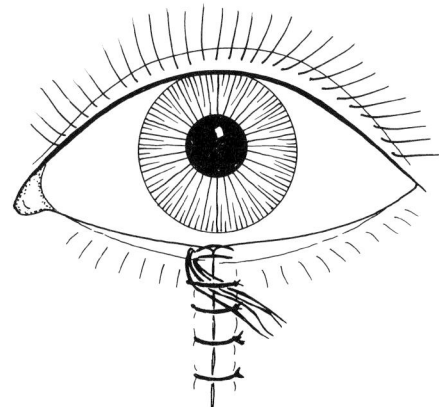

Figure 11.12 *If the eyelid laceration involves the deeper tissues, closure should be done with interrupted absorbable sutures.*

Figure 11.13 *The wound edges should be well apposed before suturing the superficial skin.*

antibiotic ointment is applied to the wound. Skin sutures are typically removed in 5 to 7 days, whereas lid margin sutures are removed after 10 to 14 days.

Orbital Wall Fractures

Orbital wall fractures are commonly seen after blunt trauma and result from the transmission of compressive forces (Fig. 11.14) (13). The thinnest bones of the orbit, the medial and inferior orbital walls, are most vulnerable to injury. Symptoms include pain, diplopia (double vision), and eyelid swelling after nose blowing. On examination, enophthalmos, infraorbital hypesthesia, subcutaneous emphysema, restriction of eye movements (see Plate 8), tenderness on palpation, and a palpable step-off of the orbital rim may be present. Radiographs (Water's and Caldwell views) or computed tomography (CT) is helpful in determining the extent of the fracture (Fig. 11.15).

Initial treatment consists of applying ice packs to the orbit for the first 24 to 48 hours to minimize swelling (Table 11.6). Broad-spectrum oral antibiotics (i.e., cephalexin 250–500 mg orally four times a day or erythromycin 250–500 mg four times a day) may be considered for 10 to 14 days in some cases. In addition, the patient may be prescribed nasal decongestants and is asked to refrain from nose blowing. A full ophthalmologic examination should be performed. Surgical repair may be considered if there is cosmetically unacceptable enophthalmos, persistent diplopia, or a large fracture. The tim-

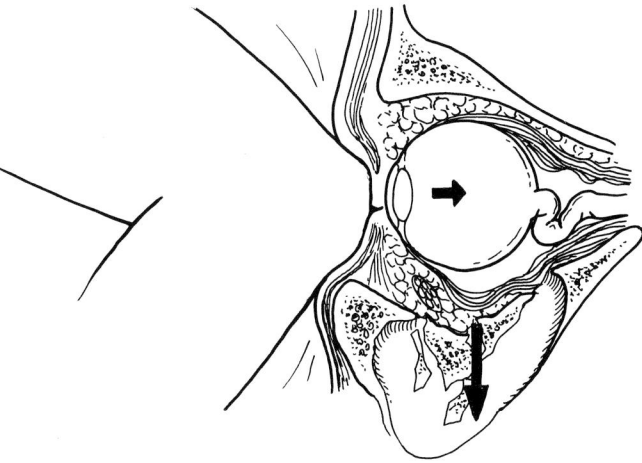

Figure 11.14 *Blunt trauma (e.g., an elbow) may transmit compressive forces to the eye, resulting in an orbital fracture.*

Anterior Segment Injuries 203

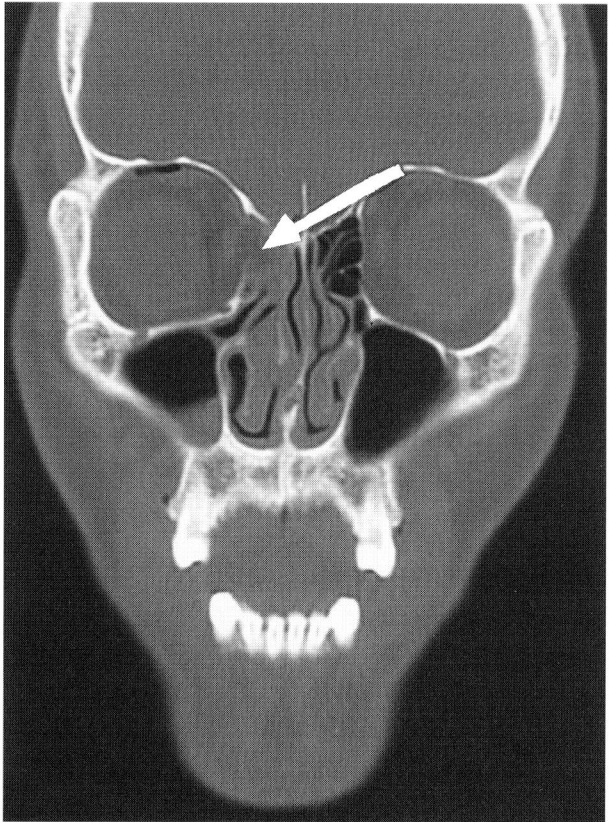

Figure 11.15 *Computerized tomogram of the patient shown in Plate 22. A medial wall fracture is present (arrow) in the right orbit.*

Table 11.6 Management of orbital wall fractures

Apply ice packs to the orbit for the first 24 to 48 hours to minimize swelling
Consider broad-spectrum oral antibiotics (i.e., cephalexin or erythromycin for 10 to 14 days)
Prescribe nasal decongestants as needed; patient should refrain from nose blowing
Take radiographs (Water's and Caldwell views) or use CT
Reevaluate patient and consider surgical repair if persistent diplopia, a large fracture, or cosmetically unacceptable enophthalmos is present

ing for surgical intervention is variable but is usually delayed until approximately 2 weeks after injury to allow orbital edema to subside.

Nonpenetrating Foreign Bodies

Foreign bodies may become lodged anywhere in the eyelids, globe, or orbit. Pain, tearing, redness, decreased vision, and foreign body sensation are common presenting symptoms. Associated findings may include corneal abrasions, subconjunctival hemorrhage, and lid or orbital lacerations. With the presence of any conjunctival or corneal foreign body, it is essential to exclude the presence of a ruptured globe. The lids should be everted (see Plate 15 and Fig. 11.9), and lid and conjunctival lacerations should be thoroughly explored after topical anesthetic is instilled. If the foreign body is nonperforating, it can be removed under a slit-lamp using a moistened cotton-tipped applicator or a 25- to 30-gauge needle after the instillation of topical anesthetic (Fig. 11.16). A complete examination of the eye should be performed to look for additional foreign bodies. Broad-spectrum topical antibiotics are prescribed after the removal of a foreign body until the corneal or conjunctival epithelial defect has healed. A pressure patch is placed if the underlying defect is large.

Penetrating Foreign Bodies and Ruptured Globe

Intraocular foreign bodies are usually associated with decreased vision and eye pain. An obvious foreign body may be present externally

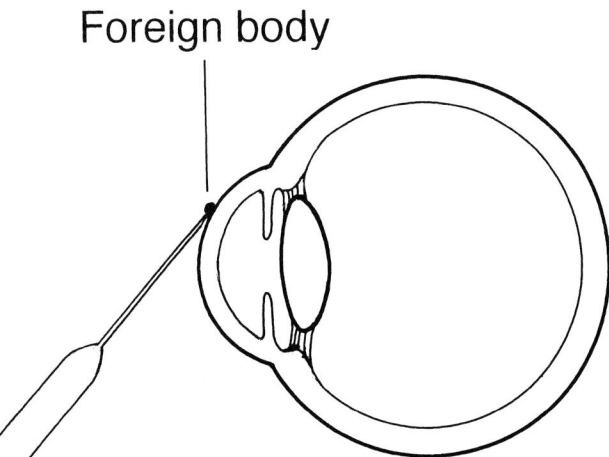

Figure 11.16 *A superficial foreign body may be removed using a 25- to 30-gauge needle under a slit-lamp.*

if large (e.g., fish hook) or may have an occult site of entry. Other signs may include subconjunctival hemorrhage, chemosis, localized corneal edema, an irregular pupil, retroillumination defect on slit-lamp examination, sectorial cataract, anterior and/or posterior segment inflammation, vitreous hemorrhage, decreased intraocular pressure, or retinal hemorrhage and tear.

A penetrating foreign body should never be removed at the scene of the injury. The primary goal of initial management is to prevent further damage from occurring (Table 11.7). Eye medications should not be given. The patient is instructed not to eat or drink anything (preoperative precautions). A protective eye shield is placed over the injured eye, and the patient is immediately transported to a medical center, where the foreign body may be removed in a controlled setting. Tetanus prophylaxis and broad-spectrum intravenous antibiotics should be considered, and the patient should take nothing by mouth in preparation for possible surgery.

Radiographic evaluation can be helpful in identifying the presence and location of a foreign body. A plain film x-ray may be helpful in determining the presence or absence of a metallic foreign body but may not identify nonmetallic foreign bodies. CT will pick up most foreign bodies unless they are composed of wood or plastic (14). CT is also more specific in terms of identifying the precise location of a foreign body in relation to other soft-tissue structures. In cases of a nonmetallic foreign body, magnetic resonance imaging may be helpful.

Lens Injuries

Contusion injuries to the eye may cause disruption of the zonules or the lens substance itself, leading to subluxation (partial displacement) (see Plate 23) or dislocation (complete displacement) of the lens and cataract formation. A traumatic cataract may occur acutely if the lens capsule has been ruptured or as a late sequela if the lens capsule remains intact.

Patients with a subluxated or dislocated lens may complain of fluc-

Table 11.7 Management of ruptured globe

Place a protective eye shield over the eye to prevent further damage (no pressure patch)
Do not instill any drops or ointment
Do not allow patient to eat or drink anything (preoperative precautions)
Consider tetanus prophylaxis and broad-spectrum antibiotics
Refer to an ophthalmologist immediately

tuating vision, blurry vision (secondary to induced myopia or astigmatism), or monocular diplopia (if the edge of the lens is in the visual axis). Zonular rupture, lens subluxation, and dislocation can be diagnosed by an ophthalmologist under a slit-lamp with a fully dilated pupil. The appropriate medical or surgical management of these cases will depend on the degree of injury and the patient's symptoms.

Traumatic cataracts may cause symptoms of glare or decreased vision, or the patient may be asymptomatic if the opacity is small and out of the visual axis. If the lens capsule is ruptured, acute inflammation and secondary glaucoma may develop. Traumatic cataracts are diagnosed by dilated slit-lamp examination and may be seen as opacities in the red reflex with an ophthalmoscope. Treatment will again depend on the degree of functional visual loss and the ability to manage the patient medically.

Retrobulbar Hemorrhage

Severe ocular trauma can result in orbital bleeding that is referred to as a retrobulbar hemorrhage (Fig. 11-17). Symptoms and signs include

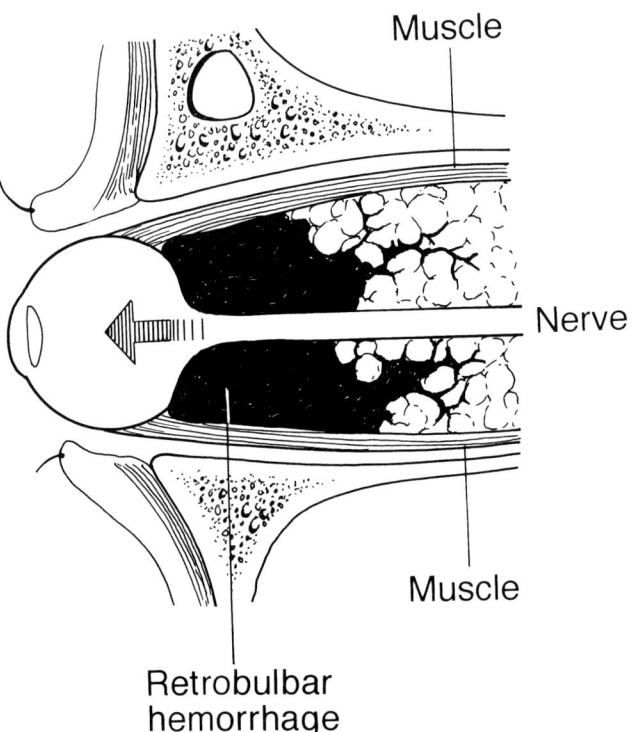

Figure 11.17 *Retrobulbar hemorrhage with a proptotic (pushed out) eye.*

Anterior Segment Injuries

Table 11.8 Management of retrobulbar hemorrhage

Determine intraocular pressure if possible
Perform a lateral canthotomy emergently
Recheck intraocular pressure
Refer to ophthalmologist

pain, proptosis with resistance to retropulsion, restriction of ocular motility, a marked elevation of intraorbital and subsequently intraocular pressure, chemosis, diffuse subconjunctival hemorrhage, and decreased vision (15). This is an ocular emergency in which the patient's vision can be preserved if immediate action is taken in the field.

Treatment is aimed at immediate decompression of the orbit (Table 11.8). A lateral canthotomy should be emergently performed by a qualified health care provider (Fig. 11.18, A–C). Local anesthesia

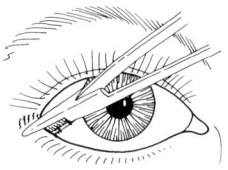

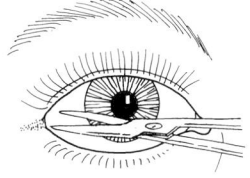

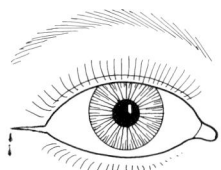

Figure 11.18 *Method for performing a lateral canthotomy. After anesthetic is injected into the lateral canthus, a hemostat is placed over the lateral canthus extending down to the fornix. A crush mark is made with the hemostat. Scissors then cut over the crush mark.*

may be applied in the area of the lateral canthus, although the procedure should not be delayed if anesthesia is unavailable. A hemostat is then placed horizontally along the lateral canthus and clamped for approximately 1 minute to decrease bleeding. A scissor is then used to make a 1-cm incision across the lateral canthal tendon. If adequate decompression is not evident, a cantholysis should then be performed by placing the scissor between the skin and conjunctiva directed slightly inferiorly to release the inferior arm of the lateral canthal tendon. A trickle of blood is usually observed, and the orbit is allowed to decompress. Marked softening of the globe should be noted. If treatment is delayed, permanent damage to the optic nerve may result from the ischemia secondary to compression by the hematoma. The patient should be immediately transferred to a medical center, where additional evaluation and treatment by an ophthalmologist can be provided.

Conclusion

Sports-related ocular trauma can result in a wide range of eye injuries. If an orderly systematic approach to evaluating these injuries is used, many conditions can be identified early and properly managed. Referral to an ophthalmologist may be required because many seemingly minor injuries may lead to permanent visual compromise if prompt attention is not given to the patient. The importance of proper eye protection should be stressed to all athletes because prevention of injury is the best solution.

References

1. Stock JG, Cornell FM. Prevention of sports-related eye injury. Am Fam Physician 1991;44:515–520.
2. National Society to Prevent Blindness. 1993 Eye injuries associated with sports and recreational products. Schaumburg, IL: National Center for Sight, 1994.
3. Zagelbaum BM, Tostanoski JR, Kerner DJ, et al. Urban eye trauma: a one year prospective study. Ophthalmology 1993;100:851–856.
4. Larrison WI, Hersh PS, Kunzweiler T, et al. Sports-related ocular trauma. Ophthalmology 1990;97:1265–1269.
5. Zagelbaum BM. Sports-related eye trauma: managing common injuries. Phys Sportsmed 1993;21:25–42.
6. Burde RM, Savino PJ, Trobe JD. Clinical decisions in neuro-ophthalmology, St. Louis: Mosby-Year Book, 1992:7–9.

7. Zagelbaum BM, Tostanoski JR, Hochman MA, et al. Topical lidocaine and proparacaine abuse. Am J Emerg Med 1994;12:96–97.
8. Hersh PS, Zagelbaum BM, Kenyon KR, et al. Surgical management of anterior segment trauma. In: Tasman W, Jaeger EA, eds. Duane's clinical ophthalmology. vol. 6. Philadelphia: Lippincott, 1994:1–19.
9. Schein OD, Hibberd PL, Shingleton BJ, et al. The spectrum and burden of ocular injury. Ophthalmology 1988;95:300–305.
10. Shingleton BJ. Eye injuries. N Engl J Med 1991;325:408–413.
11. Goldberg MF. Antifibrinolytic agents in the management of traumatic hyphema. Arch Ophthalmol 1983;101:1029–1030.
12. Shingleton BJ, Hersh PS. Traumatic hyphema. In: Shingleton BJ, Hersh PS, Kenyon KR, eds. Eye trauma. St. Louis: Mosby-Year Book, 1991:104–116.
13. Smith B, Regan WF. Blow-out fracture of the orbit. Am J Ophthalmol 1957;44:733–739.
14. Westfall CT, Shore JW. Intraorbital foreign bodies. In: Shingleton BJ, Hersh PS, Kenyon KR, eds. Eye trauma. St. Louis: Mosby-Year Book, 1991:3–24.
15. Chavis RM, Krohel GB, Perman KI. Acute proptosis in adults. In: Duane TE, ed. Clinical ophthalmology. vol. 2. Philadelphia: Lippincott, 1992:7–8.

CHAPTER 12

Posterior Segment Injuries

Stephanie A. Skolik
D. Virgil Alfaro
Peter E. Liggett

When we speak of the "posterior segment," we are referring to that portion of the eye that is posterior to the iris. This includes the retina, optic nerve, vitreous body, and choroid. Serious posterior segment ocular injuries can occur in any sport. Although anterior segment injuries tend to be more frequent, posterior segment injuries tend to be more serious and are associated with more severe and permanent visual loss. The most common mechanism is blunt trauma, and injury type may vary dramatically. Suspicion of a posterior segment injury calls for referral to an ophthalmologist for a dilated fundus examination. The earlier a posterior segment injury is diagnosed, the better the prognosis for maximizing visual potential.

Posterior segment injuries occur with higher frequency in contact sports such as boxing, in which blunt trauma may be inherent in the sport. Boxing causes more damage to the eye than any other sport. In one prospective study, 24% of boxers examined at the time of renewing their boxing licenses had previously undiagnosed retinal tears (1). Well-known highly successful professional boxers Sugar Ray Seales and Sugar Ray Leonard sustained retinal detachments and underwent surgical repair (2). Other athletes like professional basketball player Orlando Woolridge suffered retinal detachment, underwent subsequent repair, and have fortunately been able to resume playing successfully with protective goggles. Seelenfreund et al (3) described 10 patients who sustained eye injuries from a high-speed tennis ball. Seven of the patients required either retinal surgery, laser, or both for retinal detachments and/or tears.

Patient Evaluation

Important Clues to Posterior Segment Injuries

History

One of the most important parts of evaluating ocular injury is a complete and accurate history (see Chapter 11). Subjective findings are not uniformly present even with significant posterior segment injury; however, clues to the presence of posterior segment injury can often be obtained. These help to establish whether ophthalmologic consultation is urgently needed. Certain questions are particularly meaningful in determining vitreoretinal abnormalities. Inquiry as to the assessment of subjective change in visual acuity is important; however, visual acuity changes may be transient or deceptively absent even in the face of an already present or impending posterior segment problem. For example, a small retinal tear may occur with little or no symptomatology after injury, yet if left untreated a retinal detachment may develop, resulting in poor vision.

As a routine part of the ocular history regarding the posterior segment, the examiner should present the following questions to the athlete:

1. Has your vision changed in any way since the injury occurred?
2. Have you experienced any "specks" (black spots) in your vision? Commonly referred to as "floaters," these represent a change in the structure of the vitreous and may indicate coexisting retinal damage.
3. Have you noticed any "flashing lights"? The sensation of flashing lights may imply an area of vitreoretinal traction that could lead to a retinal tear or detachment.
4. Have you experienced a veil, curtain, or shade coming across your vision from any direction? This veil or curtain can be diaphanous or solid and could be the retina itself coming away from the wall of the eye.

A positive answer to any of the above questions indicates the presence of a potentially serious posterior segment injury and immediate threat to vision. This patient should have immediate evaluation by an ophthalmologist. The ophthalmologist will perform a bilateral dilated fundus examination to view the entire retina, posterior pole including optic nerve, and periphery. In patients who are unconscious, have suffered serious head trauma, or have pupillary abnormalities, a neurologic examination should be performed before dilating the pupils. It is important that the first examiner viewing the posterior segment be as delicate and thorough as possible, as any further internal hemorrhage (i.e., vitreous hemorrhage) may obscure the view and prevent further examination.

Mechanisms of Posterior Segment Injuries

The mechanisms of sports-related eye injury may be divided into the following five categories: ball-to-eye contact, racket- or bat-to-eye contact, body-to-eye contact, introduction of a foreign material into the eye, and striking the eye or head in a fall (4,5).

Pathophysiology of Posterior Segment Injuries

Blunt Trauma (Concussive Force) to Posterior Segment

Quinlan (6) found that blunt injury occurred in 49.2% of all ocular injuries. Blunt injuries have been reported to account for most sports-related eye trauma (59.2%), and nearly one-third of cases result in a perforating ocular injury (7).

In a contusional injury, the damage sustained will depend on the mass of the object, its velocity, and the resultant force imparted to the eye. It will also depend on the direction of approach of the projectile, its surface characteristics, and size. A blunt object striking the eye at high speed will cause rapid anteroposterior compression and equatorial dilatation, followed by successively smaller waves of distortion. The eye will also be moved posteriorly en masse, which can affect the integrity of the bony orbit by a piston effect.

With blunt impact to the globe, rapid distortion of the equatorial proportions of the globe may occur; this places the peripheral retina under great stress (8–11) and may result in retinal detachment. Trauma accounts for 10% of all cases of retinal detachment (8,12,13).

When a forceful object strikes the anterior surface of the eye, the indentation that results generates a wave or current within the globe (Fig. 12.1). Analogous to the coup-countrecoup injury theory that explains brain injury during a blunt impact to the head, models have demonstrated that a current wave that transmits the magnitude of the impact through the globe may render considerable force to the anterior surface of the retina (Fig. 12.2).

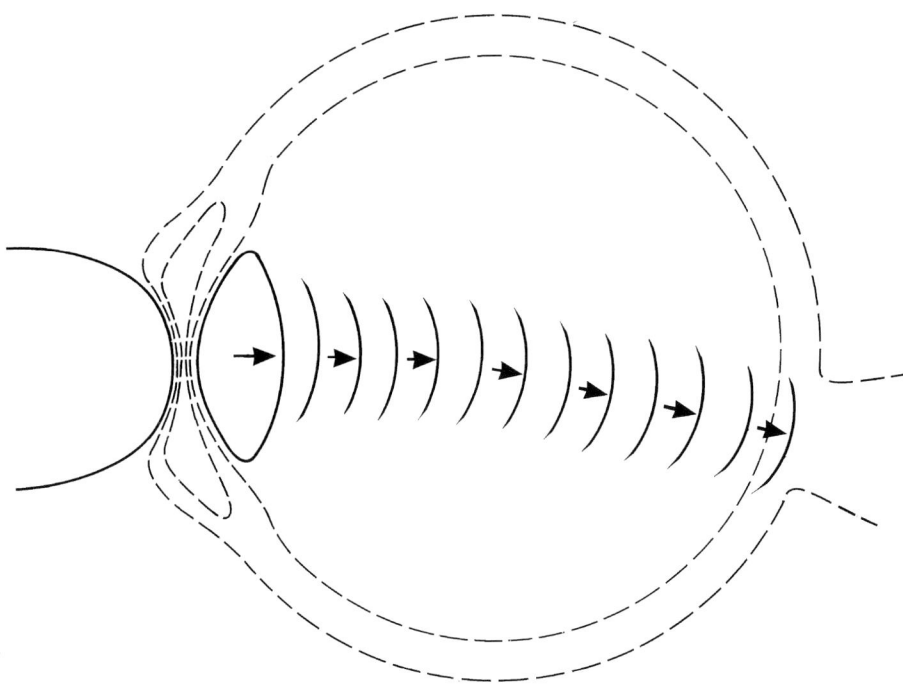

Figure 12.1 *Illustration of how the force in commotio retinae is thought to transverse the eye.*

With this contusional force, the swollen retina that results (commotio retinae) can lead to a decreased visual acuity if the macular area is involved. The serious posterior segment injuries that may occur as a result of contusional force include retinal tears, macular holes, vitreous hemorrhage, choroidal injury, retinal detachments, or rupture of the globe itself. Permanent visual impairment can result from any of these.

If blunt trauma is transmitted to the macula, disruption, such as a macular hole, may occur, giving severe and permanent visual loss. Macular holes are partial or focal full-thickness retinal holes involving the central retina (fovea) (14,15).

Posterior Segment Globe Rupture from Blunt Trauma

Penetrating ocular injury can result from blunt trauma. In a study by DuJuan et al (16), 22% of ruptured globes were from blunt trauma. Injuries from blunt force had a significantly worse prognosis. Both the location and extent of penetrating wound(s) have been

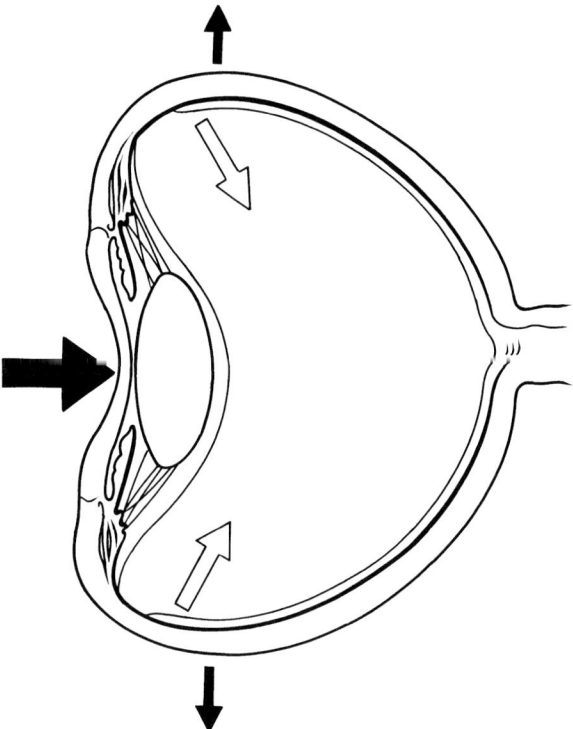

Figure 12.2 *Illustration of the equatorial expansion that occurs with an impact to the anterior globe.*

shown to correlate with visual outcome (16). Wounds limited to the cornea had a better prognosis than those involving the cornea and sclera (corneoscleral wounds).

In eyes with scleral wounds, the posterior extent and the total length of the wound correlated with the final visual result. Scleral wounds that did not extend posterior to the rectus muscle insertions had a better prognosis than those that extended further posteriorly. Eyes with wounds extending behind the rectus muscle insertions had a better visual prognosis that those extending posterior to the equator of the globe. Wounds with a total length equal to or less than 10 mm had a better prognosis than wounds greater than 10 mm in length.

Penetrating Posterior Segment Injury (Sharp Object or Missile)

Ocular injury from sharp or small high velocity objects may occur in some sporting activities (see Chapter 9). Another cause of penetrating eye injury in sports is frequently the glass fragments from breakage of eyeglasses (17,18). Eagling's (19) study showed that sports-related penetrating trauma accounts for 2% to 5% of all penetrating eye injuries. When the sclera, ciliary body, lens, or posterior structures are damaged, visual outcome is much less certain and devastating complications can ensue (16,20).

Factors Correlated with Poor Visual Outcome

Several factors have been found to have an association with poor visual prognosis, as defined by final vision of less than 5/200: 1) initial vision less than 5/200, 2) presence of an afferent pupillary defect on initial testing, 3) injuries from blunt force causing rupture of the globe, 4) wounds involving the sclera and/or extending posterior to the rectus muscle insertions and/or wounds that are greater than 10 mm in length, 5) subluxation of the lens or loss of the lens through the wound in the wall of the eye, 6) vitreous hemorrhage sufficient enough to obscure the retinal vessels and optic nerve on indirect ophthalmoscopy, and 7) injuries associated with an intraocular BB gun pellet.

Manifestations of Orbital Trauma: Posterior Segment

Commotio Retinae

Posttraumatic retinal whitening, Berlin's edema, or commotio retinae is a grayish-white discoloration of the retina that may occur when the globe receives a direct contusion (21,22). Most commonly, this occurs at the posterior pole but can involve the periphery as well (Plates 24 and 25). The retinal whitening occurs rapidly. If the involved area is the posterior pole a "pseudo-cherry red spot" may be noted. A rapid deterioration of the visual acuity to a level of 20/200 develops within several hours if the macula is involved.

Other signs of concussive injury to the anterior segment may be present. The prognosis for visual recovery to the preinjury acuity level is good. Occasionally, if the damage is extensive, the visual prognosis may be poor. Commotio retinae, as seen on dilated fundus examination, is located in the deep sensory retina and is usually directly across from the site of globe impact. Other associated injuries, such as retinal hemorrhage or choroidal rupture, may be present.

Commotio retinae represents disrupted photoreceptor outer segments. Migration of pigment within the retina sometimes occurs. Permanent visual loss may result from loss of photoreceptors (21).

Although the edema usually resolves quickly, commotio retinae may occasionally result in permanent visual loss. Often at times immediately after blunt impact to the globe, visual acuity may drop anywhere between 20/200 and counting fingers for a relatively short period (minutes to hours) but then often returns to normal (20/20 or patient's visual baseline) within a few days to weeks. If the commotio retinae is limited to the peripheral retina, the patient may be asymptomatic.

Treatment of commotio retinae involves observation and reassurance. As always, a complete ophthalmic examination should be performed to rule out other causes of decreased visual acuity and to identify additional trauma-related pathology.

Choroidal Injuries

Choroidal hemorrhage or hemorrhagic choroidal detachment may be found after blunt trauma to the eye. These may occur in the absence of choroidal rupture, presumably caused by the tearing of choroidal blood vessels from the sudden traction near their anchorage at the optic nerve head (23). Posttraumatic retinal whitening or Berlin's edema is often associated. Blood can sometimes extravasate into the subretinal space and may even break through into the vitreous cavity. As the blood resorbs, the choroidal ruptures become more apparent and appear as curvilinear or crescent-shaped yellowish lines that are concentric to the optic disc.

When the globe receives a significant compressive force, there is an indentation of the globe at the site of impact and an immediate horizontal expansion of the globe at the equator. This stretching force rendered to the globe can exceed the elastic forces inherent to the choroid, and choroidal rupture can occur. In some situations, the force may not be sufficient to rupture the choroid but is sufficient to cause breaks (ruptures) in Bruchs' membrane, which is relatively inelastic.

Choroidal ruptures often occur on the temporal side of the optic nerve and may even traverse the fovea (Plate 26). They are often crescent shaped and concentric to the optic disc. The underlying retina is usually intact; however, rupture of the choriocapillaris may result in retinal or vitreous hemorrhage.

Visual prognosis for posterior or indirect choroidal rupture is good if the fovea is not involved. Any accompanying retinal edema or intraocular hemorrhage may affect the initial visual acuity. The treatment of choroidal rupture is observation and surveillance by an ophthalmologist for secondary problems such as subretinal neovascularization (23) that may occur subsequent to the initial injury. Serosanguineous detachments of the macula after traumatic choroidal rupture have been reported many months after the initial injury (24,25).

Traumatic Macular Holes

Macular holes after contusion are a well-known sequela to severe blunt trauma to an eye. A macular hole is a full-thickness rupture of the integrity of the retina at the fovea (Plate 27). Visual acuity is generally reduced and relative to the size of the macular hole created by the impact. Usually, the visual acuity is in the 20/60 to 20/200 range in a full-thickness macular hole.

The mechanism by which the rupture occurs stems from the contussive force causing deformation of the globe in an anterior-posterior manner. As the forceful compression shortens the anterior-posterior length of the eye, the horizontal equatorial expansion transmits an anterior pulling force on the attached vitreous. The vitreous that lines the inside of the posterior segment of the eye is abruptly displaced anteriorly and can literally pull a hole in the thinnest portion of the retina known as the fovea (or macula), thus creating a traumatic macular hole.

It is recognized that traumatic macular holes can arise from an immediate concussive tear or a later breakdown of traumatically induced macular cystoid changes (26,27). The foveolar portion of the retina is extremely thin; moreover, blunt trauma may cause a full-thickness macular hole by either one or a combination of mechanisms: contusion necrosis, subfoveal hemorrhage, and vitreous traction. Holes may be present initially or soon afterward in a patient with severe Berlin's edema, with a subretinal hemorrhage caused by choroidal rupture, or in a whiplash separation of the vitreous from the retina (27).

Treatment of traumatic macular holes is controversial. Some retina specialists believe that relieving residual tractional forces by vitrectomy and membrane peeling from the macular surface may be helpful.

Peripheral Retinal Changes After Blunt Trauma Including Retinal Detachments

Traumatic retinal dialyses are a common cause of retinal detachment in all age groups and are the major cause of detachment in children and young adults (28,29). The time interval between ocular contusion and the clinical appearance of a retinal detachment is extremely variable. There is often a latent period between injury and the diagnosis of retinal detachment (13,24,28–32). Cox et al (13) found that 12% of detachments after blunt trauma occurred immediately, 30% were detached within 1 month, 50% within 8 months, and 80% within 2 years. After blunt injury, approximately 10% of cases show peripheral retinal and/or choroidal breaks. All patients that sustain blunt trauma should have a dilated retinal examination by an ophthalmologist

Posterior Segment Intraocular Foreign Bodies

To perforate the eye and end up in the posterior segment, a foreign body must have a high velocity. It can reach the posterior segment by penetrating the sclera itself or it may traverse the cornea, anterior chamber, iris, and lens before depositing posteriorly.

The damage produced by an intraocular foreign body is a result of the injuries sustained from the penetration of the object and the potential infection (endophthalmitis), toxicity, or inflammatory response that the foreign body may initiate. The composition of the foreign body is important because reactive metals may produce extensive intraocular damage, whereas inert metals may be better tolerated. The nature and location of the foreign body also dictate the decision and timing for surgical intervention.

Treatment of an intraocular foreign body includes immediate referral to an ophthalmologist and anticipation of intraocular surgery. Broad-spectrum antibiotic prophylaxis and careful follow-up are highly recommended because an intraocular infection (endophthalmitis) would have devastating visual consequences.

Vitreous Hemorrhage

Ocular trauma represents a major cause of vitreous hemorrhage, particularly among young males. Dana et al (33) found that trauma was the second most likely cause of vitreous hemorrhage. Blunt trauma was responsible in 66% of cases, projectiles were responsible in 25%, and sharp or lacerating injuries were responsible in 9% of cases. The presence of a vitreous hemorrhage can be associated with retinal pathology. The hemorrhage may obscure the view and make it difficult to view the underlying structures (Plate 28).

A variety of ancillary diagnostic modalities are useful when examining eyes with a vitreous hemorrhage. Ultrasonography is the principal test used, but CT and even magnetic resonance imaging (if a metallic foreign body is not present) are helpful in further evaluation of the retina and vitreous cavity in eyes with vitreous hemorrhages (33).

A vitreous hemorrhage will often clear within a few weeks to months. When a vitreous hemorrhage persists for greater than 6 months, ophthalmic surgical intervention (pars plana vitrectomy) is often considered. With all suspected vitreous hemorrhages, ophthalmologic evaluation is advised and long-term follow-up is required.

Preretinal Hemorrhage from Valsalva Retinopathy

Valsalva retinopathy, or "retinal vessel rupture associated with physical exertion," is a spontaneous rupture of either normal or abnormal superficial retinal capillaries associated with a sudden rise in intrathoracic or intra-abdominal pressure, particularly against a closed glottis. This is often associated in sports with lifting or straining against heavy weights against a closed glottis. Sudden loss of vision may result from hemorrhagic detachment of the internal limiting membrane, vitreous hemorrhage, or dissection of blood beneath the retina (Plate 29). This is readily evident on dilated fundus examination. Patients typically have a circumscribed, round, or dumbbell-shaped bright red mound of blood beneath the internal limiting membrane in or near the central macula (33).

Treatment involves observation by an ophthalmologist with careful follow-up. Intervention is not indicated. A fluorescein angiogram may be obtained in attempts to identify underlying retinal pathology. Visual recovery is usually the rule.

Retinitis Sclopetaria

Retinitis sclopetaria is the rupture of the choroid or retina caused by shock waves generated when a high-velocity missile passes through the orbit without directly striking the eye. It is attributed to shock waves produced by the missile itself (34). Usually a vitreous hemorrhage is seen initially and often an extensive fibrous tissue proliferation into the vitreous is observed as the hemorrhage clears. If the optic nerve is damaged, visual acuity can be profoundly affected. Treatment involves ophthalmologic consultation, observation, and follow-up.

Optic Nerve Evulsion

A blunt force to the eye can result in the backward dislocation of the optic nerve from the scleral canal (Plate 30) (27,35). There are several circumstances in which this can occur, including extreme rotation and forward displacement of the globe; penetrating orbital injury, causing a backward pull of the optic nerve; or sudden increase in intraocular pressure, causing a rupture of the lamina cribrosa. Chow et al (36) reported an 18-year-old male who sustained an optic nerve evulsion from being poked in the eye while playing basketball.

In all cases of optic nerve evulsion, there is a tear in the lamina cribrosa and the nerve fiber layer that is either partial or complete. This tear may be associated with massive intraocular hemorrhage. Visual loss is usually great. Unfortunately, there is no effective treatment.

Rupture of the Globe

An eye can be ruptured with either a sharp object (broken glass from a spectacle) or from blunt trauma. If a direct force of sufficient magnitude is applied to the globe, the rupture may occur in one of two ways. First, a direct rupture may occur in which the break is the site of the impact. Alternatively, an indirect rupture may result at a site remote from the area of direct impact. The location of this indirect rupture will vary from globe to globe, and the rupture will be found in the weakest point in the wall of the globe (37).

Indirect traumatic rupture of the globe has been found to be associated with several clinical signs: severe chemosis, hyphema, and hypotonia. In one study involving 50 traumatic ruptured globes, over 80% of scleral ruptures were at or anterior to the equator (38). More than 75% of these anterior ruptures were located in the superior half of the eye, with the superionasal quadrant being the most common location of the scleral rupture.

If one considers scleral thickness alone, it would appear that the most likely location of indirect scleral rupture would be its thinnest part, namely, the area just posterior to the recti muscle insertions. However, in one series, rupture occurred at the recti muscle insertion approximately 43% of the time (37). The most common site for the location of scleral ruptures was at or near the limbus under intact conjunctiva in 50% of cases and in the posterior pole in 7%.

Treatment involves protecting the eye from further injury and immediate ophthalmologic referral. Prompt surgical exploration by an ophthalmologist for a suspected ruptured globe is likely.

Initial Management of Suspected or Identified Posterior Segment Injury

1. Protect the eye from any further compression. Cover the orbit with a Foxx shield if available. If a Foxx shield is not available, use any ridged, oval-shaped device with the cover resting not on the eye but on the orbital bones above and below the eye. A lid of a jar or similar device will often suffice when secured in place with tape.
2. Prevent exertion. Keep patient quiet.
3. Patient should rest quietly during transport to the hospital in a 45-degree position to keep the head elevated.
4. With anticipation of possible surgical intervention, no food or drink should be ingested by the patient.
5. Avoid nausea. If nausea develops, make every attempt to avoid vomiting because this will increase the intraocular pressure. If a globe rupture is present, intraocular contents could potentially be extruded through the rupture in the globe with increased intrathoracic pressure and consequently simultaneous increased intraocular pressure. If it is available, give an antiemetic agent if patient becomes nauseated.

If the ophthalmologist confirms the suspicion of an open globe, surgical exploration and repair are likely. When posterior segment injuries are suspected, often a retinal specialist is consulted. Intraocular foreign bodies are usually promptly removed by surgery. Globe ruptures that do not involve intraocular foreign bodies are usually closed primarily. The timing of removal of traumatic vitreous hemorrhage or vitreoretinal incarceration in the wound is variable but is often addressed by a second surgery 10 to 14 days after the primary closure of the open globe. If retinal detachment is also part of the initial presentation, some retinal specialists may choose to be involved immediately (39,40).

Conclusion

Posterior segment injury presents unique and important challenges to the ophthalmologist. The rapid diagnosis of such an injury can have great impact on the visual outcome of the patient. It is essential that every patient evaluated for sports-related ocular trauma receives a complete ophthalmic evaluation, including a dilated fundus examination, where applicable, to provide the highest quality of care to athletes.

References

1. Giovinazzo VJ, Yannuzzi LA, Sorenson JA, et al. The ocular complications of boxing. Ophthalmology 1987;94:587–596.
2. Smith DJ. Ocular injuries in boxing. Int Ophthalmol Clin 1988;28:242–245.
3. Seelenfreund MH, Freilich DB. Rushing the net and retinal detachment. JAMA 1976;235:2723–2726.
4. MacEwen CJ. Sport associated eye injury: a casualty department survey. Br J Ophthalmol 1987;71:701–705.
5. MacEwen CJ. Eye injuries: a prospective survey of 5671 cases. Br J Ophthalmol 1989;73:888–894.
6. Quinlan MP. Trauma eye injury. Br J Hosp Med 1983;14:392–401.
7. Larrison WI, Hersh PS, Kunzweiller T, et al. Sports-related ocular trauma. Ophthalmology 1990;97:1265–1269.
8. Delori F, Ponerantzeff O, Cox MS. Deformation of the globe under high-speed impact: its relation to contusion injuries. Invest Ophthalmol 1969;8:290–301.
9. Courville CB. Coup-contrecoup mechanism of craniocerebral injuries. Arch Surg 1942;45:19–43.
10. Holt JE, Holt R, Blodgett JM. Ocular injuries sustained during blunt facial trauma. Ophthalmology 1983;90:14–18.
11. Wolter JR. Coup-contrecoup mechanism of ocular injuries. Am J Ophthalmol 1963;56:785–796.
12. Weidenthal DT, Schepens CL. Peripheral fundus changes associated with ocular injury. Am J Ophthalmol 1966;54:675–679.
13. Cox MS, Schepens CL, MacKenzie F. Retinal detachment due to ocular contusion. Arch Ophthalmol 1966;76:678–681.
14. Knapp H. Ueber isolierte Zerreissungen der Aderhaut in Folge von Traumen auf den Augapfel. Arch Augenh 1869;1:6–12.
15. Noyes HD. Detachment of the retina with laceration of the macula lutea. Trans Am Ophthalmol Soc 1871;1:28–90.
16. DeJuan E, Steinberg P, Michels RE. Penetrating ocular injuries: types of injury and visual results. Ophthalmology 1983;90:1318–1322.
17. Ingram DV. Ocular hazards of playing squash rackets. Br J Ophthalmol 1973;57:434–438.
18. Cole MD, Smerdon D. Perforating eye injuries caused by darts. Br J Ophthalmol 1988;72:511–514.
19. Eagling EM. Perforating injuries to the eye. Br J Ophthalmol 1976;60:732–736.
20. Shock JP, Atkins AD. Long term visual acuity after penetrating and perforating ocular injuries. Am J Ophthalmol 1978;100:714–718.
21. Shipperley JO, Quigley HA, Gass JDM. Traumatic retinopathy in primates: the explanation of commotio retinae. Arch Ophthalmol 1978;96:2267–2273.

22. Blight R, Dean Hart JC. Histological changes in the internal retinal layers produced by concussive injuries to the globe: an experimental study. Trans Ophthalmol Soc UK 1978;98:270–277.
23. Gitter KA, Sluser M, Justice J. Traumatic choroidal rupture with late serous detachment of the macula. Arch Ophthalmol 1968;79:729–732.
24. Hilton GF, Norton EWD. Juvenile retinal detachment. Mod Probl Ophthalmol 1969;8:325–327.
25. Dean Hart JC, Natsikos VE, Raistrick ER, et al. Indirect choroidal tears at the posterior pole: a fluorescein angiographic and perimetric study. Br J Ophthalmol 1980;64:59–67.
26. Ogilivie FM. On one of the results of contusion injuries of the eye ("holes" at the macula). Trans Ophthalmol Soc UK 1900;20:202–207.
27. Gass JDM. Stereoscopic atlas of macular diseases: diagnosis and treatment. vol. 2. St. Louis: Mosby, 1987:551–579.
28. Zentmayer W. Hole in the macula. Ophthalmol Rec 1912;18:472–477.
29. Tasman W. Peripheral retinal changes following blunt trauma. Trans Am Ophthalmol Soc 1972;190–198.
30. Tasman W. Juvenile retinal detachment. J Pediatr Ophthalmol 1968;5:160–166.
31. Hagler WS, North AW. Retinal dialyses and retinal detachment. Arch Ophthalmol 1968;79:376–379.
32. Hagler WS. Retinal dialysis as the cause of a special type of retinal detachment. S Med J 1965;58:1475.
33. Dana M, Werner MS, Viana MAG, Shapiro MJ. Spontaneous and traumatic vitreous hemorrhage. Ophthalmology 1993;100:1377–1383.
34. Duane TD. Valsalva hemorrhagic retinopathy. Am J Ophthalmol 1973;75:637–641.
35. Park JH, Frenkel M, Dobbie JG, Choromokos E. Evulsion of the optic nerve. Am J Ophthalmol 1971;72:969–973.
36. Chow AY, Goldberg MF, Frenkel M. Evulsion of the optic nerve in association with basketball injuries. Ann Ophthalmol 1984;16:35–37.
37. Cherry PMH. Rupture of the globe. Arch Ophthalmol 1972;88:498–507.
38. Cherry PMH. Indirect traumatic rupture of the globe. Arch Ophthalmol 1978;96:252–256.
39. Restori M, McLeod D. Ultrasound examination of the traumatized eye. Trans Ophthalmol Soc UK 1978;98:38–42.
40. Archer DB. Injuries of the posterior segment of the eye. Trans Ophthalmol Soc UK 1985;104:597–615.

CHAPTER 13

Medicolegal Aspects

John G. Classé

There are two principal sources of liability in sports vision: negligence and product liability. These two causes of action vary remarkably, in terms of both the legal basis on which a claim is brought to court and the parties who may be held responsible for injury. Product liability involves injuries from defective eyewear, such as sports frames, with the responsible party being the designer, manufacturer, or seller of the product. Negligence involves a deviation from accepted standards of practice, such as failure to prescribe the proper lens material for an athlete, with the eyecare provider being the responsible party. Although claims alleging negligence are a much more likely cause of liability for eyecare practitioners, because sports vision entails the prescribing and dispensing of eyewear, eyecare practitioners may also be involved in claims involving product liability. Therefore, it is necessary to understand both causes of action.

With an estimated 100,000 sports-related ocular injuries occurring each year in the United States, there is the very genuine possibility of a legal claim resulting from injury (1,2). Either or both theories of liability may be alleged, depending on the circumstances. The more common type of claim, however, is one of negligence (3).

Negligence

Negligence is composed of four elements, each of which must be proven by the plaintiff (the one bringing the lawsuit) to establish a prima facie case. Evidence must be offered in support of each element, and although a variety of sources are generally available to the plaintiff in providing this evidence, medical records and expert testimony are primarily relied on in claims of negligence against health care providers. The four elements of negligence follow.

Duty to Provide Due Care

By virtue of assuming the doctor-patient relationship, a practitioner is required to follow a course of conduct that is intended to minimize the risk of injury to the patient. The practitioner must provide "due care," which is an obligation to act prudently and to use reasonable levels of knowledge and skill in the diagnosis and treatment of the patient's condition.

Breach of the Standard of Care

If a practitioner does not act prudently, the result is a breach of the duty to provide due care. To establish what is considered to be reasonable care, testimony must be offered by a qualified expert witness. The determination of the standard of care and the analysis of the defendant practitioner's conduct by the expert witness are usually the most contentious aspects of a negligence case.

Injury

Plaintiffs are required to establish that a physical injury occurred; expert testimony is necessary to determine the actual injury suffered by the plaintiff. Psychological injury may be successfully alleged if there is also a physical injury.

Proximate Cause

The plaintiff must show, through the use of expert testimony, a legal link between the act or omission on the part of the defendant and the resultant injury suffered by the plaintiff.

The gist of a negligence claim is the assertion that the defendant practitioner failed to act as a reasonable practitioner would have acted under the same or similar circumstances. For that reason, it is necessary to consider the essential aspects of the assessment of patients who participate in sports. One essential aspect is the history.

Patient History

The history must be sufficiently thorough to discover not only the patient's vocation but also any avocations, such as athletic or recreational activities, that pose a risk of ocular injury. Although the frequency of participation in sporting activities is of importance and should be ascertained, it should never be forgotten that even occasional participation in some activities may pose a significant risk of injury if the incorrect eyewear is prescribed. The history should reveal both the primary use of the patient's eyewear and any secondary use, such as participation in sports, which may create a risk of injury. Based on the history, the appropriate frames and lenses should be selected.

There are three general classes of ophthalmic materials that can be dispensed to patients: dress, industrial (safety), and athletic or recreational. Although these categories may overlap somewhat in terms of individual patient needs, one of these categories represents the primary use of the eyewear. Any frames and lenses sold to a patient must be suitable for the primary purpose for which they will be worn. If the eyewear poses a risk of injury for secondary use, such as sporting activities, at a minimum the practitioner must warn the patient of the risk of injury and advise the patient of the availability of the proper protective eyewear or lens material. It is hoped that the practitioner will go beyond this minimum obligation and serve as an advocate for eye protection, impressing upon the patient the significant difference between frames and materials and prescribing only eyewear that meets the highest standards. If the improper eyewear is worn during sports activities, injury may occur, which may prompt a negligence claim to be filed against the practitioner. In such cases, the impact resistance of the ophthalmic lenses prescribed by the practitioner is often the key issue. Different impact-resistance standards exist for lenses worn for dress purposes, for industrial (safety) use, or for participation in athletic events.

Impact-Resistance Standards for Ophthalmic Lenses

U.S. standards for the impact resistance of ophthalmic lenses began with voluntary efforts initiated in the 1950s by an organization that became the American National Standards Institute (ANSI). The standards that emerged eventually became identified with the ANSI committees that created them: the Z80.1 committee for dress eyewear and the Z87.1 committee for industrial strength (safety) eyewear. In the 1970s, ANSI impact-resistance standards were adopted by the federal government, which had the effect of making them legally binding in all states and jurisdictions. The two responsible administrative agencies were the Food and Drug Administration (FDA), which adopted the impact-resistance standards of Z80.1, and the Occupational Safety and Health Administration, which adopted the impact-resistance standards of Z87.1.

Prescription Dress Lenses

The current impact-resistance requirement for prescription dress lenses, which is based on ANSI standard Z80.1–1987 (4), requires all lenses to "be capable of" passing a drop-ball test, which requires a 5/8-inch diameter steel ball to be dropped on the lens from a height of 50 inches. There are three principal exceptions to this requirement (4): allyl resin (CR-39) plastic lenses, laminated multifocals, and raised edge multifocals. For these exceptions, the manufacturer may certify that they meet the Z80.1 standard by testing statistically significant samples.

For glass lenses, the manufacturer of the spectacles performs the drop-ball test. Therefore, the dispenser does not have to perform the drop-ball test on any prescription dress lenses, unless the dispenser is also the manufacturer of the spectacles into which glass lenses have been placed.

Plano Dress Lenses

Nonprescription dress lenses are most commonly used for sunglasses, and a separate ANSI standard has been established for this classification of eyewear, the most current version of which is ANSI Z80.3-1986 (5). These standards have also been adopted by the FDA and require nonprescription dress lenses to pass the same drop-ball test as the one administered for prescription dress lenses (i.e., a 5/8-inch diameter steel ball dropped on the lens from a height of 50 inches) (5). This standard applies to plano eyewear sold within the United States, regardless of the place of manufacture. It also applies to plano sunglasses manufactured for children.

Prescription Safety Lenses

The impact-resistance requirements for safety lenses are more stringent than those for dress lenses. The current standard, which is based on ANSI standard Z87.1-1989, requires a drop-ball test for all lenses, glass or plastic, in which a 1-inch diameter steel ball is dropped from a height of 50 inches onto the lens; a minimum thickness of 3 mm for all lens materials (glass, allyl resin [CR-39] plastic, high index plastic, polycarbonate); and that the logo of the manufacturer must be etched onto the edge of the lens (6). The only exception to the above standards is a high-plus lens, which may be 2.5 mm at the edge.

In addition, to meet the industrial strength standards of safety eyewear, the lenses must be placed in a frame that meets Z87.1 standards (and which therefore contains a Z87 logo). Failure to use a safety frame means the eyewear does not meet the standards for safety glasses (6).

Plano Safety Lenses

Nonprescription industrial strength lenses must meet the same Z87.1 requirements as prescription lenses, and plastic (allyl resin [CR-39], high index, and polycarbonate) lenses must pass a needle penetration test (6). There is also a separate drop-ball test that is used to ensure that lenses will not chip, dislodge from the frame, or eject from it. The tests must be administered by the manufacturer of the eyewear.

Athletic Frames and Lenses

The federal government has not adopted standards for athletic eyewear. Therefore, no uniform impact-resistance requirements exist. Performance standards for selected eyewear, such as racquetball goggles and protective shields for Little League baseball and ice hockey, have been established by the American Society of Testing and Materials (ASTM) (7–9), but there are no governmental standards for any sports. Eyewear meeting ASTM standards for racket sports must be made of polycarbonate plastic and must meet performance standards designed to withstand the high velocity impacts of ball and racket (7). This standard, ASTM F803.94, would seem to offer the best protection for participants of sports that pose a risk of injury, including nonracket sports such as baseball, football, and basketball. It should be considered the applicable standard when prescribing eyewear for participants of these and other high-risk sports (10).

Whether for dress, industrial, or athletic use, the choice of polycarbonate plastic greatly improves the impact resistance of the ophthalmic lenses worn by the patient.

Impact Resistance of Polycarbonate Plastic

The conventional materials available for use as ophthalmic lenses have been glass and allyl resin (CR-39) plastic. Testing of the impact resistance of these two materials demonstrates some interesting differences (Fig. 13.1) (11,12).

Heat-tempered glass is unquestionably the least impact resistant, and chemically tempered glass offers a slight advantage when a larger slower moving projectile strikes the lens (11,12). Allyl resin (CR-39) plastic provides somewhat of an advantage when small rapidly moving projectiles strike the lens (which is most often the case) (11,12).

However, impact resistance is also dependent on the reliability of materials to withstand impact, and for that reason the variability of an ophthalmic material's impact resistance is another important consideration (Fig. 13.2) (11,12).

Heat-tempered glass offers a wide range of impact resistance, which means its variability is great. It provides the least impact resistance of any material. Chemically tempered glass is also widely variable, even though it may provide considerably more protection than heat-tempered glass and allyl resin (CR-39) plastic. The chief advantage of allyl resin (CR-39) plastic is its reliability; it offers a predictable range of impact resistance. Furthermore, when it shatters, it tends to break into rounder, less injurious, fragments than glass,

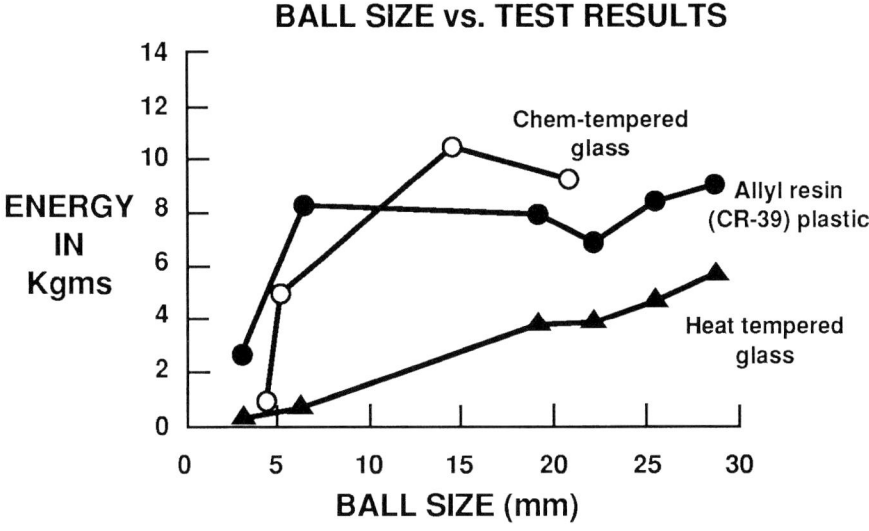

Figure 13.1 *Comparison of impact resistance of heat-tempered glass, chemically tempered glass, and allyl resin (CR-39) plastic for different sized objects and velocities.* (SOURCE: Davis JK. Perspectives on impact resistance and polycarbonate lenses. Int Ophthalmol Clin 1988;28:215–218; Davis JK. Lenses for sports vision. In: Pizzarello LD, Haik BG, eds. Sports ophthalmology. Springfield, IL: Charles C Thomas, 1987:9–43.)

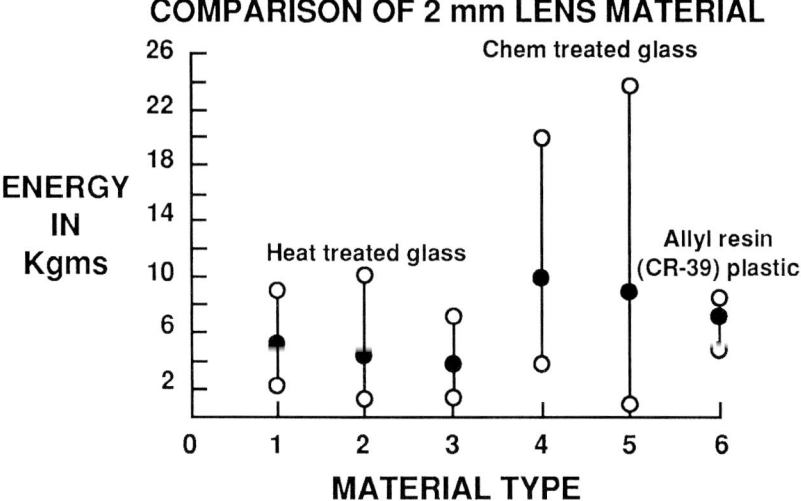

Figure 13.2 *Variability of impact resistance for heat-tempered glass, chemically tempered glass, and allyl resin (CR-39) plastic. ○, range; ●, mean. (SOURCE: Davis JK. Perspectives on impact resistance and polycarbonate lenses. Int Ophthalmol Clin 1988;28:215–218; Davis JK. Lenses for sports vision. In: Pizzarello LD, Haik BG, eds. Sports ophthalmology. Springfield, IL: Charles C Thomas, 1987:9–43.)*

which often shatters into sharp shards that can cause severe ocular injury.

When these materials are compared with polycarbonate plastic, it is apparent that the differences in impact resistance between glass and allyl resin (CR-39) plastic are minor, whereas the differences between these same materials and polycarbonate are significant (11,12). This difference is apparent for both dress (i.e., 2 mm) and safety (i.e., 3-mm) lenses (Table 13.1).

Although there is little published data on the impact resistance of high index materials, it is alleged by lens manufacturers that these materials possess a higher degree of impact resistance than glass or allyl resin (CR-39) plastic (13). Even so, high index materials do not offer anything near the impact resistance of polycarbonate plastic (Fig. 13.3).

Polycarbonate has a significantly greater capacity to withstand impact from both large and small projectiles, whether the projectiles are moving rapidly or not and regardless of whether dress or safety (i.e., 3-mm) lenses are used. Because of the enormous advantage in impact resistance offered by polycarbonate, it is the lens material of choice whenever ocular protection is a key clinical consideration.

Table 13.1 Differences In Impact Resistance

TYPE OF IMPACT	MISSILE SIZE (INCHES)	IMPACT ENERGY LEVEL CAUSING LENS BREAKAGE		IMPACT ENERGY LEVEL (FT-LB) CAUSING FRACTURE OF 2-MM LENSES[a]			IMPACT ENERGY LEVEL (FT-LB) CAUSING FRACTURE OF 3-MM LENSES[a]		
		KG-CM	FT-LB	CHEMICALLY TREATED GLASS	ALLYL RESIN	POLYCARBONATE	HEAT-TREATED GLASS	ALLYL RESIN	POLYCARBONATE
Pitched baseball	>1	281	21	0.66	0.66	>120	2.1	1.28	>120
Softball	>1	228	17	0.66	0.66	No failures	2.1	1.28	No failures
Volleyball	>1	40–80	3–6	0.66	0.66	in published	2.1	1.18	on 9 ft-lb
Fist assault	>1	27–52	2–4	0.66	0.66	tests	2.1	1.18	
Flying gravel									
30 mph	1/8	4	0.3	0.07	0.22	4.7	0.07	0.37	—
50 mph	1/8	11	0.8	0.07	0.22	4.7	0.07	0.37	—
Automobile collisions	>1	911	67	0.66	0.66	—	2.1	1.28	—
Falls	>1	68–204	5–15	0.66	0.66	>120	2.1	1.28	>120

[a]There are no published tests of lenses impacted with balls greater than 1 inch in diameter. Heat-treated 3-mm safety lenses, properly mounted, might withstand some large missiles.

Unpublished test of a 40-lb steel plate dropped 3 feet, with the lens bridging two separated 2 × 4 timbers.

One-eighth inch is an estimate of the effective radius of the edge of a pea stone that is approximately 3/8 inch in diameter. Probably, the edge is sharper than 1/8 inch.

Calculations assumed a 5-lb head striking a part of the vehicle at 20 mph.

Calculations assumed a 5-lb head falling 1 to 3 feet before striking an object.

Adapted from Pizzarello LD, Haik BG. Sports Ophthalmology. Springfield, IL: Charles C Thomas, 1987.

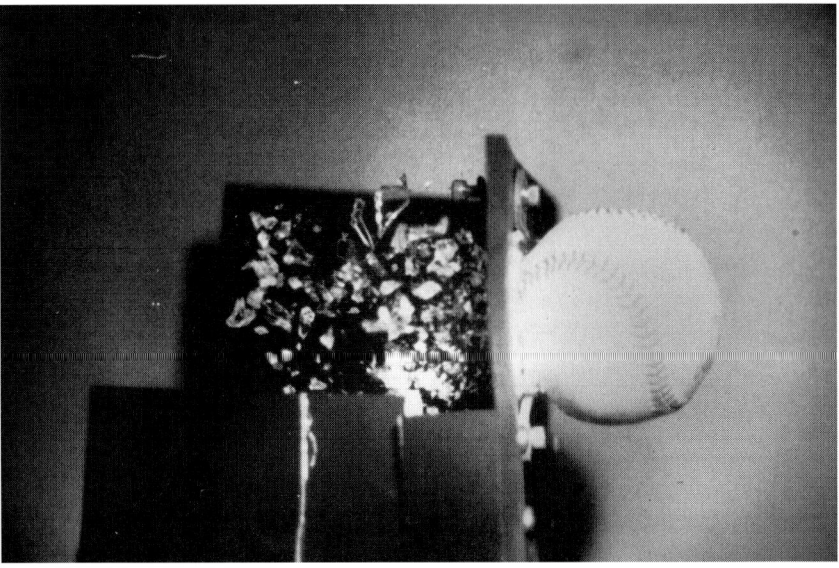

Figure 13.3 *High index lens shattering during testing of impact resistance. High index materials do not possess significant impact resistance and should not be prescribed for ocular protection.* (Photograph courtesy of Paul Vinger, M.D.)

For athletes, the selection of polycarbonate is essential. Refusals on the part of patients who participate in athletics, even on an occasional basis, to obtain polycarbonate plastic should be documented in the patients' record of care.

Claims of Negligence

Sports vision-related claims brought against eyecare practitioners include failure to prescribe the material of choice (i.e., polycarbonate), failure to warn of the risk of injury from alternative materials (i.e., glass, allyl resin plastic, high index plastic), failure to inspect and verify the ophthalmic materials dispensed, and failure to properly manage sports-related ocular trauma or its sequelae (14,15). In each of these situations, the basic question being posed by the court is, "What would a reasonable practitioner have done under the same or similar circumstances?"

Failure to Prescribe the Material of Choice

The suitability of polycarbonate for ocular protection is such that it is clearly the lens material of choice when protection is a key clinical consideration (16). The major decision facing practitioners is when protection from injury is required. The individuals most likely to require protection are monocular patients, athletes, persons whose occupations place them at special risk for injury (e.g., policemen), children, and persons with compromised eyes (i.e., by surgery, injury) (17) (Fig. 13.4).

For athletes, polycarbonate is the material of choice. Failure to prescribe polycarbonate, even for occasional athletes, may result in liability for the practitioner.

A myopic young man was examined by an optometrist and fitted with glass lenses and a dress frame. While participating in a basketball game, a player struck one of the lenses with his elbow, causing it to shatter into splinters of glass that penetrated the eye. Despite treatment, the young man suffered a 25% loss of acuity in the eye. He sued the optometrist for negligence, alleging that the impact resistance of the lenses was inadequate (18).

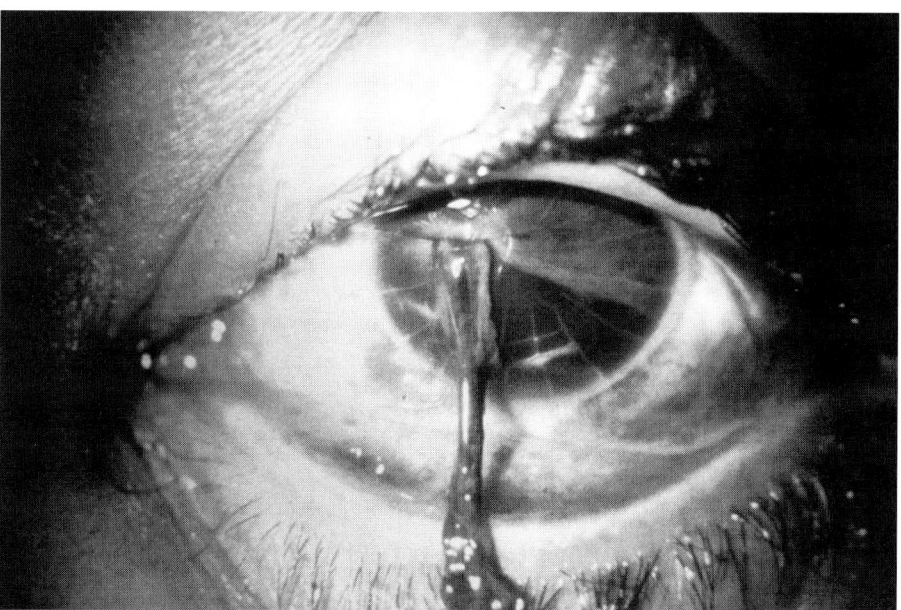

Figure 13.4 *Rupture of cornea along incision lines with iris prolapse in an eye with previous radial keratotomy that was struck by a fist.* (Photograph courtesy of Paul Vinger, M.D.)

If polycarbonate is the lens material of choice, it should be specified ("polycarbonate plastic only") on any prescription that is to be filled by a third-party dispenser. If technicians or assistants order and dispense lenses for a practitioner, they should be aware of the need to provide ocular protection for patients such as athletes. If a patient refuses polycarbonate, this decision should be documented by the technician or assistant.

Failure to Warn of the Risk of Injury from Alternative Lens Materials

If glass, allyl resin (CR-39) plastic, or high index plastic is to be dispensed to an athlete or sports occasional, the patient must be warned of the diminished impact resistance of these materials compared with polycarbonate.

> *A myopic social worker was prescribed spectacles by an optometrist, which he wore while participating in a pick-up baseball game. While at bat he checked his swing, causing the pitched ball to strike the spectacles and shatter one of the glass lenses, lacerating his cornea in three places. He sued the optometrist for the injury, alleging that he had not been adequately warned of the inadequate impact resistance of glass lenses (19).*

Any warnings concerning the reduced impact resistance of alternative materials should be documented in the patient's record.

Inadequate Inspection and Verification

Because a practitioner may also be the seller of a product, there is a duty to inspect the product before dispensing it to the patient. Probably the most common omission is failure to inspect safety eyewear to ensure that it meets Z87.1 standards (particularly lens-thickness requirements). If technicians or assistants are responsible for the inspection of ophthalmic materials, they should possess a clear understanding of the applicable standard, because the employer is responsible for negligence that occurs while employees are acting within the line and scope of their duties.

> *A young man obtained an examination from an optometrist for the purpose of obtaining safety glasses to wear while hunting. He was subsequently involved in an accident, during which one of the lenses shattered, seriously injuring an eye. Analysis of the lens afterward demonstrated that it was not a safety lens. It was discovered that the optometrist's assistant had failed to mark the order correctly and had not dispensed safety lenses to the patient. He filed a lawsuit against the optometrist for his injuries (20).*

Improper Management of Sports-Related Ocular Trauma

The usual issues in these cases are failure to examine adequately an injured patient or failure to warn a patient of the sequelae of injury (i.e., infection, retinal detachment, glaucoma). The examination of an injured patient must meet the standard of care (21,22). Adequate follow-up must also be provided. If a risk of subsequent injury is present, it must be communicated to the patient and documented in the record.

> *A woman struck in the face with a fist was examined by an ophthalmologist and found to have a hyphema and a depressed fracture of the orbit. After 2 months of treatment her problems resolved and she was dismissed from his care, but 8 months later she experienced a retinal detachment. Because he had not warned her of the symptoms of detachment, she did not immediately seek treatment. After unsuccessful surgery to restore her vision, she sued the ophthalmologist on the basis of a failure to warn (23).*

Blunt trauma to the eye can result in secondary injury (such as the rebleeding of a hyphema during the days immediately after injury), complications that arise well after the injury (such as retinal detachments, which may require months to evolve from traumatic retinal dialysis), or even long-term disease (such as unilateral glaucoma occurring years after the injury due to extensive angle recession). Patients injured by blunt trauma require careful education and long-term follow-up.

Product Liability

Product liability is as much social theory as law, for its intent is to place the burden for economic loss from a defective product on the party best able to bear it: the producer of the product. The rationale offered by the courts is that the producer can make the cost of insurance part of the sales price of the product, whereas the consumer bears the cost of the injury—medical bills, lost time from work, disability, pain and suffering—alone.

Product liability law generally holds that if a consumer is using a product (such as an ophthalmic lens) for its intended purpose without substantial alteration and the consumer is injured by a defect in the product, then the designer, manufacturer, or seller of the product is liable for the consumer's injuries, regardless of the care that went into the design, manufacture, or sale of the product (24).

Optometrists, ophthalmologists, and opticians get drawn into product liability cases because they are the sellers of ophthalmic products. But the usual issue is the design or manufacture of the product.

> *The manager of a racquetball court purchased a lensless eye guard to wear during play. He was injured when a ball penetrated the lensless opening and struck his eye, causing a traumatic cataract. He filed a lawsuit against the manufacturer, offering proof from a testing agency that the eye guard design was defective because it permitted penetration of the ball through the lensless opening (25).*

Although there are numerous cases that have been brought to court because of eye injuries from defective eyewear, the most common claims have involved sports frames; lensless eye guards for racket sports have been a leading example. Failure to fit sports eyewear properly or to instruct the wearer in its proper use can also lead to a liability claim.

> *An emmetropic racquetball player purchased an athletic eye guard for use during play. Nothing on the package or in the package insert indicated that a lens had to be placed in the eye guard to ensure protection, and the player was not told at the time of purchase that lenses had to be used. He was injured when a racquetball penetrated the lensless opening and struck his eye. He sued both the manufacturer and the seller for damages (26).*

Showing that a product (the eyewear) is defective is the most difficult legal challenge facing the plaintiff. Proof is obtained by demonstrating that the product did not measure up to appropriate design standards and thus was unreasonably dangerous for the purpose for which it was sold. Expert testimony is necessary to establish the defect in the product's design or manufacture.

If a product is inherently dangerous, it is necessary to warn the purchaser. Failure to do so, if an injury results, can create liability for the manufacturer.

> *A high school baseball player practicing for a game misjudged a fly ball, causing it to carom off his glove and strike his flipped-down plano baseball sunglasses. The impact shattered the lens, driving shards of glass into the youngster's eye and causing the eye to be enucleated 9 days later. The sunglasses were advertised as "just perfect for active and spectator sports—world's finest sunglasses." Although they resembled ordinary sunglasses, the*

center thickness of the lenses was only 1.5 mm, and the lenses were not tempered for impact resistance. The youngster sued the manufacturer of the lenses, alleging that they were unreasonably dangerous for the purpose sold. The manufacturer defended the claim by asserting that the lenses were an inherently unsafe product. The court held the manufacturer liable, however, asserting that such products had to be accompanied by a warning, which had not been provided for the sunglasses (27).

Product liability has not been applied by the courts to contact lenses (28). Cases involving extended-wear lenses, however, could change this (29).

Record Keeping

Accurate, complete records are essential to the defense of a liability claim. Whereas a well-kept record can provide an excellent shield against liability, a poorly documented record can become an Achille's heel. Therefore, eyecare practitioners should observe legal guidelines intended to achieve adequate record keeping and documentation.

Problem-oriented record keeping is well accepted in both the medical and legal professions and is the generally preferred method for the organization of data being recorded. Entries or findings should be descriptive whenever possible; rather than using words without content, such as "normal," "clear," or "unremarkable," the practitioner should describe the pertinent details of the structure being observed. Negative findings, where clinically relevant, should also be recorded.

If a dilated examination is performed, the pharmacologic agents used should be recorded as well as instrumentation used to examine the eye. Erroneous entries should be corrected by drawing a line through the error, writing in the correct information, and initialing and dating the change. If an explanation of the correction is needed, it should be provided. All referrals and recalls should be documented. If a patient must be referred, the appointment should be scheduled with the practitioner to whom the patient is being referred and documented in the patient's record.

Copies of prescriptions for spectacles, contact lenses, and pharmacologic agents for treatment should always be retained in the record of care. In some states, statutes require that patient records be maintained for a specific period of time. For eyecare practitioners in states that have not enacted these statutes, the records should be retained for as long as practicable. Records should not be discarded until after applicable statutes of limitations have run; these statutes vary from state to state in length, depending on the cause of action (i.e., tort, contract). If necessary, legal counsel may be consulted to ascertain the periods of time involved in a specific state.

The importance of adequate record keeping in the defense of liability claims cannot be overemphasized.

Conclusion

It is well documented that sports-related injuries to the visual system have remained at an unacceptable level, despite the development of eyewear and materials that greatly reduce the likelihood of injury (30). Clearly, eyecare practitioners are not adequately advocating and providing eye protection for persons who participate in sporting activities, and lawsuits are an inevitable result of this clinical shortcoming on the part of all three eyecare professions. Greater emphasis needs to be given to this problem, so that practitioners can better appreciate the necessity for prescribing polycarbonate lenses and athletic frames, even for occasional athletes.

The result of such a process would be wider use of protective eyewear, an opportunity to decrease the appalling number of eye injuries, and an inevitable decline in sports-related litigation. Not coincidentally, it would also improve the eyecare professions' service to the public, by heightening awareness of the need for eye protection when participating in sports and leisure activities.

References

1. Vinger P. The incidence of eye injuries in sports. Int Ophthalmol Clin 1981; 21(4):21–45.
2. Vinger P, Horner EF. Sports injuries: the unthwarted epidemic. 2nd ed. Littleton, MA: PSG Publishing, 1986:1–21.
3. Classé JG. A review of 50 malpractice claims. J Am Optom Assoc 1989;60: 694–706.
4. American National Standards Institute. Recommendations for impact resistance of prescription ophthalmic lenses, standard Z80.1-1987. New York: American National Standards Institute, 1987.
5. American National Standards Institute. Recommendations for nonprescription sunglasses and fashion eyewear, standard Z80.3-1986. New York: American National Standards Institute, 1986.
6. American National Standards Institute. Practice for occupational and edu-

cational eye and face protection, standard Z87.1-1989. New York: American National Standards Institute, 1989.
7. American Society of Testing and Materials. Standard specification for eye protectors for use by players of racket sports, standard F910.94. Philadelphia: American Society for Testing and Materials, 1988.
8. American Society of Testing and Materials. Qualifications for faceguards in youth baseball, standard F910.86. Philadelphia: American Society for Testing and Materials, 1985.
9. American Society of Testing and Materials. Eye and face protective equipment for hockey players, standard F513.80. Philadelphia: American Society for Testing and Materials, 1980.
10. Classé JG. Legal aspects of sports vision. Optom Clin 1993;3(1):27–32.
11. Davis JK. Perspectives on impact resistance and polycarbonate lenses. Int Ophthalmol Clin 1988;28:215–218.
12. Davis JK. Lenses for sports vision. In: Pizzarello LD, Haik BG, eds. Sports ophthalmology. Springfield, IL: Charles C Thomas, 1987:9–43.
13. Woods TA. Ophthalmic lenses for athletes and sportsmen. Optom Clin 1993;3(1):33–55.
14. Classé JG. Legal aspects of prescribing for athletes and sportsmen. J Am Optom Assoc 1987;58:674–679.
15. Classé JG. Legal aspects of sports-related ocular injuries. Int Ophthalmol Clin 1988;28(3):211–214.
16. Vinger PF. Principles of protection. Int Ophthalmol Clin 1981;21(4):149–161.
17. Classé JG, Scholles JR. Liability for ophthalmic materials. J Am Optom Assoc 1986;57:470–477.
18. *Westerman v State Optical Co., Ltd.*, 15 ATLA News Letter 458 (1972).
19. *Corey v Robinson*, 19 ATLA News Letter 245 (1976).
20. Classé JG. Legal aspects of optometry. Boston: Butterworths, 1989:348.
21. Bettman JW. How to reduce medicolegal involvement in cases of trauma. Ophthalmology 1980;87:432–434.
22. Bettman JW. Seven hundred medicolegal cases in ophthalmology. Ophthalmology 1990;97:1379–1384.
23. Bettman JW. A review of 412 claims in ophthalmology. Int Ophthalmol Clin 1980;20(4):131–142.
24. Section 402A, Second Restatement of Torts.
25. *Soutee v Pro-Tec, Inc.*, 25 ATLA Law Reporter 375 (1982).
26. *Whitacre v Optical Products, Inc., and Optical Dispensary*, 501 So 2d 994 (La App 1987).
27. *Filler v Rayex Corp.*, 435 F 2d 336 (7th Cir 1970).
28. *Barbee v Rogers*, 425 SW 2d 342 (Tex 1968).
29. *Beaman v Schwartz*, 738 SW 2d 632 (Tenn App 1986).
30. Vinger PF. The eye and sports medicine. In: Duane TD, ed. Clinical ophthalmology. vol. 5. Hagerstown, MD: Harper & Row, 1991:1–51.

CHAPTER 14

Visual Training

David B. Granet
Richard W. Hertle

Despite what seems to be an obvious connection, the role the visual system plays in sports performance has never been clear. This is best illustrated in the game of baseball. The catcher, for example, sees more pitches than any other player yet usually is not one of the best hitters on the team. The shortstop, making decisions based on the complicated visual input of a bouncing ball coming off a rounded bat, generally is one of the weakest hitters on the team. In fact, there are no catchers and only three shortstops represented in the top 100 major league batting averages of all time (1). However, every one of the all-time top 10 outfielders and second basemen are in this top 100. All of these players are elite performers with years of practice at complicated visual tasks; yet the discrepancy exists. If the visual system is such a key component in sports, the question remains, why should this be?

Rationale for screening the athlete's visual system include various studies (2–6). For example, at the 1986 National Olympic Festival, 20% of athletes had visual acuity less than 20/20, with 6% having uncorrected myopia and 13% having uncorrected astigmatism as measured by autorefraction (2). In addition, one quarter of athletes who wore a "habitual" distance prescription did not use this correction for athletic use. The conclusion was that an unmet need for vision care exists in athletes. These results could just as easily be interpreted as elite athletes demonstrating superb performance regardless of screening failures. Does this mean that all athletes can throw their glasses away?

Mass screenings of visual performance have attempted to distinguish those factors that separate an athlete's visual sensory system from that of nonathletes (2–6). Using a 95% confidence interval, one could find a difference on one test out of 20 that appeared statistically significant but was not. Shotgunning makes it easier to hit a target but also means that unintended hits may occur as well. Indiscriminate and inconsistent tests may not be the best approach in discovering differences in an athlete's visual system.

Despite these inconsistencies, it is reasonable to postulate that the visual system is a major contributor in the development of the elite athlete's ability to compete in virtually all sports. When an athlete accepts this assumption, he or she may then ask, "If the visual system is so important, can I get better on the field by improving my visual system off the field?" Athletes are already training their muscles and skills on a host of machines in the gym. Trainers and coaches stress these off-field activities as being crucial to future performance. Keep in mind that only the truly elite performers ever reach the professional ranks. For example, there are only about 700 major league baseball players. It is no surprise that athletes involved in a Darwinian survival of the fittest selection process would be receptive to the possibility of improving performance through training of another part of their body. The impact of offering a certain regimen that will make one a better performer, and the fear of being at a disadvantage if not partaking in these training regimens, is strong motivation to these athletes. However, as scientists, we must first identify the different aspects of the elite athlete's visual system. Then we must find out whether these differences cause the athletes to be better or if they are just coincidentally related.

An example in which training of the visual system seemed appropriate outside of sports is the treatment of dyslexia. Dyslexia is an idiopathic difficulty in reading by persons of otherwise normal intelligence (7,8). Many methods of "visual training" have been advocated to help these patients. In 1993, Menacker et al (8) reported a rigorous study evaluating tinted lenses purported to improve reading skills in dyslexia. They demonstrated no improvement in reading skills. As part of this study, children were subjectively asked to select the tinted lens that improved reading ability. Interestingly, their selection did not correlate with actual reading performance. This is similar to an athlete believing that a specific therapy improved performance *regardless* of actual results. Imagine the response of a family in hearing about a practitioner that could improve reading performance without their knowing that these techniques do not help reading disabilities (9). This would be parallel to the athlete that is desperately looking for the "edge" and willing to try anything, but not having the expertise to evaluate what is truly valuable.

Many training programs are the results of studies that are poorly designed. The major problem is control of tester bias. To avoid these problems, scientists use double-blind techniques. In this way, tester bias cannot influence the results unintentionally (10). Bias can have an effect in various ways. For example, sugar pills and saline injections have been shown to decrease pain in certain subjects (11). There is no doubt that this placebo effect is a real and powerful one (11,12). However, no physician routinely prescribes these so-called medicines because the mechanism by which they work is now understood. All drug studies now must prove that they are more effective than placebo before being accepted as efficacious. Just as we do not allow a drug treatment program on the basis of anecdotal evidence or as a placebo, we should not permit other treatment programs without proper study.

Current Concepts

Because "sports vision training" is generally the purview of behavioral optometrists, the terms most often applied come from the optometric literature. For those unfamiliar with these terms, an explanation and discussion follow.

Static Visual Acuity

Static visual acuity is the most common measure of vision. Snellen's eye chart (first designed in 1862) is the predominant testing method. Other techniques are also available. This measure of acuity is generally accepted as important in sports.

No studies have been done demonstrating a decrease in performance related to a change in vision. In fact, Applegate et al (13) showed that for shooting a basketball, decreasing visual acuity, in steps from 20/20 to 20/400, did not significantly change performance. Fremion et al (14) showed in their evaluation of world class tennis players that the athletes as a group had better visual acuity than the age-matched controls. However, they went on to conclude that "neither superior visual acuity nor other visual functions, monocular or binocular, seem either requisite or limiting in reaching advanced tennis skills. . . ."

Dynamic Visual Acuity

Dynamic visual acuity is defined as that acuity obtained during relative motion of either optotypes (symbols) or the observer (15). Because much of sports takes place in motion, it is believed that acuity measured in this fashion would be more representative of the on-field tasks. Methods for stimulus presentation have not been standardized.

Studies have shown that motion reduces dynamic visual acuity compared with static acuity (16,17). Although they were not comparing groups, Demer et al (18) showed that retinal image motion in the vertical direction affects visual acuity. Dynamic visual acuity has been shown to correlate with a catching task (19). Others have even suggested that dynamic visual acuity may be trainable (20).

Contrast Sensitivity

This is the ability to visually discriminate shades of grey and black from white. Contrast sensitivity testing generally uses black and white gratings of different sizes and shades. Research has previously shown separate brain pathways specifically sensitive to this type of stimulus (21). There are standard stimulus techniques, including Vistech charts, Mentor B-VAT (Fig. 14.1), and Pelli-Robson charts (22).

The role of contrast sensitivity in athletic performance is unclear. Contrast sensitivity testing may more accurately reflect real world conditions than other measures of acuity. For example, Campbell et al (23) evaluated the effect of decreasing illumination on cricket batting and showed reaction time decreased as contrast decreased.

Depth Perception

Gross depth perception is an estimate of the distance from the observer to an object or the relative distance of two or more targets (24). Stereopsis can be thought of as fine depth perception and requires binocular function. Gross depth perception has been studied using the Howard Dolman apparatus (a device with no external reference cues that requires the subject to align two rods). The Brock string (Fig. 14.2) is also used to administer tests in this area.

There are clearly two sets of clues for orientation in space: monocular, which are experiential in nature, and binocular, which are based on intrinsic physiologic arrangements (25). Unfortunately, depth perception and stereopsis are sometimes used interchangeably in the sports vision literature (26). Although gross depth perception would seem to be a requirement in elite athletes, the role of stereopsis

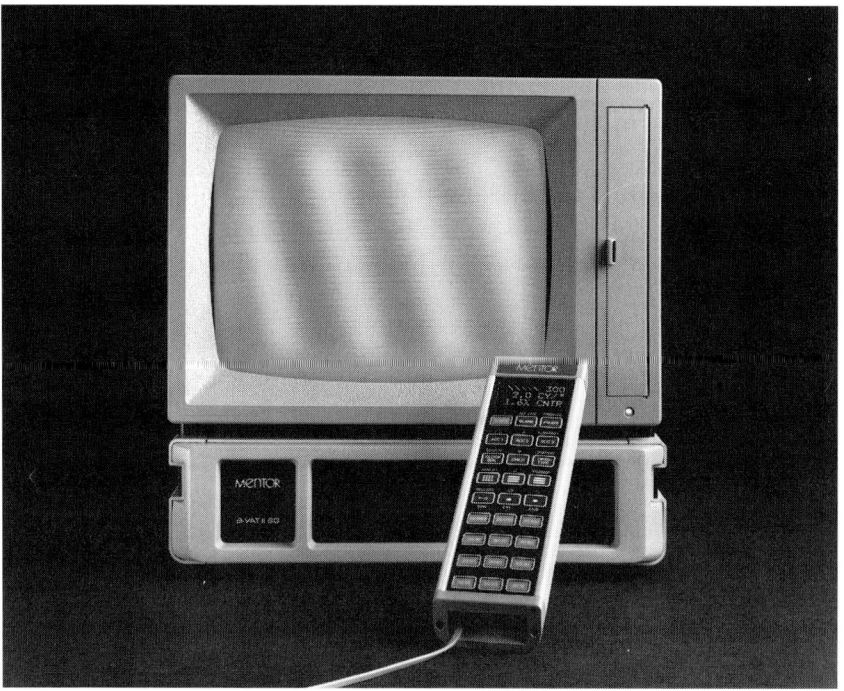

Figure 14.1 *The Mentor B-VAT. Contrast sensitivity and other visual functions can easily be tested on this precalibrated machine.* (Courtesy of Mentor, Inc.)

is not clear. Some elite athletes have suffered from poor stereopsis and less well developed binocular cooperation.

Eye Movements

The brain controls vestibulary stabilized eye movements via separate pathways for slow movements (pursuit, convergence, and divergence) and fast movements (saccades). Electrophysiologic testing of eye movements (oculography) (Fig. 14.3) is the precise method of studying these systems. Often saccades are clinically evaluated for their speed and accuracy. In some studies, subjects hold their heads still and report letters being projected while being timed (King-Devick test).

Tracking an object and stabilizing the eyes during head and body movements (smooth pursuit) and refixating (saccades) are necessary oculomotor functions used during athletic competition (27). Athletes can use parts of trajectories to predict future locations in space in a task of vernier acuity (28), and altering the exposure duration to a

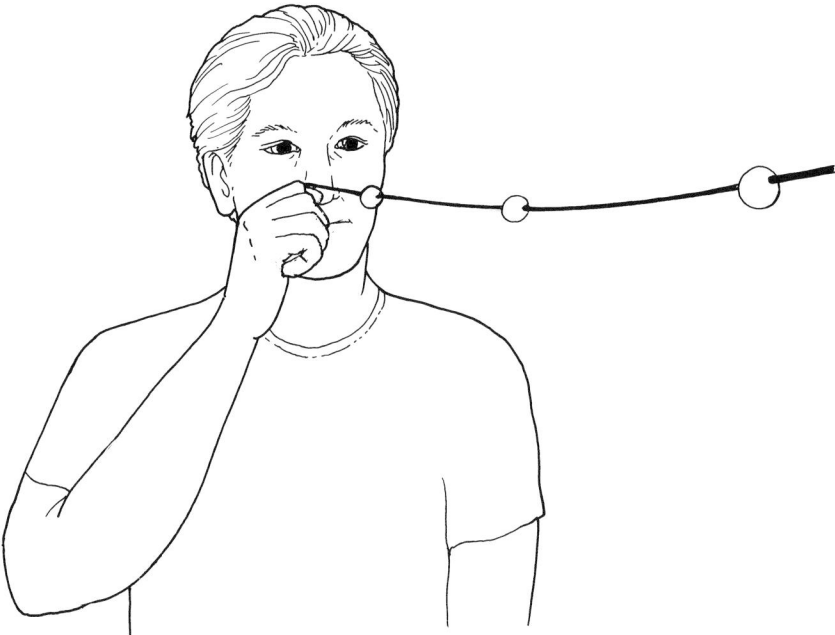

Figure 14.2 *The Brock string. Balls are located at intervals. The athlete is asked to identify where the strings appear to cross.*

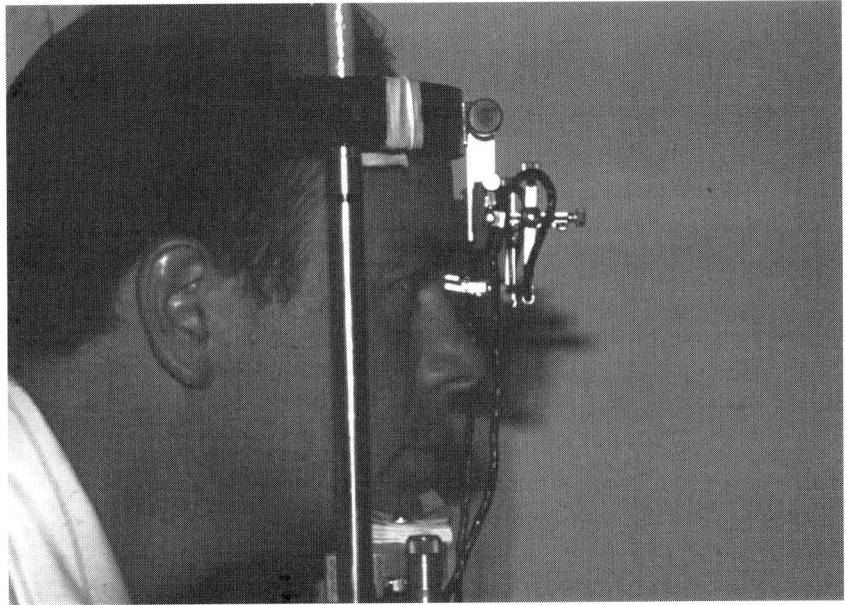

Figure 14.3 *Infrared oculography. Infrared detectors track eye movements and record the signal for quantitative analysis.*

moving target will affect vernier acuity ability (29). Using oculography, Ripoll (30) analyzed the visual-search pattern of table tennis players and showed that these patterns varied in drills (practice) versus match play. However, in either setting, only the first part of the trajectory was tracked. Other variables involved in tracking have been studied as well (31). Unfortunately, quantitative techniques are not generally used by those doing sports vision research (2,3). Smooth pursuit (tracking) is often measured inadequately (2–4).

Accommodation and Vergence

Accommodation is the process whereby the refractive power of the eye is altered to ensure a clear retinal image (25). Vergence is when the visual axes of the eyes move in opposite directions. To refixate or continue fixation on moving targets, these systems must be working accurately.

Testing is clinically easy and reliable. There is widespread evidence that this system is trainable (32). Vigorous exercise was shown to decrease visual acuity and extend the near point of accommodation (33). Athletes in sports such as baseball, hockey, and tennis must track objects that place high demands on both accommodation and vergence.

Central and Peripheral Recognition

Central and peripheral recognition involve the speed and accuracy in recognizing letters projected to either the central or peripheral field. Although perimetry, the formal testing of peripheral vision (Fig. 14.4), should be used in evaluations of visual field, it is not included in most studies (34).

The role of this aspect of visual function in sports would correlate to the athlete's ability to concentrate on a central task or be cognizant of a peripheral one. Such ability has been noted as split-vision (35). In fact, this is only partially a visual task and involves more complex cortical functions, some of which are unrelated to the visual system.

Eye-Hand Coordination

Sensory information from the retina and position of the eye in the orbit is processed, and a motor signal drives the hand (or foot). In sports, coordinated, instinctual, and learned responses should be linked to input from the visual system. The Wayne Saccadic Fixator (Fig. 14.5) and the AcuVision tester are examples of the equipment used for eye-hand coordination testing and training. This equipment

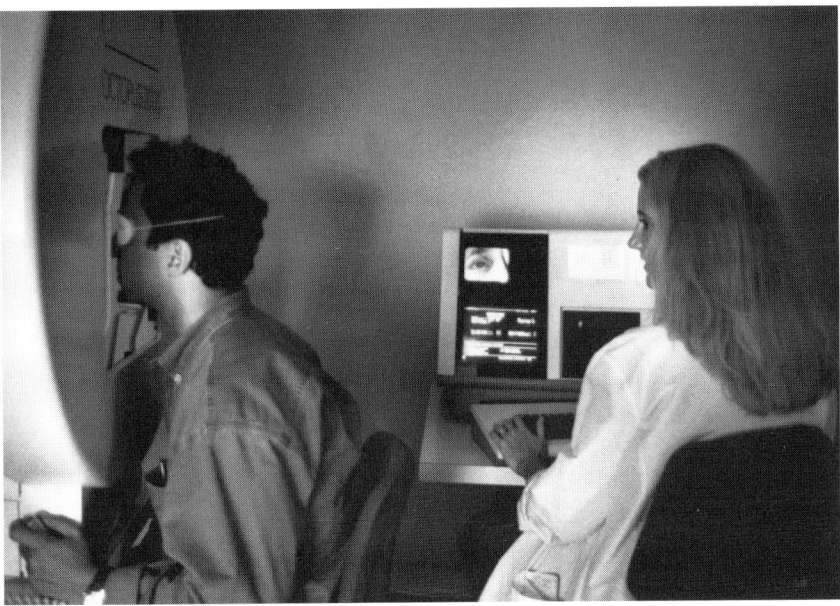

Figure 14.4 *Octopus perimeter. Formal testing of peripheral vision. Quantitative analysis is computer driven.* (Courtesy of Tom Clark.)

has switches spread along a board that when lit must be depressed. This essentially combines testing of the sensory and motor systems together.

Various reports have described connections between manual pointing and visual stimulus (36–38). These studies and legions of video game players would probably claim that the evidence is overwhelming that one can improve hand-eye coordination through practice.

Logic

To accept training of the visual system as a plausible method of improving performance, a number of assumptions must be made: 1) elite athletes have different visual systems than nonathletes, 2) sports performance is affected by these differences, 3) these differences can be isolated and tested adequately, 4) improvement of the visual system is possible, and 5) improvement on a test translates to better on-field performance.

There is scientific support behind the belief that the visual system functions differently in athletes. As far back as 1942, Winograd (39) discovered differences in ability to perform a number of visual tasks

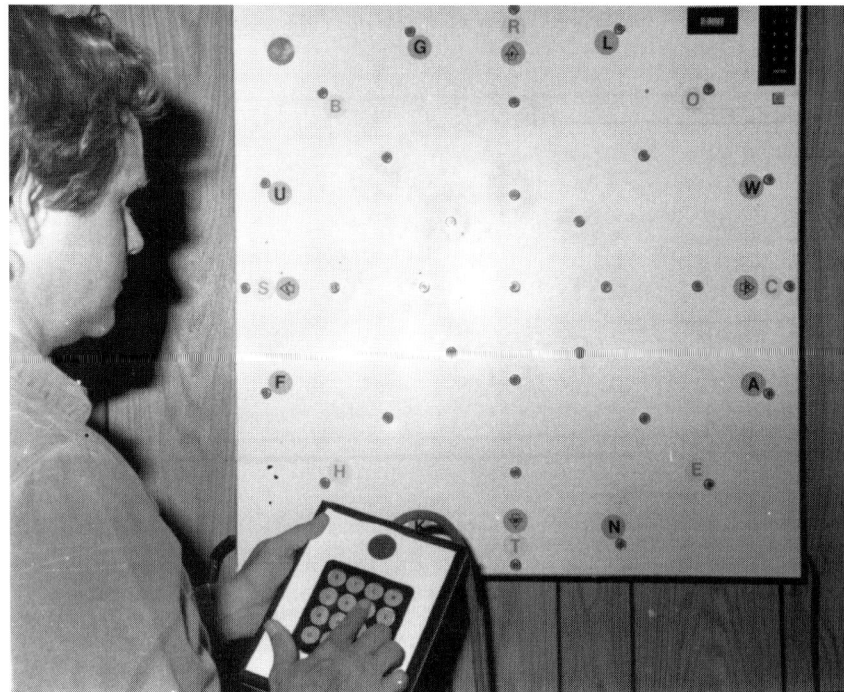

Figure 14.5 *Wayne Saccadic Fixator. The athlete is asked to tap the lit button. In this way the area of deficit can be identified.* (Courtesy of Wayne Engineering.)

among collegiate varsity athletes, rejected candidates for the same varsity teams, and normal controls. Graybiel et al (40), working in the Soviet Union in 1955, showed that, as a group, skilled tennis players perceived depth more accurately than those less proficient on the court. In 1956, Olson (41) was able to demonstrate an increased span of recognition (peripheral vision) in both varsity and intramural athletes compared with a control population of nonathletes. Bahill et al (27) demonstrated the ability of a baseball player to generate smooth pursuit eye movements at more than twice the normal rate. Professional baseball players have also been shown to perform appreciably better under certain conditions at a vernier acuity task with motion than medical student controls (27). Interestingly, baseball players have a higher incidence of crossed ocular dominance than the normal population (42,43). Presumably, this is because hitters have the contralateral eye presented to the pitcher. Others, using large screenings, have reported differences as well (2–6). In general, experts at a task have been shown to have many differences from novices in their approach to practice, performance, and learning (44,45). Brain electrical activity has even been used as a measure of pliability and skill acquisition in sports (46).

Scientific support also exists denying differences between athletes and controls. Beer et al (47) did not show any differences even in eye color of horseshoe winners at a county fair. Dunham (48) compared adolescent baseball players with nonplayers for estimates of a pitched ball crossing the plate and found no differences. Abernathy (49) evaluated visual-search characteristics of expert and novice squash players and could find no differences. Kruk et al (50) found no differences in absolute visual thresholds (earliest detection of an object) between flying and nonflying personnel. McLeod (51) in 1989 could not demonstrate any difference between experienced and inexperienced cricket players in the level of tachistoscopic performance. Even in this brief review of those studies done to compare athletes with controls, it becomes difficult to draw conclusions. Quite often the study design or analysis has been poor (11,52,53). The examiners are not blinded and may be biased. As with any research, studies must be read carefully to determine whether the conclusions drawn are warranted.

Next, it is necessary to determine whether those aspects of the visual system contributing to athletic performance can be isolated and tested adequately. Visual acuity, dynamic visual acuity, contrast sensitivity, smooth pursuit, saccades, and vergence can all be tested in a repeatable standardized way, as noted earlier in this chapter. How much or even if they contribute to on-field performance is difficult to ascertain because athletic performance is dependent on a number of factors.

To understand the difficulty in separating out the various components that make up athletic performance, let us analyze one task from baseball. Hitting a baseball was termed by Ted Williams as "the single most difficult thing in sport" and appears to require the visual system to perform at its extreme (54). Just to determine a ball's location in space, one must know his or her own position, the location of the object image on the retina, and the relation of body position to eye position (55–57). Baseball players must perform this task, constantly updating the position of the ball and then move an object (the bat) into place to interrupt the ball's anticipated future location (Fig. 14.6). All this is done while receiving minimal visual input as to the trajectory of the ball in about 0.2 to 0.5 seconds (Fig. 14.7)

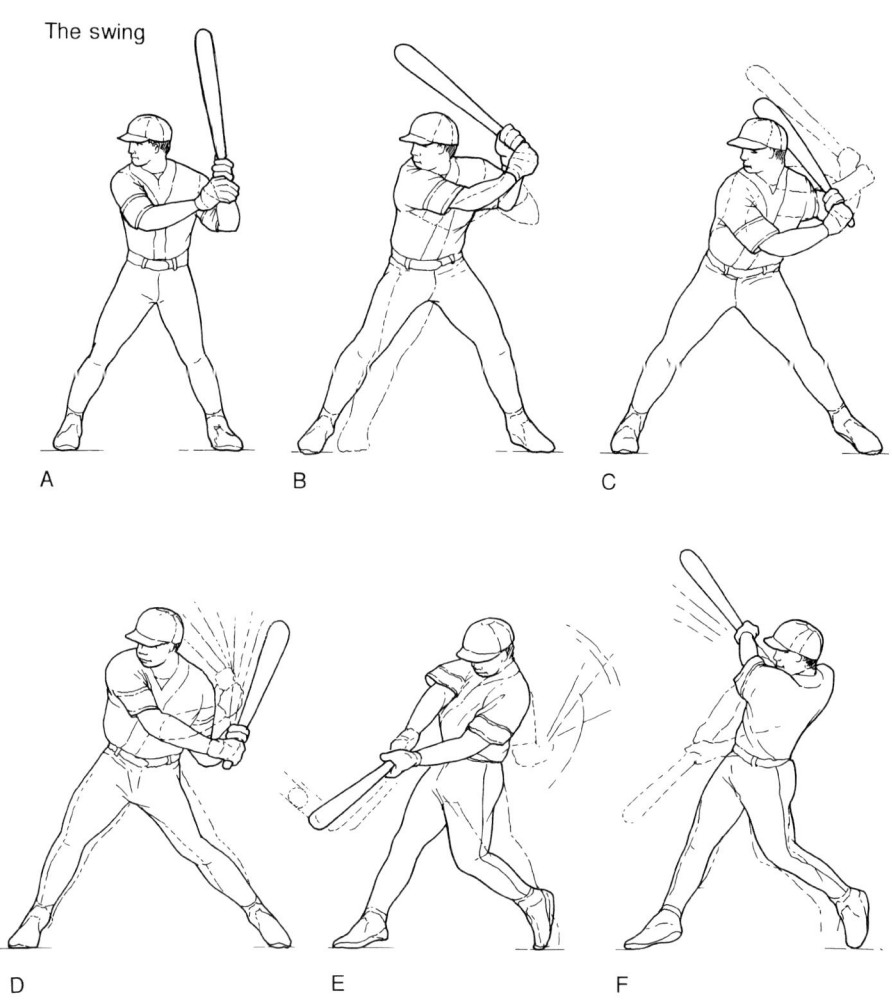

Figure 14.6 *Schematic of tasks involved in hitting a baseball.* (Redrawn by permission from Ward J. The art of hitting. New York Times. March 27, 1994:20.)

(26,27). This takes place with presumed pseudocontinuous adjustments of the reaching movement (58). Moreover, the player must not just determine where but also when the ball crosses the plate (59).

Clearly, this complicated task does not lend itself to simplistic explanations. Where does dynamic visual acuity or contrast sensitivity fit in? How do we calculate what percent of this task to ascribe to each subsystem? What role does the motor system play? Well-designed scientific studies with control groups and elimination of tester bias are key factors in appropriately approaching the evaluation of these issues.

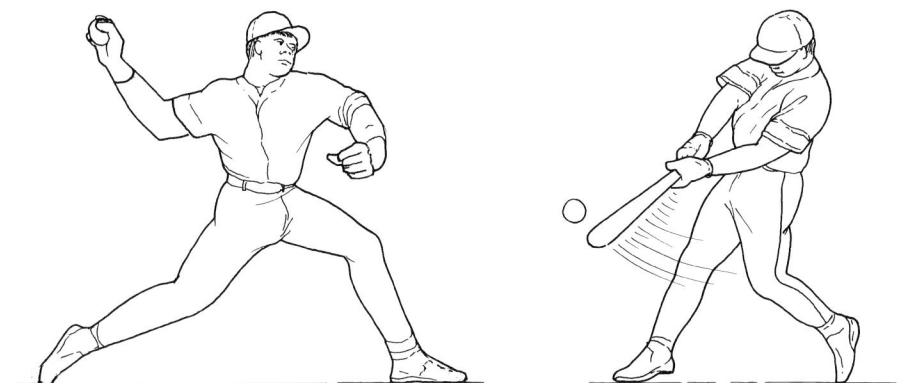

Figure 14.7 *Schematic of the first 0.4 seconds while at bat.* (Redrawn by permission from Ward J. The art of hitting. New York Times. March 27, 1994:20.)

Proven methods to affect the human sensory-motor system include amblyopia therapy and treatment of convergence insufficiency and increasing fusional amplitudes (25). These are successful when implemented in the younger age groups (under 8 years of age). Intervention at an older age is less effective because of maturation of the visual system.

When evaluating results of research on training the visual system for athletics, we must separate the practice effects, learning curves, and placebo effects. McKee et al (60) reported that observers improve their results at a visual task simply by practicing. Schalen (61) further demonstrated that training can activate the smooth pursuit and saccadic system to perform voluntary visual tracking with desired precision. The authors have noted asymmetric smooth pursuit in a college baseball player correlating with the direction he tracked a pitched ball. Clearly, athletes who perform spatial and tracking tasks from an early age have had an enormous amount of practice in the game they play. Then, are differences innate or learned?

Balance training is advocated in some optometric methodologies (2–5). Physical therapists, athletic trainers, and other students of the physical education sciences have worked on balance and proprioception for years. Their literature is complete with multiple studies in this field, and as such this review of visual training does not discuss this in depth (62,63).

Imaging and visualization techniques used by sports psychologists have powerful impacts when administered correctly (64,65). It appears as if motivation, belief, learning, creativity, decision making, and memory are key factors in sports performance (66). In 1985, Harper et al (67), in an attempt to control for the psychological effects of training, randomized elite marksmen to receive either optometric training or imagery training. They could not demonstrate an improvement over control. It seems as if the psychological aspect of one-on-one training and the confidence it engenders may be responsible for the improvements seen in some sports vision training programs (12,68).

It is accepted that activities that improve stamina and strength (e.g., weight lifting and aerobics) often improve athletic performance. If the visual system is able to be improved away from the sport (our final assumption), can this also improve performance?

Stories abound of locker room speeches by coaches that spur their players on to monumental feats. We have noted that practice can help improve performance as can off-field tasks (62,63). Athletic performance is also affected at least by size, quickness, psychological status, experience, and coaching (69). Technically then, we encounter a difficult problem. What parameter does one use for measuring improvement? Is the outcome making the team? Is it winning and losing? Is it improved statistical performance? Can you improve one phase of athletic performance but not improve as a player? Improvement, for scientific purposes, must be defined as more than just athletes' thinking they are better.

As currently formulated, vision training for the athlete relies on "constant emphasis to the athlete that sports vision therapy will enhance the efficiency of their visual system, which then may help in achieving maximal athletic potential" (2). Further, it has been recommended that being aware of the nonverbal communication to the athlete is crucial to the "athlete's positive enthusiasm toward therapy" (2). These techniques, although successfully helping the athlete perform better, may not rely on the visual system for their effects. In 1982, Stine et al (69), after their review of the literature, stated, "the belief that it makes no difference whether the visual training or something else [i.e., placebo effect] is responsible for the improvement after visual training, so long as there is improvement, *may be acceptable to the coach but to the optometric profession, it is unsatisfactory.*"

With regard to training influencing the visual system, Hitzeman et al (70) noted "there is little evidence demonstrating that a regimen of visual training will achieve an improvement in the visual skills of athletes." In an editorial, Stein et al (71) concurred, stating "we strongly feel that at present the relationship between sports vision training and athletic performance is unknown." It is even possible that giving a sense of confidence without a corresponding improvement in performance could lead to eventual negative impact (71,72). The belief that training in the laboratory can enhance performance has yet to be proven.

Areas for Future Study

A primary interest should be investigation of the elite athlete's visual system. Careful selection of study groups is essential. Different sports, flying planes, playing video games, and so on present varied challenges to participants. Lumping these together confuses the investigator. Future studies must be designed and carried out using standard scientific approach and statistical analysis.

Correlated events do not always mean one causes the other. For example, heart attacks might be correlated to number of cars in a country that cost over $50,000. No one would suggest that the cars were the cause of heart attacks or attempt to train members of a community to purchase less costly vehicles. However, it would not be unreasonable to infer that industrialized societies where fat intake, cigarette use, and stress contribute to heart attacks also lead to the purchase of expensive cars. By analogy, vision scientists must be careful about drawing conclusions regarding cause and effect. The same systems that allow superb balance, coordination, and prioritization may appear to result in a better visual system without the vision being the cause of elite athletic performance. Again, proper study design can help answer these questions.

Studies of peripheral visual fields, for example, should use standardized perimetry. Refractive errors should be determined not by autorefracting machines but by cycloplegic retinoscopy (regardless of difficulty). Visual acuity, stereoacuity, and contrast sensitivity all can be tested using devices like the Mentor B-VAT with easy repeatability. Smooth pursuit and saccadic evaluation, both of extreme interest in this field, must be evaluated by oculography. Perhaps the study of visually handicapped athletes would be of interest as well.

Training of athletes to perform better by taking advantage of mental strategies or improving confidence is the province of sports psychologists (12,68). Protocols evaluating well-designed visual training paradigms based on the results of our improved understanding of the visual system may one day allow active participation by vision specialists (73). For now, these attempts should take a back seat to learning more about the role of the visual system in sports.

The effect of athletics on the health of the visual system is also of general interest. The effects of exercise on intraocular pressure and visual acuity have been reported (74–78). They showed that exercise affected both parameters. Exercise has even been shown to induce ocular motility disorders (79). There is enough evidence to warrant further study of the effects of exercise, both positive and negative, on the function of the eyes.

Recommendations

Athletes should have complete examinations by a vision expert. It is reasonable to ensure proper refractive correction for sports performers given our current state of knowledge. Alerting an athlete to a potential problem like glare recovery may allow him or her to compensate using other strategies (e.g., sunglasses).

The risks of damage to the eyes from participation and trauma in sports are discussed elsewhere in this volume and represent a well-studied area (80–86). If for no other reason, athletes should be examined to evaluate the health of the eye and be counseled as to proper protective eyewear. The only psychological impact from the ocular examination should be reassurance that the eyes (once checked) are not the cause of poor performance.

The opportunity to affect the visual system is of course greatest during childhood. According to the recommendations of the American Academy of Ophthalmology, all children should have an evaluation to detect eye and vision abnormalities during the first few months of life and again at about age 3 (87). This is in addition to screening by the pediatrician. In this way, early identification of eye abnormalities facilitates optimum treatment (88). Young athletes should be examined routinely to evaluate the eyes for trauma-related issues. Naturally, teaching athletes safety at a young age is advantageous.

Summary

Elite athletes, by definition, demonstrate an empirically superior ability to perform certain complicated tasks. For this, society rewards them with celebrity status, fame, and fortune. For some, athletic success is the ticket to an education and the cornerstone upon which a new life is built. Even athletes performing at the small college, high school, Little League, or the local level reap varying levels of rewards. Parents take great interest and become emotionally invested in the participation and the outcome of their children's athletic endeavors. For many people, their self-esteem is linked to the quality of their athletic competition. It is no surprise that sports performers are always searching for ways to improve.

Many sports require what appears to be key input from the visual system for optimal performance. For example, hitting a baseball is so difficult that a professional may fail 70% of the time (i.e., hitting .300) and be considered successful. Moreover, a small change in this rate, failing 75% of the time, can mean the difference between rising to the professional ranks and perhaps millions of dollars. It would appear that the visual system is crucial in other sports, like tennis, hockey, basketball, archery, and pool. In addition, arguments could be made that sports like football, soccer, gymnastics, and even track and field require a superior visual system. It is with a sense of hope and anticipation then that an uninformed athlete would embark on a trial of visual training.

Some people are bound to report feeling an improvement after such visual training (8). Although interesting, these reports are not scientific. Although this type of anecdotal evidence does not serve as an adequate basis for diagnosis and treatment, it can provide part of the background rationalization for future study.

Reichow et al (2) state that maximum athletic performance is related to multiple factors, including 1) intelligence, 2) confidence, 3) coaching, 4) nutrition, 5) desire, 6) conditioning, 7) physical attributes, 8) concentration, 9) natural ability, 10) practice and experience, 11) speed of response, and 12) vision. The role any given visual subsystem plays must then be further diminished. Therefore, if the goal of therapy is to bolster an athlete's confidence, concentration, or desire, the behavioral experts best suited to this task would be sports psychologists and not vision experts.

Once again let us use dyslexia as an analogy for sports performance. The American Academy of Ophthalmology, the American Association for Pediatric Ophthalmology and Strabismus, and the American Academy of Pediatrics issued a joint statement regarding its treatment:

> *No known scientific evidence supports claims for improving the academic abilities of dyslexic or learning disabled children, or modification of delinquent or criminal behavior, with treatment*

based on: 1) visual training, including muscle exercises, ocular pursuit or tracking exercises, or glasses (with or without bifocals or prisms); and 2) neurologic organizational training (laterality training, balance board, perceptual training).

Furthermore, such training frequently yields deleterious effects. A false sense of security is created, which may delay or prevent proper instruction or remedial therapy. The teaching of dyslexic and learning disabled children and adults is a problem of educational science (89).

This logic should apply to sports until or if future studies provide different data.

It is therefore the responsibility of the scientific community to *prove* these hypotheses regarding the visual system. Before coaches proceed with testing and training athletes to improve performance, a comprehensive and scientifically rigorous examination of the visual system should be mandated. Until vision specialists first understand and elucidate the role of the visual system in sports, it seems reasonable for the athlete to turn his or her energy toward more traditional methods of improving performance. To paraphrase, the teaching of athletes is a problem of physical education and coaching sciences.

Conclusion

If there truly are aspects of the visual system that vary from group to group and affect the ability to perform tasks, it does seem that athletes would be an excellent model to study. The visual tasks involved in sports appear to demand a severe selection process. Eventually, the systematic study of athletes should generate an enhanced understanding of the way in which the visual system functions. Armed with this knowledge, ophthalmologists and vision specialists would be better able to advise, assist, and care for all of their patients.

References

1. Thorn J, Palmer P. Total baseball: the ultimate encyclopedia of baseball. 3rd ed. New York: Harper Perennial, 1993.
2. Reichow AW, Stoner MW, eds. Sports vision: introduction to behavioral optometry. Santa Ana, CA: Optometric Extension Program Inc., 1991.
3. Berman AM. Clinical evaluation of the athlete. Optom Clin 1993;3:1–26.

4. Coffey B, Reichow AW. Optometric evaluation of the elite athlete. Probl Optom 1990;2:32–59.
5. Christenson GN, Winkelstein AM. Visual skills of athletes versus nonathletes: development of a sports vision testing battery. J Am Optom Assoc 1988;59:666–675.
6. Revien L, Gabor M. Sports vision. New York: Workman Publishing Co., 1981.
7. Rutter M. The concept of specific reading retardation. J Child Psychol Psychiatry 1975;16:181–197.
8. Menacker SJ, Breton ME, Breton ML, et al. Do tinted lenses improve the reading performance of dyslexic children? Arch Ophthalmol 1993;111:213–218.
9. Metzger RL, Werner DB. Use of visual training for reading disabilities: a review. Pediatrics 1984;73:824–828.
10. Connelly RJ. Deception and the placebo effect in biomedical research. IRB: a review of human subjects research. 1987;9:5–7.
11. Price L. Art, science, faith and medicine: the implications of the placebo effect. Soc Health Illness 1984;6:61–73.
12. Mrna B, Skrivanek A. Placebo effect on healthy volunteers-athletes. Presented at the 26th Annual Psychopharmocological Meeting: Activitas Neurvosa Superior, 1985.
13. Applegate RA, Applegate RA. Set shot performance and visual acuity in basketball. Optom Vis Sci 1992;69:765–768.
14. Fremion AS, Demyer WE, Helveston EM, et al. Binocular and monocular visual function in world class tennis players. Binocular Vision 1985;1:147–154.
15. Miller JW, Ludvigh EJ. The effect of relative motion on visual acuity. Surv Ophthalmol 1962;7:83–116.
16. Ludvigh E, Miller JW. Study of visual acuity during the ocular pursuit of moving test objects. I. Introduction. J Optom Soc Am 1958;48:799–802.
17. Reading VM. Visual resolution as measured by dynamic and static tests. Pflugers Arch 1972;333:17–26.
18. Demer JL, Amjadi F. Dynamic visual acuity of normal subjects during vertical optotype and head motion. Invest Ophthalmol Vis Sci 1993;34:1894–1906.
19. Sanderson FH, Whiting H. Dynamic visual acuity and performance in a catching task. J Motil Behav 1974;6:87–94.
20. Long R, Riggs C. Training effects on dynamic visual acuity free-head viewing. Perception 1991;20:363–371.
21. Campbell FW, Robson JG. Application of Fourier analysis to the visibility of gratings. J Physiol 1968;197:551.
22. Pelli DG, Robson JG, Wilkins AJ. The design of a new letter chart for measuring contrast sensitivity. Clin Vision Sci 1988;2:187.
23. Campbell FW, Rothwell SE, Perry MJ. Bad lights stop play. Ophthal Physiol Optics 1987;7:165–167.
24. Katz M. The human eye as an optical system. In: Tasman W, ed. Duane's textbook of clinical ophthalmology. 1991:1:33;31.
25. Von Norden GK. Binocular vision and ocular motility. St. Louis: C. V. Mosby, 1990.
26. Coffey BC, Reichow AW. Optometric evaluation of the elite athlete. Probl Optom 1990;2:32–59.

27. Bahill AT, LaRitz T. Why can't batters keep their eyes on the ball? Am Sci 1984;72:249–253.
28. Granet DB. Vernier acuity in motion: a comparison of athletes and non-athletes. Thesis, Yale University School of Medicine, 1987.
29. Morgan MJ, Watt RJ, McKee SP. Exposure duration affects the sensitivity of vernier acuity to target motion. Vision Res 1983;23:541–546.
30. Ripoll H. Uncertainty and visual strategies in table tennis. Percept Mot Skills 1989;68:507–512.
31. Lanman J, Bizzi, Allum J. The coordination of eye and head movement during smooth pursuit. Brain Res 1978;153:39–53.
32. Haynes HM, McWilliams LG. Effects of training on near-far response time as measured by the distance rock test. J Am Optom Assoc 1979;50:715–718.
33. Ishigaki H, Miyao M, Ishiahara S, et al. The deterioration of visual acuity by exercise under a mesopic vision environment. J Sports Med Phys Fitness 1991;31:272–276.
34. Bjurwill C. Perceptual-motor behavior in sport: the double reaction. Percept Mot Skills 1991;72:137–138.
35. Drance SM. Visual field defects. In: Tasman WM, ed. Duane's textbook of ophthalmology. 1991:1–23.
36. Soechting JF, Flanders M. Sensorimotor representations for pointing to targets in three-dimensional space. J Neurophysiol 1989;62:582–594.
37. Soechting JF, Helms Tillery SI, Flanders M. Transformation from head-to-shoulder centered representation of target direction in arm movements. J Cogn Neurosci 1990;2:32–43.
38. Prablanc C, Pelisson D, Goodale MA. Visual control of reaching movements without vision of the limb. Exp Brain Res 1986;62:293–302.
39. Winograd S. The relationship of timing and vision to baseball performance. Res Q Am Assoc Health Phys Educ 1942;13:481–493.
40. Graybiel A, Jokl E, Trapp C. Russian studies in vision related activity and sports. Res Q Am Assoc Health Phys Educ 1955;26:212–223.
41. Olson EA. Relationship between psychological capacity and success in college athletics. Res Q Am Assoc Health Phys Educ 1956;27:79–89.
42. Teig D. Major league baseball research project. Ridgefield, CT: Institute for Sports Vision, 1980.
43. McLean JM, Ciurczak FM. Bimanual dexterity in major league baseball players: a statistical study. N Engl J Med 1982; 1278–1279.
44. Ferrari M, Pinard A, Reid L, Bouffard-Bouchard T. The relationship between expertise and self-regulation in movement performance: some theoretical issues. Percept Mot Skills 1991;72:139–150.
45. Glaser R. Thoughts on expertise. In: Schooler C, Schaie W, eds. Cognitive functioning and social structure over the life course. Norwood, NJ: Ablex 81–94.
46. Gioux M, Arne P, Paty J, Bensch C. Cognitive potentials and skill acquisition in sports. N Y Acad Sci 465–469.
47. Beer J, Beer J. Relationship of eye color to winning horseshoe pitching contests. Percept Mot Skills 1989;68:136–138.
48. Dunham P Jr. Coincidence-anticipation performance of adolescent baseball players and nonplayers. Percept Mot Skills 1989;68:1151–1156.
49. Abernathy B. Expertise, visual search, and information pick-up in squash. Perception 1990;19:63–77.

50. Kruk R, Regan D, Beverley KI, Longridge T. Correlations between visual test results and flying performance on the advanced simulator for pilot training. Aviat Space Environ Med 1981;455–460.
51. McLeod P. Visual reaction time and high-speed ball games. Perception 1989; 18:789–792.
52. Dippner R. The relation between basketball ability and visual acuity in the unicorn. Am J Optom Arch Am Acad Optom August 1973.
53. Lasky DI, Lasky AM. Stereoscopic eye exercises and visual acuity. Percept Mot Skills 1990;71:1055–1058.
54. Williams TS, Underwood J. The science of hitting. New York: Simon and Schuster, 1971.
55. Carpenter RHS. Movements of the eyes. London: Pion Limited, 1977.
56. Matin L, Pearce DG, Kibler G. Role of local sign and ocular proprioception in the determination of visual direction during eye movements. J Optom Soc Am 1964;54:1398.
57. Shakhnovich AR. The brain and regulation of eye movements (translated by Basil Haigh). New York: Plenum Press, 1977.
58. Pelisson D, Prablanc C, Goodale MA, Jeannerud M. Visual control of reaching movements without vision of the limb. II. Exp Brain Res 1986;62: 303–311.
59. Tynan PD, Sekuler R. Motion processing in peripheral vision: reaction time and perceived velocity. Vision Res 1982;22:61–68.
60. McKee SP, Westheimer G. Improvement in vernier acuity with practice. Percept Psychophys 1978;24:258–262.
61. Schalen L. Quantification of tracking eye movements in normal subjects. Acta Otolaryngol 1980;90:404–413.
62. Voss DE, Ionta MK, Myers BJ. Proprioceptive neuromuscular facilitation. 3rd ed. Philadelphia: Harper & Row, 1985:xi–xviii.
63. Kisner C, Colby LA. Therapeutic exercise. 2nd ed. Philadelphia: F. A. Davis Company, 1990:402–407.
64. Silva JM, Weinberg RS. Psychological foundation of sport. Champaign, IL: Human Kinetics, 1984.
65. Kubistant T. The use of visualization in sports medicine. Sportsmed Dig 1982;4:5–6.
66. Daus AT, Wilson J, Freeman WM. Predicting success in football. J Sports Med Phys Fitness 1989;29:209–212.
67. Harper WS, Landers DM, Wang MQ. The role of visual training exercises in visual abilities and shooting performance. In: Psychology of motor behavior and sport. Abstracts of the North American Society for the Psychology of Sport and Physical Activity. School of Health, Physical Education, Recreation and Dance, Louisiana State University.
68. Olson EA. Relationship between psychological capacities and success in college athletics. Res Quart Am Assoc Health Phys Educ 1956;27:79–89.
69. Stine CD, Arterburn MR, Stern NS. Vision and sports: a review of the literature. J Am Optom Assoc 1982;53:627–633.
70. Hitzeman SA, Beckerman SA. What the literature says about sports vision. Optom Clin 1993;3:145–159.
71. Stein R, Squires G, Pashby T, Easterbrook M. Can vision training improve athletic performance? Can J Ophthalmol 1989;24:105–106.
72. Leibowitz HW, Vinger PF, Landers DM. Can visual training improve ath-

letic performance? Proceedings of the United States Olympic Academy XII, The Pennsylvania State University, University Park, 1988.
73. Vinger P. Vision training study. In: Tasman WM, ed. Duane's textbook of ophthalmology. 1985:46–47.
74. Haynes WL, Johnson TJ, Alward WLM. Effects of jogging exercise on patients with the pigmentary dispersion syndrome and pigmentary glaucoma. Ophthalmology 1992;99:1096–1103.
75. Passo MS, Goldberg L, Elliot DL, Van Buskirk EMV. Exercise conditioning and intraocular pressure. Am J Ophthalmol 1987;103:754–757.
76. Passo MS, Goldberg L, Elliot DL, Van Buskirk EMV. Exercise training reduces intraocular pressure among subjects having glaucoma. Arch Ophthalmol 1991;109:1096–1098.
77. Ashkenazi I, Melamed S, Blumenthal M. The effect of continuous strenuous exercise on intraocular pressure. Invest Ophthalmol Vis Sci 1992;33:2874–2877.
78. Ishigaki H, Miyao M, Ishiahara S, et al. The deterioration of visual acuity by exercise under a mesopic vision environment. J Sports Med Phys Fitness 1991;31:272–276.
79. Osterele CS. Exercise induced esotropia. J Pediatr Ophthalmol Strabismus 1989;26.
80. Giovinazzo V, Yannuzzi LA, Sorenson JA, et al. The ocular complications of boxing. Ophthalmology 1987;94:587–595.
81. Zagelbaum B, Hersh P, Donnenfeld E, Perry H. Major league baseball eye trauma. New Engl J Med 1994;330:1021–1023.
82. Zagelbaum B, Starkey C, Hersh P, et al. The National Basketball Association (NBA) eye injury study. Arch Ophthalmol 1995;113:749–752.
83. Zagelbaum B. Sports-related eye trauma: managing common injuries. Phys Sports Med 1993;21:25–42.
84. Larrison WI, Hersh PS, Kunzweiler T, Shingleton BJ. Sports-related ocular trauma. Ophthalmology 1990;97:1265–1269.
85. Belongia EA, Goodman JL, Holland EJ, et al. An outbreak of herpes gladitorium at a high school wrestling camp. N Engl J Med 1991;325:906–910.
86. Vinger P. The eye and sports medicine. In: Tasman WM, ed. Duane's textbook of ophthalmology. 1985;5:46–47.
87. Pediatric Ophthalmology Panel Members. Comprehensive pediatric eye evaluation. Preferred practice pattern. San Francisco, CA, 1992:2.
88. Pediatric Ophthalmology Panel Members. Amblyopia. Preferred practice pattern. San Francisco, CA, 1992:8.
89. American Academy of Ophthalmology, American Academy of Pediatrics, American Association for Pediatric Ophthalmology and Strabismus. Policy statement on learning disabilities, dyslexia and vision. In: Pediatric ophthalmology and strabismus: basic and clinical science course. 1990;6:196–197.

Index

Abdul-Jabbar, Kareem, basketball goggles and, 53–54
Accommodation, in visual training, 246
Adnexa, injury and, 186–187, *187–188*
Afferent Pupillary Defect (APD), 190
Air gun injuries, 135–143
Allyl resin
 chemically tempered glass, comparison, *229*
 heat tempered glass, comparison, *229*
Amblyopia, 185
American Amateur Racquet Association, 77
American Baseball Cap Company, 34
American Legion Helmet, baseball, 35
American National Standards Institute, 7, 226
American Society for Testing and Materials, safety standards, 6, 7
Anatomy, 154–183
 apex, orbital, *168*
 arteries, superficial, *165*
 bones, orbit, *155*
 bony orbit, 154–159, *155–160*
 cranial nerve, fifth, ophthalmic division of, *170*
 eyelid
  anatomic landmarks, *177*
  lymphatic drainage of, *167*
  soft tissues, 176–179, *177–178*, *180*
 fascia, orbital, 161–163
 frontozygomatic suture, fracture at, *156*
 globe, 161, *162*
 lacrimal system, 180–182, *181*
 muscles
  extraocular, *162*
  of orbit, *162*, 172–176, *174–175*
 nerves, orbital, 167–172, *168*, *170*
 ophthalmic artery, major branches of, within orbit, *163*
 orbicularis oculi muscle, *178*
 orbit
  contents, 160–182
  floor, *159*
  right, *174*
  roof, *157*
  structures, anterior, *175*
   lateral, *160*
   medial, *158*
 periorbita, 160
 septum, orbital, *180*
 tripod fracture, *156*
 venous drainage, of orbit, *166*
 vessels, orbital, *163*, 163–167, *165–167*
 zygomaticomaxillary suture, fracture at, *156*
Anesthesia
 for ocular injuries, 195
 for lid injuries, 201
 topical, 195
Angle abnormalities, boxing and, 96–97
Anhydrase inhibitors, hyphema, 198
ANSI. *See* American National Standards Institute
Anterior segment injury, 184–209
 anterior chamber, estimating depth of, *193*
 blunt trauma, 199, 202
 canthotomy, lateral, *208*
 cataract, traumatic, *206*
 clinical evaluation, 184–185
 conjunctival lacerations, 197
 corneal abrasion, *194*, 194–196, 195t, *196*
 diagnosis, 194–207
 examination, 185–191, *187*
  adnexa, 186–187, *187–188*
  cornea, *187*
  external examination, 185–187
  eyelids, 185–186
  face, 185–186
  globe, *187*
   ruptured, suspicion of, *188*
  near card, *189*
  ocular surface, 186–187, *187–188*
  pupil, 189–190, *190*, 190–191
   constriction, *191*
  visual acuity, 187–189, *189*
 extraocular movements, 191
 eyelid, laceration, 200–202, *201*, 201t
 first-aid kit, 186t
 fluorescein stain, *193*
 foreign body, 194
  nonpenetrating, *194*, 204, *204*
  penetrating, 204–205, 205t
 globe, ruptured, 204–205, 205t
 hemorrhage
  retrobulbar, 207, 207t, *208*
  subconjunctival, 197
 hyphema, 198–200, *199*, 200t
 intraocular pressure, 193–194
 iritis
  management of, 197t
  traumatic, 197t, 197–198

Anterior segment injury (*Continued*)
  lens injuries, 205–206, *206*
  management, 195–207
  nonpenetrating, removal of, *204*
  orbital wall fractures, *202–203*, 202–204, 203t
  overview, 207–209
  patient history, 185, 186t
  pressure patch, *196*
  relative afferent pupullary defect, testing for, 190
  visual acuity and, 187–189, *189*
  wound edges, suturing superficial, *201*
Anticoagulants, hyphema, 198
Apex, of orbit, *168*
Artery
  ophthalmic, major branches of, within orbit, *163*
  superficial, *165*
ASTM. *See* American Society for Testing and Materials
Athletic participation, guidelines for, 10

Badminton, 72–73, *73*, 74t
Balance training, 251
Ball
  golf, *124*
  speed, in racquetball, 79, 79t
  velocity, racquetball, 79
Bandage Contact lens, 195
Base, baseball, sliding into, 32
Base runner, baseball, injury to, 27–32, *32*
Baseball, 23–42, 34, 41
  age, injury and, 23
  American Baseball Cap Company, 34
  American Legion Helmet, 35
  ball, 33–34, *35*
  base, sliding into, 32
  base runner, 27–32, *32*
  bat, 33–34, *34*
  at bat, first 0.4 seconds, schematic of, *251*
  batter, 24–26, *25*
    swing of, *25*
  batting helmet, 34–36, *35*
  C-flap, 38, *40*
  catcher, 27, *28–31*
  catcher's mask
    of 1930's, *30*
    modern, *31*
    of nineteenth century, *28–29*
  contact lenses, 40–41
  Dixie Youth baseball, 36–37
  dugout, 24
  equipment, 33–36
  eyeglasses, 37
  face guard, *39*, 39, 37–39
  fielder, 27
  helmet, batting, 34–36, *35*
  hitting, components of act, 249–250
  infielder, 27
  injury from, 34
  level of experience, injury and, 24
  Little League, 36
    rulebook, 36
  Louisville Slugger, 33
  Major League, 24, 37
  on-deck circle, 24
  outfielder, 27
  pitcher, 26
  popularity of, 23
  spectators, 33
  sunglasses, 39–40
  tasks involved in hitting, visual training and, 250
  umpire, 32–33
    police, comparison, 32
Baseball Hall of Fame, 32
Basketball, 43–55, *44*
  Abdul-Jabbar, Kareem, 53–54
  activity, of athlete, at time of injury, 48
  ball, as mechanism of injury, 47–48
  blunt trauma, 48t, 48–50, *49–51*
  defensive player, arm, hand extension, *50*
  develoment of, Naismith, Rev. James, 43
  examination of eye, preparticipation, 54
  eyewear, 52–54, *53*
  goggles, 52–53, *53*
  history of, 43–44
  injury database, National Collegiate Trainers' Association, 45
  mechanisms of injury, 47–50
    center position, 47
    forward position, 47
    guard position, 47
  National Basketball Association
    eye trauma, frequency of, 46, *46*
    mechanism of eye injury, 48, *48*
  National Basketball Association Eye Injury Study, 45–47, *46*, 46t
  NCAA Guideline 4B, eye safety in sports, 52
  overview, 54
  prevalence, of injuries, 45
  prevention of eye injury, 50–54, 52t
  projectile mechanisms, 47–48
  protective equipment, rules mandating use of, 44–45
    National Collegiate Athletic Associaton, 44–45
  rebounding, arm, finger, extension, *49*
  sports frames, 52–53, *53*
  "warding off" of opponent, *51*
Bat
  baseball, injury from, 32–33, *34*
  first 0.4 seconds, schematic of, *251*
Batter, baseball
  injury to, 24–26, *25*
  swing of, *25*
Batting helmet, baseball, injury from, 34–35, *35*
BB gun, 135–141, *138*, *140*
  BB, on CT, *138*t
Bishop, Pat, 83, 86
Blind patients
  sports and, 11–12
  U.S. Association for Blind Athletes, 11–12
Blood, in eye. *See* Hyphema

Blunt trauma
  anterior segment, *199, 202*
  posterior segment injury, 212–213, *213–214*
Bones of orbit, *155*
Bony orbit, anatomy of, 154–159, *155–161*. See also Orbit
Boxing, 90–107, 90–107t, *91–92*
  angle abnormalities, 96–97
  contact lenses, 102–103
  contrecoup, 93–94, *94*
    lesions, at tissue interfaces, *94*
  coup, 93, *93*
  cutaneous lacerations, treatment of, 101
  diagnosis of injuries, 99–101, *100*
  equatorial expansion, 94, *95*
    with globe compression, *95*
  examination of boxer, 104–105
  eyelids, local damage to, from coup-type injury, *95*
  frequency of injuries, 96t
  gloves, 103, *104*
    thumb-locked, *104*
    thumbless, *104*
  gouging of eye, by thumb, *92*
  guidelines, 104–106
  lens, injuries to, 97
  macula, injuries to, 97
  mechanisms of injury, 92–94
  New York State Athletic Commission, 91
  ocular examination, 100
  postcataract surgery, 103
  postretinal detachment surgery, 102
  prevention of injury, 103–106
  reform, 103–106
  regulations, 105–106
  retina
    peripheral, injuries to, 98t, 98–99
      tears, 98–99, 101
        risk factors, 98t
        treatment of, 101
  safety equipment, 105
  special situations, 101–103
  taking aim at opponent, *91*
  treatment of injury, 99–101, *101*
  types of injury, 95–99
  vision-threatening injuries, 95, 96t
Brock String, visual training, *245*
Browning, Pete, Louisville Slugger and, 32

C-flap, 39, *40*
CAHA. See Canadian Amateur Hockey Association
Canadian Amateur Hockey Association, 58
Canadian Ophthalmological Society, data collection, 4
Canaliculus, 182, *181*
Canthotomy, lateral, anterior segment, *208*
Canthus, 207–208
Carbonic anhydrase inhibitors, hyphema, 198
Carcinoma, from ultraviolet, 15

Cataract
  traumatic, *206*
  ultraviolet light, 15
Cataract surgery, boxing after, 103
Catcher, baseball, injury to, 27, *28–31*
Catcher's mask, baseball
  of 1930's, *30*
  modern, *31*
  of nineteenth century, *28–29*
Center position, basketball, mechanism of injury, *47*
Central recognition, visual training and, 246, *247*
Certification of equipment, councils, 9–10
Chemically tempered glass
  resin, glass, comparison of, *229*
Chemicals, eye injury from, in football, 114
Chemosis, 197
Chlorine, contact lens, 13
Choroidal injury, posterior segment, 216–217
Ciliary arteries, 164
Club, for golf, fit into orbit, *124*
Coach, role in sports safety, 21–22
Commotio retinae, 215–216
  force, illustration of, *213*
Conigliaro, Tony, 37
Conjunctiva
  edema of, 197
  evaluation of, 197
  of eyelid, 179
Conjunctival lacerations, 197
Consumer Product Safety Commission, data collection, 3
Contact lenses, 40–41
  boxing and, 101–102
  chlorine, 13
  pool contaminants, 13
  in sports, 13–14
  ultraviolet light, 13
Contents of orbit, 160–182
Contrast sensitivity, visual training and, 243, *244*
Contrecoup injury, in boxing, 93–94, *94*
  lesions from, *94*
Cornea
  abrasion, *194*, 194–196, 195t, *196*
    foreign body, 194
    pain, 195
    pressure patch, 195
    treatment of, 194–196
  injury, *187*
  rupture, along incision lines, *233*
COS. See Canadian Ophthalmological Society
Councils, for certification of equipment, 9–10
Coup injury, in boxing, 93, *93*
Court sports, 72–89, *77–78, 78*
  ball
    speed, 79, 79t
    velocity, 79
  data collection, 74t, 78–79
  eye guard, 81–88, 87t
    on Alderson headform, *85*
    certification, 85–88

Court sports (*Continued*)
    hinged, with polycarbonate, 85
    for nonprescription wearers, 85
    open, *81–82*, 81–83, *82*, *84*, 84t
        injuries sustained, 84
        lenseless, *81*
    overview, 88
    polycarbonate
        with antifog coat, 86
        nonprescription, 85
            with antifog coat, *85*
    prescription, 83, 85–86, 87t
    voluntariness, 85
    wearing of, 83–85
  glasses, streetwear, 80
  lenses, polycarbonate protective, 80
  mechanism of injury, 79
  penetrating orbit, 78
CPSC. *See* Consumer Product Safety Commission
CR39 lenses, 52t
Cranial nerves, 167–168
  fifth, ophthalmic division of, *170*
Crick, Edward, baseball helmet, 34

Data collection, sports-related injury, 3–5
  Canadian Ophthalmological Society (COS), 4
  Consumer Product Safety Commission (CPSC), 3
  National Athletic Injury/Illness Reporting System (NAIRS), 3
  National Electronic Injury Surveillance System (NEISS), 3
  National Eye Trauma System (NETS), 4
  National Society to Prevent Blindness (USEIR), 5
  United States Eye Injury Registry, 4
Decompression, water sports and, 150–151
Defensive player, in basketball, arm, hand extension, 50
Depth perception, visual training and, 243–244, *245*
Designers, of American Society for Testing and Materials, 6
Desjardins, Gerry, 66
Dilation, 190
Diving, after ocular surgery, 151
Dixie Youth baseball, injuries, 36–37
Dress lenses, prescription, impact-resistance standards, 227
Due care, duty to provide, 226
Dyslexia
  defined, 241
  training, results of, 241

Economics, of injury, sports-related, National Institutes of Health, funding, 5–6
Engineers, of American Society of Testing Materials, 6
Equatorial expansion, boxing, 94, *95*
  with globe compression, *95*

Equipment certification councils, 9–10
Examination, of eye
  external, anterior segment, 185–187
  before participation, in basketball, 54
Extraocular movements, and anterior segment injury, 191
Eye, black, 111
Eye guard, for court sports, 81–88, 83–85, 87t, 88
  Alderson headform, *84*
  certification of, 85–88
  hinged, with polycarbonate, 85
  for nonprescription wearers, 85
  open, *81–82*, 81–83, *82*, *84*, 84t
    injuries sustained, 84
    lenseless, *81*
    original, 75
  polycarbonate
    with antifog coat, 86
    nonprescription, 85
        with antifog coat, 85
  prescription, 83, 85–86, 87t
  voluntariness, 85
Eye-hand coordination, visual training and, 246–247, *246–247*, *248*
Eye movements, visual training and, 244–246, *245*
Eyeglasses
  in baseball, 37–38
  for courtsports, streetwear, 80. *See also* Prescription, Eye guard
Eyelid
  anatomic landmarks, *177*
  conjunctiva, 179
  examination, 185–186
  laceration, 200–202, *201*, 201t
  local damage to, from coup-type boxing injury, *93*
  lymphatic drainage of, *167*
  soft tissues, 176–179, *177–178*, *180*
Eyewear. *See* Eyeglasses, Eye guard

Face, examination, anterior segment injury and, 185–186
Face protector. *See under* specific sport
Failure to prescribe material of choice, 232–234, *233*
Failure to warn, injury from alternative lens materials, 234
Fascia, of orbit, 161–163
Fenway Park, 37
Fielder, baseball, injury to, 27
First-aid kit, and anterior segment injuries, 186t
Fish hook, penetrating eye, *146*
Floor, of orbit, *159*
Fluorescein staining, anterior segment injury and, *193*
Football, 108–118
  chemical, eye injury from, *114*
  eye injuries, overview, 110–111, *110–112*
  faceguard, hands sliding under, *110*

Football (*Continued*)
  facemask, grabbing of, *112*
  foreign body, eye injury from, *114*
  helmet, 113–114, *115*
  Helmet Specs, *116*
  history, 108–109
  lineman, "cage-like" mask, with visor, *115*
  mechanisms of injury, 111–113, *114*
  one-eyed player, 116–117
  penetration, 113–116
  placekicker, opening in facemask, *115*
  polycarbonate shield, 114–116, *116*
  protection, 113–116
  quarterback, giving opponent "straight arm," *111*
  running back, giving opponent "straight arm," *111*
  visor, polycarbonate, *116*
  visual enhancement, 117
  visual performance, 109–110
  visual training, 117
Foreign body
  eye injury from, in football, *114*
  intraocular, posterior segment, 218
  nonpenetrating, *194*, 204, *204*
  penetrating, 204–205, 205t
Forward position, basketball, mechanism of injury, 47
Frames, impact-resistance standards, 228
Frontozygomatic suture, fracture at, *156*

Globe, 161, *162*
  impact, equatorial expansion, *214*
  rupture, 18, 204–205, 205t, 220–221
    from blunt trauma, 214
    from golfing trauma, 125t
    suspicion of, 188
Gloves, boxing, 103, *104*
  thumb-locked, *104*
  thumbless, *104*
Goaltenders, hockey injury, 64–68, *65–67*
Goalie, hockey, mask, 67
Goggles
  for basketball, 52–53
  for racquetball, 87t
  for football, 113
  for shooting sports, 134
Golf, 119–124, 120t, 122t, *124–125*
  ball, *124*
  club, fit into orbit, *124*
  injuries, 122t
    causes of, 120t
  origin of, 119
  Royal and Ancient Golf Club, St. Andrews, Scotland, 119
  ruptured globe, computerized tomography of, *125t*
Green, Hugh, football shield, 115
Guard position, basketball, mechanism of injury, 47
Guidelines, for athletic participation, 10

Hale, Creighton, Little League, 36
Handball, 74, *75*
Heat-tempered glass
  chemically tempered glass, comparison, 229
  impact resistance, 230
HECC. *See* Hockey Equipment Certification Council
Helmet
  American Legion, baseball, 35
  baseball, batting, 33–35, *35*
  batting, baseball, injury from, 33–35, *35*
  football, 113–114, *115*
  with polycarbonate protector, hockey, *59*
Helmet Specs, football, *116*
Hemorrhage
  retrobulbar, 207, 207t, *208*
  subconjunctival, 197
History (ocular), 185
Hitting, baseball, components of act, 249–250
Hockey, 56–71
  Canadian Amateur Hockey Association, 58
  Canadian Ophthalmological Society, 57
  eye injury
    overview, 57–64, 58t, *59*, 61t
    types of, 61
  face protector
    polycarbonate, attached to helmet, *59*
    wire, *59*
      updated, *59*
  goaltenders, 64–68, *65–67*
  goalie, mask, *65*, 67
  history of, 56–57
  Hockey Equipment Certification Council (HECC), 60
  International Organizations for Standardization, 68
  Johns Hopkins University, 57
  mechanisms of eye injury, 58
  National Hockey League, 57
  overview, 68–70, *69*
  Plante, Jacques, 67
    custom moulded mask, *66*
  polycarbonate visor, original, *59*
  protective equipment, certified, *69*
  rulebook, 64
  Yale University, 57
Hockey Equipment Certification Council, 9, 60
Hyphema, 198–200, *199*, 200t
  anticoagulants and, 198
  carbonic anhydrase inhibitors, 198
  pain, 198
    management of, 200t

Imaging, in visual training, 251
Impact resistance
  high index lens, 232
  polycarbonate plastic, 228–232, 229–230, 231t, *232*
  standards, 226–228, 231t
    athletic frames, lenses, 228
Infection, ocular, water sports and, 144–145
Infraorbital artery and nerve, 164–165

Injury, sports related
  anatomy and, 154–183
  to anterior segment, 184–209
  athletic participation, guidelines for, 10
  from baseball, 23–43
  from basketball, 43–55
  blind patients, 11–12
  from boxing, 90–107
  contact lens, 13–14
    chlorine, 13
    pool contaminants, 13
    ultraviolet light, 13
  from court sports, 72–89
  data collection, 3–5
  disease, eye, prior, athletes with, 18
  economics, 5–6
    National Institutes of Health, funding, 5–6
  equipment certification councils, 9–10
  from football, 108–118
  globe, rupture, 18
  from golf, 119–124
  from hockey, 56–71
  legal issues, 20–21
  medicolegal issues, 224–239
  one-eyed athlete, 10–11
  penetrating, 204–205
  to posterior segment, 210–223
  professionals, roles of, in safety, performance, 21–22
  protector designs, 6–9
  from racket sports, 72–89
  safety standards, 6–9
    American National Standards Institute, 7
    American Society for Testing and Materials, 6, 7
    Hockey Equipment Certification Council, 9
    Sports Equipment Certification Council, 9–10
    Z series, eyewear, 7
  from shooting sports, 132–143
  from soccer, 125–129
  social cost, 5
  sunglasses, 14–18
  surgery, eye, prior, athletes with, 18
  U.S. Association for Blind Athletes, 11–12
  visual training, 19–20, 213–260
  from water sports, 154–151
Inspection, inadequate, 234
  legal issues, 234
International Organizations for Standardization, hockey, 68
International Standard Organization Committee, need for, 68
Intraocular pressure, 193–194
Iris, 187–188
Iritis, 197–198
  management of, 197t
  traumatic, 197t, 197–198
Irritation, ocular, water sports and, 144–145

Jellyfish sting, ocular injury, 147–149, *148*
Johns Hopkins University, hockey, 57

Keratitis, 131
Keratopathy, ultraviolet light and, 15
Keratotomy, radial, 18

Lacerations, 185–186
Lacrimal system, 180–182, *181*
Lateral Canthus,
Legal issues, 224–239
  allyl resin, glass, comparison of, *229*
  American National Standards Institute, 226
  cornea, rupture, along incision lines, *233*
  due care, duty to provide, 225
  failure to prescribe material of choice, 232–234, *233*
  failure to warn, injury from alternative lens materials, 234
  heat tempered glass
    chemically tempered glass, comparison of, *229*
    impact resistance for, *230*
  high index lens, impact resistance, *232*
  impact-resistance standards, 226–228, 231t
    athletic frames, lenses, 228
    plano dress lenses, 227
    plano safety lenses, 228
    prescription dress lenses, 227
    prescription safety lenses, 227–228
  inspection, inadequate, 234
  management, sports-related ocular trauma, 235
  negligence, 224–225, 232–238
  overview, 238
  patient history, 225–226
  polycarbonate plastic, impact resistance of, 228–232, *229–230*, 231t, *232*
  prescribing eyewear, 20
  product liability, 235–237
  proximate cause, 225
  record keeping, 237–238
  standard of care, breach of, 225
  verification, inadequate, 234
Lens
  for courtsports, polycarbonate protective, 80
  impact-resistance standards, 228
  injury to, 205–206, *206*
    in boxing, 98
Light, ultraviolet, 143
Lineman, football, "cage-like" mask, with visor, *115*
Little League
  baseball injury, 36
  popularity of, 23
  rulebook, 36
Lockwood's ligament, 173
Louisville Slugger, 33

Macula
  holes, traumatic, 217
  injuries to, in boxing, 97
Major league baseball, injuries, 24, 37
Mask, for goalie, in hockey, 65

Material of choice, failure to prescribe, 232–234, *233*
Maxillary nerve, 171
McDougal, Gil, 37
Maxillary bones, 126
Medical History, 185
Medical records, 185
Medicolegal issues, 224–239. *See also* Legal issues
Melanoma, malignant, from ultraviolet, 15
Mentor B-Vat, visual training and, *244*
Muller's tarsal muscle, 174, 176
Muscle
  extraocular, *162*
  orbicularis oculi, *178*
  of orbit, *162*, 172–176, *174–175*
Muse, Charles, baseball helmet, 34
Mydriasis, traumatic, 190

NAIRS. *See* National Athletic Injury/Illness Reporting System
Naismith, Rev. James, develoment of basketball, 44
Nasolacrimal drainage system, 181
National Athletic Injury/Illness Reporting System, data collection, 3
National Basketball Association
  eye trauma, frequency of, 48, *48*
  mechanism, of eye injury, 48, *48*
National Basketball Association Eye Injury Study, 45–47, *46*, 46t
National Collegiate Athletic Associaton, rules mandating protective equipment, 44–45
National Collegiate Trainers' Association, injury database, 45
National Electronic Injury Surveillance System (NEISS), data collection, 3
National Eye Trauma System, data collection, 4
National Hockey League, 57
National Institutes of Health, funding, 5–6
National Society to Prevent Blindness, data collection, 5
NCAA Guideline 4B, eye safety in sports, 52
Near card, anterior segment injury exam, *189*
Neeld, Greg, 64
Neeld Shield, 64
Negligence, 224–225, 232–238
NEISS. *See* National Electronic Injury Surveillance System
Nerves, orbital, 167–172, *168*, *170*
NETS. *See* National Eye Trauma System
Nettle, sea, ocular injury from, *148*
New York State Athletic Commission, 91
NSPB. *See* National Society to Prevent Blindness

Oblique muscles, 173
Octopus perimeter, visual training and, *247*
Ocular examination, for boxing, 100
Ocular squeeze, from water sports, 149–150

Ocular surface, anterior segment injury, 186–187, *187–188*
Oculography, infrared, visual training and, *245*
One-eyed athlete, 10–11
  football, 116–117
Ophthalmic artery, 163–164
  major branches of, within orbit, *163*
Ophthalmic vein, 166
Optic nerve, 167
Optic nerve evulsion, posterior segment, 220
Orbicularis oculi muscle, *178*
Orbit
  anatomy of, 154–159, *155–160*
  anterior structures, *175*
  apex, 168
  bones of, *155*
  ciliary arteries, 164
  contents of, 160–182
  cranial nerves, 167–168
  fascia, 161–164
  floor, 158, *159*
  fractures, 186
  infraortbital artery, 164–165
  lateral wall of, *160*
  Lockwood's ligament, 173
  maxillary nerve, 171
  medial wall of, *158*
  Muller's tarsal muscle, 174, 176
  oblique muscles, 173
  ophthalmic artery, 163–164
  ophthalmic vein, 166
  rectus muscles, 172–173
  right, *174*
  rim, 154–155
  roof of, *157*
  supratrochlear artery, 164
  venous drainage, *166*
  walls, 156–158, *158–160*
    fracture, *202–203*, 202–204, 203t
  Whitnall's ligament, 173
O'Toole, Joseph, baseball helmet, 34

Paganica, 119
Paintball, used in war games, *142*
Palmeteer, Mike, 66
Parent, Bernie, 66
Participation. *See* Athletic participation
Patching for corneal abrasion, 195–196
Pellet gun, 135–141, *138*, *140*
  pellet within orbit, *138*
Penetrating injury, posterior segment, 215
Penlight examination, 191, *192*, *193*
Periorbita, 160
Peripheral recognition, visual training and, 246, *247*
Peripheral visual fields, studies of, 253
Pitcher, baseball, injury to, 26
Placekicker, football, opening in facemask, 115
Plano dress lenses, impact-resistance standards, 227

Plano safety lenses, impact-resistance standards, 228
Plante, Jacques, custom moulded mask, 64, 65, 66
Police, umpire, comparison, 32
Polycarbonate plastic, impact resistance of, 228–232, 229–230, 231t, 232
Pool contaminants, contact lens, 13
Posterior segment injury, 210–223
   blunt trauma, 212–213, 213–214
   choroidal injuries, 216–217
   clues to, 211–212
   commotio retinae, 215–216
     force, illustration of, 213
   globe
     impact, equatorial expansion with, 214
     rupture, 220–221
       from blunt trauma, 214
   intraocular foreign body, posterior segment, 218
   macular holes, traumatic, 217
   management, initial, 220
   manifestations of, 215–221
   mechanisms of, 212
   optic nerve evulsion, 220
   overview, 222
   pathophysiology of, 212–215
   patient evaluation, 211–212
   patient history, 211–212
   penetrating injury, 215
   preretinal hemorrhage, from valsalva, 219
   retinal detachments, 218
   retinitis sclopetaria, 219–220
   visual outcome, poor, 215
   vitreous hemorrhage, 218–219
Preretinal hemorrhage, from valsalva, 219
Prescription. *See* Legal issues
Prescription dress lenses, impact-resistance standards, 227
Prescription safety lenses, 20
   impact-resistance standards, 227–228
Pressure patch
   with anterior segment injury, *196*
   for corneal abrasion, 195
Product liability, 235–237
Professionals, roles of, in safety, performance, 21–22
Protective equipment. *See also under* specific device
   safety standards, 6–9
Proximate cause, as legal issue, 225
Pterygium, ultraviolet light and, 15
Pupello, Frank, football shield visor, 114–115
Pupil, examination, 189–190, *190*, 190–191, *191*

Quarterback, giving opponent "straight arm," *111*

Racket sports, 72–89, 80
   badminton, 72–73, *73*, 74t
   ball
     speed, 79, 79t
     velocity, 79
   contact lenses, 80
   data collection, 74t, 78–79
   eye guard, 81–88, 87t
     on Alderson headform, *84*
     certification, 85–88
     hinged, with polycarbonate, 85
     nonprescription, 83, 85–86, 87t
     for nonprescription wearers, 85
     open, *81–82*, 81–83, *82*, *84*, 84t
       injuries sustained, 84
       lenseless, *81*
       original, 75
     overview, 88
     polycarbonate
       with antifog coating, 86
       nonprescription, 85
         with antifog coating, 85
       prescription, 83, 85–86, 87t
     standards for, 87–88
     voluntariness, 85
     wearing of, 83–85
   glasses, streetwear, 80
   handball, 74, *75*
   injuries, 74
   lenses, polycarbonate protective, 80
   mechanism of injury, 79
   racket
     speed, 79, 79t
     velocity, 79
   racquetball, 77–78, *78*
     penetrating orbit, *78*
   shuttlecock, for badminton, *73*
   squash, 75–77, *76*
     ball, *76*
     racket, *76*
   tennis, 73–74
Racquetball, 77–78, *78*
   ball
     speed, 79, 79t
     velocity, 79
   data collection, 74t, 78–79
   eye guard, 81–88, 87t
     on Alderson headform, *84*
     certification, 85–88
     hinged, with polycarbonate, 85
     for nonprescription wearers, 85
     open, *81–82*, 81–83, *82*, *84*, 84t
       injuries sustained, 84
       lenseless, *81*
     overview, 88
     polycarbonate
       with antifog coat, 86
       nonprescription, 85
         with antifog coat, 85
       prescription, 83, 85–86, 87t
     voluntariness, 85
     wearing of, 83–85
   glasses, streetwear, 80
   lenses, polycarbonate protective, 80
   mechanism of injury, 79
   penetrating orbit, *78*

Radial keratotomy, 18
Radiography, 18
Radiation, ultraviolet, excessive, water sports and, 143–144
RAPD. *See* Relative afferent pupullary defect
Rebounding, in basketball, arm, finger, extension, 49
Record keeping, legal aspects of, 237–238
Rectus muscles, 172–173
Reform, of boxing, 103–106
Relative afferent pupullary defect, testing for, 190
Retina
  blunt trauma to, 217–218
  commotio, 215–216
  detachments, 218
  edema, 216
  peripheral, injuries to, from boxing, 98t, 98–99
  tear, 98–99, 101
    from boxing, treatment of, 101
    boxing risk factors, 98t
Retinitis sclopetaria, 219–220
Retrobulbar hemorrhage and management, 206–208
Rim, of orbit, 154–155
Roof, of orbit, *157*
Royal and Ancient Golf Club, St. Andrews, Scotland, 119
Rule book, hockey, 64
Running back, football, giving opponent "straight arm," *111*
Ruth, Babe, eye, ear functioning, 38

Safety lenses, prescription, impact-resistance standards, 227–228
Safety performance, roles of professionals in, 21–22
Safety standards
  American National Standards Institute, 7
  American Society of Testing Materials, 6, 7
  Hockey Equipment Certification Council, 9
  for protective devices, 6–9
  Sports Equipment Certification Council, 9–10
  sports-related injury and, 6–9
  Z series, of eyewear, 7
Scuba diving, 149–151
Sea nettle, ocular injury from, *148*
SECC. *See* Sports Equipment Certification Council
Senter, Nick, Dixie Youth baseball, 37
Septum, orbital, *180*
Shield, polycarbonate, for football, 114–116, *116*
Shooting sports, 132–143
  air guns, 135–143
  BB gun, 135–141, *138*, 138t, *140*
  pellet guns, 135–141, *138*, *140*
  pellet within orbit, *138*
  shotgun sports, ocular injuries from, 132–135
  war games, 141–143, *142*

paintball used in, *142*
Shotgun sports, ocular injuries from, 132–135
Shuttlecock, for badminton, 72, *73*
Soccer, 125–129
  Trinity College, Cambridge, England, 125
Social cost, of eye trauma, 5
Spectators, baseball, injury to, 33
Sports Equipment Certification Council, 9–10
Sports frames, 53
Sports-related injury. *See also* Injury
  data collection
    Canadian Ophthalmological Society, 4
    Consumer Product Safety Commission, 3
    National Electronic Injury Surveillance System (NEISS), 3
    National Eye Trauma System, 4
    National Society to Prevent Blindness, 5
    United States Eye Injury Registry, 4
Squash, 75–77, *76*
  ball, *76*
  racket, *76*
Standard of care, breach of, 225
Standards
  impact-resistance, 226–228, 231t
    athletic frames, lenses, 228
    plano dress lenses, 227
    plano safety lenses, 228
    prescription dress lenses, 228
    prescription safety lenses, 227–228
  safety, sports-related injury and, 6–9
"Straight arm," in football, injury from, *111*
Subconjunctival hemorrhage, 197
Sun, ocular problems related to, 143–145
Sunglasses, 14–18, 40–41
  ideal, characteristics of, 17–18
  impact resistance and, 16–17
  ultraviolet light, 14–18
Supratrochlear artery, 164
Surgery, eye, prior, athletes with, 18
Swimming, 143

Tears. *See* Lacrimal system
Tennis, 73–74
  Wingfield, Major Walter Clopton, 73
Tentacles, of sea nettle, ocular injury from, *148*
Torporcer, George, 38
Training, visual, sports and, 19–20
Trap shooting, 134
Tretinal detachment surgery, boxing after, 102
Trinity College, Cambridge, England, soccer, rules of, 125
Tripod fracture, *156*

Ultraviolet light
  cataract, 15
  contact lens, 13
  keratopathy, 15
  pterygium, 15
  sports sunglasses, 14–18
  water sports and, 143–144

Umpire
    baseball, injury to, 32–33
    police, comparison, 32
USABA. *See* U.S. Association for Blind Athletes
United States Association for Blind Athletes, 11–12
United States Eye Injury Registry, data collection, 4
United States Racquetball Association
USEIR. *See* United States Eye Injury Registry
UV. *See* Ultraviolet radiation
UV light. *See* Ultraviolet light

Valsalva, preretinal hemorrhage from, 219
Venous drainage, of orbit, 166
Vergence, visual training and, 246
Verification, inadequate, as legal issue, 234
Vessels, orbital, 163, 163–167, 165–167
Vision-threatening injuries, in boxing, 95, 96t
Visor
    football, polycarbonate, 116
    polycarbonate, for hockey, original, 59
Visual acuity
    and anterior segment injury, 187–189, 189
    dynamic, visual training and, 243
    static, visual training and, 242
Visual outcome, poor, 215
Visual performance, in football, 110–111
Visual training, 19–20, 240–260, 247–253, 250–251, 253–254
    accommodation, 246
    balance training and, 251
    at bat, first 0.4 seconds, schematic of, 251
    Brock String, 245
    contrast sensitivity, 243, 244
    depth perception, 243–244, 245
    dyslexia, as example, 241
    eye-hand coordination, 246–247, 246–247, 248
    eye movements, 244–246, 245
    football, 117
    imaging and, 251
    logic, 247–253, 250–251
    Mentor B-Vat, 244
    octopus perimeter, 247
    oculography, infrared, 245
    overview, 254–256, 256
    peripheral visual fields, studies of, 253
    recognition, central, peripheral, 246, 247
    recommendations, 255
    tasks, involved in hitting baseball, schematic of, 250
    vergence, 246
    visual acuity
        dynamic, 243
        static, 242
    visualization techniques, 251
    Wayne Saccadic fixator, 248
Visualization techniques, in visual training, 251
Vitreous hemorrhage, 218–219

Walker, Wesley, amblyopia, performance with, 117
Wall, of orbit
    lateral, 160
    medial, 158
War games, 141–143, 142
    paintball used in, 142
"Warding off" of opponent, in basketball, 52
Warn, failure to, injury from alternative lens materials, 234
Water, ocular problems related to, 143–145
Water sports, 143–151
    decompression effects, 150–151
    diving, after ocular surgery, 151
    fishing
        fish hook, penetrating eye, 146
        ocular injuries in, 145–147, 146
    infection, ocular, 144–145
    irritation, ocular, 144–145
    jellyfish sting, ocular, 147–149, 148
    ocular squeeze, 149–150
    optical correction, 149
    overview, 151–152
    scuba diving, 149–151
    sea nettle, tentacles of, 148
    sun, ocular problems related to, 143–145
    ultraviolet radiation, excessive, 143–144
    water, ocular problems related to, 143–145
Wayne Saccadic fixator, visual training and, 248
Whitnall's ligament, 173
Williams, Ted, 249
Wingfield, Major Walter Clopton, 73
Wound edges, suturing superficial, with anterior segment injury, 201

Yale University, hockey, 57

Z series, of eyewear, standards for, 7
Zygoma, fracture of, 158
Zygomaticomaxillary suture, fracture at, 156